Antioxidant Role of High-Density Lipoprotein

Antioxidant Role of High-Density Lipoprotein

Guest Editor

Paul Durrington

MDPI

Basel • Beijing • Wuhan • Barcelona • Belgrade • Novi Sad • Cluj • Manchester

Guest Editor
Paul Durrington
Faculty of Biology Medicine
and Health
University of Manchester
Manchester
UK

Editorial Office
MDPI AG
Grosspeteranlage 5
4052 Basel, Switzerland

This is a reprint of the Special Issue, published open access by the journal *Antioxidants* (ISSN 2076-3921), freely accessible at: https://www.mdpi.com/journal/antioxidants/special_issues/32K8N0691X.

For citation purposes, cite each article independently as indicated on the article page online and as indicated below:

Lastname, A.A.; Lastname, B.B. Article Title. *Journal Name* **Year**, *Volume Number*, Page Range.

ISBN 978-3-7258-8201-4 (Hbk)
ISBN 978-3-7258-8202-1 (PDF)
https://doi.org/10.3390/books978-3-7258-8202-1

Contents

About the Editor

Paul Durrington

Paul Durrington is Professor of Medicine at the University of Manchester and Consultant Physician at Manchester Royal Infirmary. He graduated with degrees in Physiology and Medicine at the University of Bristol and trained in general medicine, diabetes mellitus and metabolic disorders. Early in his career, he developed immunoassays for apoB and then, at the University of California, reported that the action of insulin on hepatic VLDL secretion was inhibitory, rather than stimulatory as had earlier been believed. Later, he pioneered cascade family screening for familial hypercholesterolaemia and described the genetic basis of some rarer disorders of lipoprotein and fat metabolism. His research interests centre on disorders of lipoprotein metabolism, atherogenic modification of lipoproteins, insulin resistance, diabetes and the translation of clinical trial evidence into practice. His most important contribution to diabetes management was in the design, conduct and laboratory coordination of a multicentre randomised controlled trial demonstrating the prevention of atherosclerotic cardiovascular disease (ASCVD) by statin therapy (Collaborative Atorvastatin Diabetes Study). His group was also the first to reveal the capacity of HDL to protect LDL against atherogenic modifications, such as oxidation and glycation, and to propose that this was largely due to the presence on HDL of paraoxonase 1, the activity of which is inversely associated with ASCVD incidence. In the prevention of ASCVD generally, he devised widely used charts and computer programmes for the estimation of cardiovascular disease risk and mathematical models for the rational deployment of cholesterol-lowering drugs. Recently, he reported on the metabolic effects of bariatric surgery. His numerous publications include 'Hyperlipidaemia: Diagnosis and Management', 3rd Edition (2007), and with Allan Sniderman, 'Hyperlipidemia', 6th Edition (2021).

antioxidants

MDPI

Editorial

Antioxidant Role of High-Density Lipoprotein

Paul N. Durrington

Cardiovascular Research Group, Faculty of Biology, Medicine and Health, University of Manchester, Manchester M13 9NT, UK; pdurrington@manchester.ac.uk; Tel.: +44-161-275-1201; Fax: +44-161-275-1183

1. Introduction

Low-density lipoprotein (LDL) is the primary cholesterol-carrying lipoprotein in the circulation, where it is a significant contributor to atherosclerosis and delivers cholesterol to the tissues [1]. The role of high-density lipoprotein (HDL) is, however, far from certain.

2. HDL in Lipid Transport

In the human foetus, an apolipoprotein E-rich HDL (apoE-rich HDL) delivers cholesterol to cells via the LDL receptor (also known as the apoB100/apoE receptor, because it binds both the apolipoprotein B100 (apoB100) and apoE ligands) [1,2]. HDL is the dominant lipoprotein in the foetus and in cord blood, but within a few days of birth, both the apoE content of HDL and its contribution to serum cholesterol diminish as cholesteryl ester transfer protein (CETP) activity and circulating LDL cholesterol concentrations rise. LDL is then often regarded as being the dominant lipoprotein species in the blood circulation, supplying cholesterol, particularly to growing and repairing tissues and to those with a high requirement for steroidogenesis [1]. In the human CNS, however, apoE-rich HDL continues as the major cholesterol-carrying lipoprotein in the CSF [3]. Nonetheless, as clinicians are well aware, the serum HDL cholesterol concentration in humans, except in neonates, is almost invariably less than that of LDL. However, in terms of the serum concentration of their principal proteins, in healthy adults, the apolipoprotein A1 (apoA1) of HDL typically exceeds that of apoB100 in LDL. Furthermore, because of its smaller size, HDL crosses capillary endothelia more readily than LDL and thus, in terms of concentration of protein and of cholesterol, is the dominant lipoprotein in the tissue fluid. HDL cannot, therefore, be regarded as some minor lipoprotein with little significance. Alcover and colleagues summarise much of the current thinking about the formation and metabolism of HDL in Contribution 1 of this volume.

In many animals, apoE-rich HDL rather than LDL continues to be the major supplier of cholesterol throughout life [4]. In the rare human disorder abetalipoproteinaemia, where apoB is not produced and LDL is absent, apoE-rich HDL continues to supply cholesterol to tissues, albeit not compensating entirely for the absence of LDL, allowing red blood cells to become acanthocytes (due to lack of cholesterol in their cell membranes) and not fulfilling the role of apoB48 in the intestinal absorption of dietary fat and fat-soluble vitamins [1]. Clearly, in most human circumstances, however, HDL is no longer apoE-rich and after birth has no, or very little, role in delivering cholesterol to the tissues. This is strongly supported by the fact that most of the LDL receptors outside the liver and adrenals are likely to be saturated once the concentrations of LDL cholesterol levels exceed 2 mmol/L [5], which is the case in most adult humans, even when receiving a traditional Asian diet. The typical higher adult levels of LDL cholesterol appear to serve no useful purpose but do predispose to ASCVD and impose a requirement for the cholesterol transported out of the liver to be returned. HDL was for many years considered to be crucial in this futile, and potentially harmful, vicious cycle. This was thought to explain the inverse relationship between HDL cholesterol and ASCVD incidence reported in epidemiological studies [6]. However, as we discuss in Contribution 2, although the apparently protective role of HDL against ASCVD is indisputable, evidence that this is due to HDL playing some rate-limiting function in reverse cholesterol transport has not really been forthcoming, and the contention is fraught with anomalies.

3. HDL as a Protective Molecule

The investigation of HDL proteomics has revealed more than 100 protein components [7]. Many of these are present in only trace amounts, but those which stand out both in concentration and as being involved directly in pathogenesis or in susceptibility to a variety of diseases are apoA1, apolipoprotein A11 (apoA11), clusterin (also known as apolipoprotein J (apoJ), serum amyloid A (SAA), and lecithin (cholesterol acyltransferase (LCAT), myeloperoxidase and paraoxonase 1 (PON1)). Phospholipase A2 is present on HDL, but is mainly located on LDL. Its apparent activity on HDL is largely due to the presence of PON1 [8]. ApoA1 is an essential structural component of HDL and acts as a strong detergent, permitting the transport of lipids otherwise highly insoluble in water. It is a cofactor of LCAT, also located on HDL, which, particularly in humans, converts gram-range quantities of free cholesterol to cholesteryl esters, usually transferring to cholesterol the fatty acyl group in the Sn-2 position of phosphatidyl choline, in which HDL is rich [1]. The product of this reaction is the highly toxic lysophosphatidyl choline, which, if released into the circulation, would cause widespread damage to cell membranes. However, it remains safely confined to HDL, whence it is cleared by the liver. Although LCAT deficiency, whether genetic or acquired, for example, in extreme liver failure, is associated with disease complications associated with cholesteryl ester deficiency, its overexpression is not a cause of ASCVD [9]. However, its activity does serve to illustrate the capacity of HDL to protect the body from exposure to harmful substances. PON1 was discovered as a defence against synthetic organophosphate toxicity. This role also involves defending against exposure to naturally occurring organophosphates, such as those produced by blue-green algae. PON1 has proved to have an enormous range of hydrolytic substrates, many potentially harmful, such as lipid peroxides produced as a consequence of oxygen species reacting with phospholipids, an essential component of cell membranes and lipoproteins [10,11]. The evolution of aerobic respiration, although it brought many benefits in terms of the rate at which energy can be generated and exerted, was a hazardous business as reactive oxygen species leaking from processes, such as respiratory chain phosphorylation or from mechanisms to transport oxygen, are damaging to other biochemical processes, proteins, and tissues. Paraoxonases may well have evolved as lactonases before organisms developed aerobic metabolism. This lactonase activity may well continue to this day to contribute to their protective function against tissue damage by naturally generated lactones. Jakubowski and colleagues discuss this in detail in Contribution 3. However, this is not to deny their contribution to the antioxidative role of HDL in the case of PON1 and the intracellular antioxidative role of another family member, paraoxonase 2.

In Contribution 4, attention is drawn by Birkowitz-Fiebich and colleagues to the lower levels of lipid peroxides in HDL when higher HDL levels prevail, particularly in women.

The presence of clusterin (apoJ) on HDL, along with PON1, immediately suggests a major role for HDL in protecting the outer cell membranes and potentially their contents against damage that might otherwise result in disease or worsening of disease. Clusterin is a glycoprotein that protects against the toxicity of effete and damaged proteins [12]. We

https://doi.org/10.3390/antiox15020186

observed the increasing localisation of apoA1, PON1, and clusterin within atheromatous plaques as they progressed [13].

4. HDL in Disease Prevention

The notion that HDL has a protective role is further strengthened when one considers the wide range of diseases associated with low PON1 activity. In conditions predisposing to ASCVD and its partner in crime, aortic stenosis due to atheromatous narrowing of a congenitally bicuspid valve, discussed by Kwatiatkowska and colleagues in Contribution 5, HDL has a clearly emerging role. The same may be said in metabolic syndrome, hepatic steatosis, and diabetes [14]. Acute and chronic infections are also associated with decreased antioxidative capacity of HDL, as signalled by lower activity of PON1 [14,15], discussed by Reichert et al. in Contribution 6 in the case of HIV infection. The same may be true of several psychiatric and neurological conditions [14,16], such as depression, bipolar disorder, schizophrenia, and neuropsychiatric symptoms due to industrial organophosphate exposure [17], cerebral infarction, Alzheimer's disease, Parkinson's disease [14], and multiple sclerosis. The latter is reviewed in Contribution 7 by Damiza-Detmer and co-workers. Neoplastic disease is also associated with decreased HDL levels and low PON1 activity [14], as it now seems may also be the case for mast cell tumours of dogs reported by Ginoudis et al. in Contribution 8. Inflammatory arthritides and other acute and chronic inflammatory disorders are also associated with lower PON1 [18].

In many diseases associated with decreased serum PON1 activity, the circulating HDL particle size is decreased in comparison to HDL in health. There is decreased PON1 activity. This may be substrate-specific, but it also applies when a substrate like phenyl acetate, to which genetic isoforms of PON1 display equal activity, is used in the PON1 assay. Nonetheless, individuals may also display varying rates of hepatic synthesis and secretion, contributing to lower levels. However, a major cause of diminished PON1 activity appears to be the result of compositional change in HDL in diseases associated with low PON1 activity. Thus, in HDL, apparently predisposing to disease, myeloperoxidase is frequently elevated [10,19]. So also are apoA11 and SAA, both of which displace PON1 from HDL [10]. On the other hand, apoA1, essential for PON1 to be active against more hydrophobic substrates, is diminished. This gives rise to the concept of pro-inflammatory, pro-atherogenic HDL in disease states and anti-inflammatory, anti-atherogenic HDL in health. PON1 is an easily measured indicator of the type of HDL likely to be present (see later). The anti-inflammatory, anti-atherogenic type of HDL is also more effective in promoting the uptake of cholesterol from macrophage cells in tissue culture [20]. This cholesterol efflux capacity is related to ASCVD risk [21]. However, this is not to gainsay the earlier comments in this introduction about HDL and how little it is responsible for reverse cholesterol transport, because most of the cholesterol secreted by the liver in VLDL is cleared from the circulation with LDL via hepatic LDL receptors and thus short-circuits the tissues in which, in any case, LDL receptors are down-regulated. For cholesterol to cross the arterial endothelium (as opposed to capillary endothelia) and be incorporated into atheromatous lesions, LDL must first be modified, say by oxidation and/or glycation, so that it binds to scavenger receptors (see Contribution 2). Whilst this process is clearly related to the height of habitual circulating LDL cholesterol levels, not even in the most hypercholesterolaemic individuals can it be said to be a major fate for the enormous quantities of LDL cholesterol produced each day in humans [5].

5. Antioxidant Role of HDL

That high-density lipoprotein (HDL) could prevent the oxidative modification of proteins was discovered as the result of experiments involving the incubation of low-density

https://doi.org/10.3390/antiox15020186

lipoprotein with and without HDL under oxidising conditions. In the absence of HDL, changes in the physical properties of LDL, such as electrophoretic mobility, occurred, which were abolished or ameliorated [10]. Later, it was found that co-incubation of HDL with LDL in the presence of an oxidising agent such as copper ions prevented the accumulation of lipid peroxidation products [22] and the fragmentation of the apolipoprotein B component of LDL. This apoB fragmentation could otherwise lead to failure of LDL binding to the physiological LDL receptor of Goldstein and Brown, but rapid uptake of LDL by endothelial and macrophage cells via their scavenger receptors [11,23]. It was further realised that this cellular uptake could hasten the passage of LDL across the arterial endothelium (transcytosis) into the subintima, and once there, macrophage foam cell formation (see Contribution 2). Conjugated diene formation is the first stage in lipid peroxidation when unsaturated fatty acyl groups are exposed to oxygen-free radicals. The formation of alternating double/single carbon bonds is the consequence of hydrogen abstraction from unsaturated fatty acids present in phospholipids. It is easy to detect by ultraviolet spectroscopy and is opposed by fat-soluble vitamins present on LDL [24]. In contrast to fat-soluble antioxidant vitamins, which had largely failed to prevent atherosclerosis in clinical trials, the protection of LDL against oxidative modification by HDL and PON1 was unrelated to conjugated diene formation but was associated with decreased generation of lipid peroxidation products occurring downstream [10,11,24]. It is likely that this is due to hydrolytic removal of peroxidised unsaturated acyl groups at position Sn-2 on phosphatidyl choline and on cholesteryl esters by PON1 and sequestration by HDL of lysophosphatidyl choline and the ketone and aldehyde products of the breakdown of the peroxidised fatty acyl groups released. Some evidence suggests that the latter may be metabolised to harmless fatty acids [11,25], but in any case, they, together with lysophosphatidyl choline, will be removed during the passage of HDL through the liver.

6. The Place of HDL in the Clinic

The measurement of HDL cholesterol in clinical practice, usually to enter into an ASCVD risk algorithm as the term total serum cholesterol to HDL cholesterol concentration ratio or non-HDL to HDL cholesterol concentration ratio, is well established [26]. Monitoring responses to lipid-lowering medication by non-HDL cholesterol is also widely recommended, although there is an increasing tendency for guidelines to recommend direct apoB assays for this purpose [26]. There is a loose correlation between PON1 activity and HDL cholesterol, most evident in the general population [27]. However, there is discordance between the two, mostly in diabetes, established ASCVD, and dyslipidaemia [19,28,29]. The question thus arises whether anything of clinical value could accrue from measuring PON1 rather than, or in addition to, HDL cholesterol as a marker of whether the HDL present is pro-inflammatory and pro-atherogenic and therefore deficient in its antioxidant capacity. In general, this is controversial. However, in diabetes and established ASCVD, knowledge of PON1 activity may add to the assessment of the likelihood of future ASCVD events [28,29]. This might signal the need for more intensive intervention with, for example, lipid-lowering, antihypertensive, or anti-coagulant treatment. Given the range of diseases associated with decreased PON1 activity, its possible value in determining therapy in these conditions should also be explored.

Of course, there is also the issue of whether increasing serum PON1 activity could have therapeutic value. Few traditional therapeutic approaches to raising PON1 levels have emerged thus far. Extracts of pomegranate may, however, lead the way forward [30]. There has also been considerable interest in the production of PON1 by recombinant DNA technology, largely to combat or ameliorate organophosphate toxicity due to military and industrial exposure or to self-harm [17]. The biopharmaceutical versions of PON1 are

https://doi.org/10.3390/antiox15020186

modified in their manufacture to be water-soluble, which means they have therapeutic potential against water-soluble PON1 substrates, but not those for which the lipid solubility of naturally occurring PON1 embedded in HDL is critical for hydrolysis. Unless this can be overcome, the most profitable step forward is likely to be the development of a means of boosting the hepatic synthesis of PON1 whilst retaining the physiological mechanism by which it enters the hydrophobic lipid domains of HDL. An alternative is to increase cofactors of PON1. Unfortunately, raising apoA1 levels by overexpressing *APOA1* has proved disappointing unless several copies are expressed [31]. On the other hand, decreasing the expression of myeloperoxidase or of proteins that displace PON1 from HDL, such as SAA or apoA11, may prove therapeutic.

7. Conclusions

The antioxidant role of HDL is well-established. The concept of pro- and anti-inflammatory and pro- and anti-atherogenic HDL is of considerable interest and appears to be driven by the capacity of HDL to interfere with the oxidative modification of proteins, which is itself largely due to PON1 and to the hydrophobic, protective environment provided by HDL.

Conflicts of Interest: The author declares no conflicts of interest.

List of Contributions:

1. Alcover, S.; Ramos-Regalado, L.; Girón, G.; Muñoz-García, N.; Vilahur, G. HDL-Cholesterol and Triglycerides Dynamics: Essential Players in Metabolic Syndrome. *Antioxidants* **2025**, *14*, 434. https://doi.org/10.3390/antiox14040434.
2. Durrington, P.N.; Bashir, B.; Soran, H. How Does HDL Participate in Atherogenesis? Antioxidant Activity Versus Role in Reverse Cholesterol Transport. *Antioxidants* **2025**, *14*, 430. https://doi.org/10.3390/antiox14040430.
3. Jakubowski, H. The Molecular Bases of Anti-Oxidative and Anti-Inflammatory Properties of Paraoxonase 1. *Antioxidants* **2024**, *13*, 1292. https://doi.org/10.3390/antiox13111292.
4. Berkowitz-Fiebich, L.; Flaherty, S.M.; Kitayama, S.; Karasawa, M.; Kawakami, N.; Rigotti, A.; Coe, C.L. Healthier Lipid Profiles of Japanese Adults, Especially in Women with Elevated High-Density Lipoprotein Cholesterol (HDL-C), Are Associated with Low HDL-C Peroxide Content. *Antioxidants* **2024**, *13*, 1434. https://doi.org/10.3390/antiox13121434.
5. Kwiatkowska, M.; Mickiewicz, A.; Krzesińska, A.; Kuchta, A.; Jankowski, M.; Gruchała, M.; Fijałkowski, M. The Role of Paraoxonase-1 Activity, Apolipoprotein B Levels, and Apolipoprotein B/Apolipoprotein A-I Ratio as Risk Markers for Aortic Stenosis in Patients with a Bicuspid Aortic Valve. *Antioxidants* **2025**, *14*, 167. https://doi.org/10.3390/antiox14020167.
6. Reichert, C.O.; Levy, D.; Maselli, L.M.F.; da Cunha, J.; Gualandro, S.F.M.; Bydlowski, S.P. PON-1 and PON-2 Polymorphisms and PON-1 Paraoxonase Activity in People Living with HIV-1. *Antioxidants* **2025**, *14*, 209. https://doi.org/10.3390/antiox14020209.
7. Damiza-Detmer, A.; Pawełczyk, M.; Głąbiński, A. Protective Role of High-Density Lipoprotein in Multiple Sclerosis. *Antioxidants* **2024**, *13*, 1276. https://doi.org/10.3390/antiox13111276.
8. Ginoudis, A.; Pardali, D.; Mylonakis, M.E.; Tamvakis, A.; Tvarijonaviciute, A.; Lymperaki, E.; Ceron, J.J.; Polizopoulou, Z. Oxidative Status and Lipid Metabolism Analytes in Dogs with Mast Cell Tumors: A Preliminary Study. *Antioxidants* **2024**, *13*, 1473. https://doi.org/10.3390/antiox13121473.

References

1. Durrington, P.N. *Hyperlipidaemia: Diagnosis and Management*, 3rd ed.; Hodder Arnold: London, UK, 2007; p. 399.
2. Nagasaka, H.; Chiba, H.; Kikuta, H.; Akita, H.; Takahashi, Y.; Yanai, H.; Hui, S.P.; Fuda, H.; Fujiwara, H.; Kobayashi, K. Unique character and metabolism of high density lipoprotein (HDL) in fetus. *Atherosclerosis* **2002**, *161*, 215–223. [CrossRef] [PubMed]
3. Mahley, R.W. Central Nervous System Lipoproteins: ApoE and Regulation of Cholesterol Metabolism. *Arterioscler. Thromb. Vasc. Biol.* **2016**, *36*, 1305–1315. [CrossRef] [PubMed] [PubMed Central]

4. Goldstein, S.; Chapman, M.J. Comparative immunochemical studies of the serum low-density lipoprotein in several animal species. *Biochem. Genet.* **1976**, *14*, 883–896. [CrossRef] [PubMed]
5. Brown, M.S.; Kovanen, P.T.; Goldstein, J.L. Regulation of plasma cholesterol by lipoprotein receptors. *Science* **1981**, *212*, 628–635. [CrossRef] [PubMed]
6. Miller, G.J.; Miller, N.E. Plasma-high-density-lipoprotein concentration and development of ischaemic heart-disease. *Lancet* **1975**, *1*, 16–19. [CrossRef] [PubMed]
7. Gomes, F.A.; Souza Junior, D.R.; Holzer, M.; Ronsein, G.E. Proteomic analysis of HDL isolates reveals method-driven variability: An interlaboratory approach. *J. Lipid Res.* **2025**, *67*, 100957. [CrossRef] [PubMed]
8. Rodrigo, L.; Mackness, B.; Durrington, P.N.; Hernandez, A.; Mackness, M.I. Hydrolysis of platelet-activating factor by human serum paraoxonase. *Biochem. J.* **2001**, *354*, 1–7. [CrossRef]
9. Calabresi, L.; Franceschini, G. Lecithin:cholesterol acyltransferase, high-density lipoproteins, and atheroprotection in humans. *Trends Cardiovasc. Med.* **2010**, *20*, 50–53. [CrossRef] [PubMed]
10. Durrington, P.; Soran, H. Paraoxonase 1: Evolution of the enzyme and of its role in protecting against atherosclerosis. *Curr. Opin. Lipidol.* **2024**, *35*, 171–178. [CrossRef] [PubMed] [PubMed Central]
11. Durrington, P.N.; Bashir, B.; Soran, H. Paraoxonase 1 and atherosclerosis. *Front. Cardiovasc. Med.* **2023**, *10*, 1065967. [CrossRef] [PubMed] [PubMed Central]
12. Du, X.; Chen, Z.; Shui, W. Clusterin: Structure, function and roles in disease. *Int. J. Med. Sci.* **2025**, *22*, 887–896. [CrossRef] [PubMed] [PubMed Central]
13. Mackness, B.; Hunt, R.; Durrington, P.N.; Mackness, M.I. Increased immunolocalization of paraoxonase, clusterin, and apolipoprotein A-I in the human artery wall with the progression of atherosclerosis. *Arterioscler. Thromb. Vasc. Biol.* **1997**, *17*, 1233–1238. [CrossRef] [PubMed]
14. Steenackers, E.; Van Hul, W. The Paraoxonase (*PON*) Gene Family in Health, Metabolic Dysfunction-Associated Steatotic Liver Disease (MASLD) and Other Diseases. *Int. J. Mol. Sci.* **2025**, *26*, 11054. [CrossRef] [PubMed]
15. Draganov, D.; Teiber, J.; Watson, C.; Bisgaier, C.; Nemzek, J.; Remick, D.; Standiford, T.; La Du, B. PON1 and oxidative stress in human sepsis and an animal model of sepsis. *Adv. Exp. Med. Biol.* **2010**, *660*, 89–97. [CrossRef] [PubMed]
16. Morris, G.; Puri, B.K.; Bortolasci, C.C.; Carvalho, A.; Berk, M.; Walder, K.; Moreira, E.G.; Maes, M. The role of high-density lipoprotein cholesterol, apolipoprotein A and paraoxonase-1 in the pathophysiology of neuroprogressive disorders. *Neurosci. Biobehav. Rev.* **2021**, *125*, 244–263. [CrossRef] [PubMed]
17. Cherry, N.; Mackness, M.; Durrington, P.; Povey, A.; Dippnall, M.; Smith, T.; Mackness, B. Paraoxonase (PON1) polymorphisms in farmers attributing ill health to sheep dip. *Lancet* **2002**, *359*, 763–764. [CrossRef] [PubMed]
18. Razmjou, A.A.; Kremer, J.M.; Pappas, D.A.; Curtis, J.R.; Wang, J.; Shahbazian, A.; Elashoff, D.A.; Guo, R.; Meriwether, D.; Sulaiman, D.; et al. Disease response in rheumatoid arthritis across four biologic therapies associates with improvement in paraoxonase-1 activity and oxylipins. *RMD Open* **2024**, *10*, e004829. [CrossRef] [PubMed] [PubMed Central]
19. Variji, A.; Shokri, Y.; Fallahpour, S.; Zargari, M.; Bagheri, B.; Abediankenari, S.; Alizadeh, A.; Mahrooz, A. The combined utility of myeloperoxidase (MPO) and paraoxonase 1 (PON1) as two important HDL-associated enzymes in coronary artery disease: Which has a stronger predictive role? *Atherosclerosis* **2019**, *280*, 7–13. [CrossRef] [PubMed]
20. Rosenblat, M.; Volkova, N.; Aviram, M. HDL3 stimulates paraoxonase 1 antiatherogenic catalytic and biological activities in a macrophage model system: In vivo and in vitro studies. *Biofactors* **2014**, *40*, 536–545. [CrossRef] [PubMed]
21. Ogura, M. How can cholesterol efflux capacity be used as a risk factor for atherosclerotic cardiovascular disease? *Expert Rev. Cardiovasc. Ther.* **2025**, *23*, 647–653. [CrossRef]
22. Mackness, M.I.; Arrol, S.; Durrington, P.N. Paraoxonase prevents accumulation of lipoperoxides in low-density lipoprotein. *FEBS Lett.* **1991**, *286*, 152–154. Erratum in *FEBS Lett.* **1991**, *292*, 307. [CrossRef] [PubMed]
23. Boullier, A.; Bird, D.A.; Chang, M.K.; Dennis, E.A.; Friedman, P.; Gillotre-Taylor, K.; Hörkkö, S.; Palinski, W.; Quehenberger, O.; Shaw, P.; et al. Scavenger receptors, oxidized LDL, and atherosclerosis. *Ann. N. Y. Acad. Sci.* **2001**, *947*, 214–222, discussion 222–223. [CrossRef] [PubMed]
24. Mackness, M.I.; Abbott, C.; Arrol, S.; Durrington, P.N. The role of high-density lipoprotein and lipid-soluble antioxidant vitamins in inhibiting low-density lipoprotein oxidation. *Biochem. J.* **1993**, *294*, 829–834. [CrossRef] [PubMed] [PubMed Central]
25. Ahmed, Z.; Ravandi, A.; Maguire, G.F.; Emili, A.; Draganov, D.; La Du, B.N.; Kuksis, A.; Connelly, P.W. Multiple substrates for paraoxonase-1 during oxidation of phosphatidylcholine by peroxynitrite. *Biochem. Biophys. Res. Commun.* **2002**, *290*, 391–396. [CrossRef] [PubMed]
26. Soffer, D.E.; Marston, N.A.; Maki, K.C.; Jacobson, T.A.; Bittner, V.A.; Peña, J.M.; Thanassoulis, G.; Martin, S.S.; Kirkpatrick, C.F.; Virani, S.S.; et al. Role of apolipoprotein B in the clinical management of cardiovascular risk in adults: An Expert Clinical Consensus from the National Lipid Association. *J. Clin. Lipidol.* **2024**, *18*, e647–e663. [CrossRef] [PubMed] [PubMed Central]

https://doi.org/10.3390/antiox15020186

27. Kunutsor, S.K.; Bakker, S.J.; James, R.W.; Dullaart, R.P. Serum paraoxonase-1 activity and risk of incident cardiovascular disease: The PREVEND study and meta-analysis of prospective population studies. *Atherosclerosis* **2016**, *245*, 143–154. [CrossRef] [PubMed]
28. Mahrooz, A.; Khosravi-Asrami, O.F.; Alizadeh, A.; Mohmmadi, N.; Bagheri, A.; Kashi, Z.; Bahar, A.; Nosrati, M.; Mackness, M. Can HDL cholesterol be replaced by paraoxonase 1 activity in the prediction of severe coronary artery disease in patients with type 2 diabetes? *Nutr. Metab. Cardiovasc. Dis.* **2023**, *33*, 1599–1607. [CrossRef] [PubMed]
29. Leocádio, P.C.L.; Goulart, A.C.; Santos, I.S.; Lotufo, P.A.; Bensenor, I.M.; Alvarez-Leite, J.I. Lower paraoxonase 1 paraoxonase activity is associated with a worse prognosis in patients with non-ST-segment elevation myocardial infarction in long-term follow-up. *Coron. Artery Dis.* **2022**, *33*, 515–522. [CrossRef] [PubMed]
30. Zamanian, M.Y.; Sadeghi Ivraghi, M.; Khachatryan, L.G.; Vadiyan, D.E.; Bali, H.Y.; Golmohammadi, M. A review of experimental and clinical studies on the therapeutic effects of pomegranate (*Punica granatum*) on non-alcoholic fatty liver disease: Focus on oxidative stress and inflammation. *Food Sci. Nutr.* **2023**, *11*, 7485–7503. [CrossRef] [PubMed] [PubMed Central]
31. Mackness, M.; Boullier, A.; Hennuyer, N.; Mackness, B.; Hall, M.; Tailleux, A.; Duriez, P.; Delfly, B.; Durrington, P.; Fruchart, J.C.; et al. Paraoxonase activity is reduced by a pro-atherosclerotic diet in rabbits. *Biochem. Biophys. Res. Commun.* **2000**, *269*, 232–236. Erratum in *Biochem. Biophys. Res. Commun.* **2000**, *270*, 676. [CrossRef] [PubMed]

antioxidants MDPI

Review

HDL-Cholesterol and Triglycerides Dynamics: Essential Players in Metabolic Syndrome

Sebastià Alcover [1,2], Lisaidy Ramos-Regalado [1,2], Gabriela Girón [1,3], Natàlia Muñoz-García [1,2] and Gemma Vilahur [1,4,*]

1 Research Institute Sant Pau (IR SANT PAU), 08041 Barcelona, Spain; salcover@santpau.cat (S.A.); lramosr@santpau.cat (L.R.-R.); ggiron@santpau.cat (G.G.); nmunoz@santpau.cat (N.M.-G.)
2 Facultat de Biologia, Universitat de Barcelona, 08028 Barcelona, Spain
3 Facultat de Biociències, Universitat Autònoma de Barcelona, 08193 Barcelona, Spain
4 Centro de Investigación Biomédica en Red Enfermedades Cardiovasculares, Instituto de Salud Carlos III, 28029 Madrid, Spain
* Correspondence: gvilahur@santpau.cat; Tel.: +34-935537100

Abstract: Metabolic syndrome (MetS) is a complex cluster of interrelated metabolic disorders that significantly elevate the risk of cardiovascular disease, making it a pressing public health concern worldwide. Among the key features of MetS, dyslipidemia—characterized by altered levels of high-density lipoprotein cholesterol (HDL-C) and triglycerides (TG)—plays a crucial role in the disorder's progression. This review aims to elucidate the intricate interplay between HDL-C and TG within the context of lipid metabolism and cardiovascular health, while also addressing the detrimental impact of various cardiovascular risk factors and associated comorbidities. The dynamics of HDL-C and TG are explored, highlighting their reciprocal relationship and respective contributions to the pathophysiology of MetS. Elevated levels of TGs are consistently associated with reduced concentrations of HDL-C, resulting in a lipid profile that promotes the development of vascular disease. Specifically, as TG levels rise, the protective cardiovascular effects of HDL-C are diminished, leading to the increased accumulation of pro-atherogenic TG-rich lipoproteins and low-density lipoprotein particles within the vascular wall, contributing to the progression of atheromas, which can ultimately result in significant ischemic cardiovascular events. Ultimately, this paper underscores the significance of HDL and TG as essential targets for therapeutic intervention, emphasizing their potential in effectively managing MetS and reducing cardiovascular risk.

Keywords: triglycerides; HDL; metabolic syndrome; lipid metabolism; reverse cholesterol transport; antioxidant activity; insulin resistance; atherosclerosis; cardiovascular disease

1. The Metabolic Syndrome: Epidemiology and Introduction

The earliest associations between comorbidities, including visceral obesity, hypertension, and atherosclerosis, among others, date back to the eighteenth century [1]. However, it was not until the twentieth century that the term metabolic syndrome (MetS) was coined [2] and was defined as the cluster of at least three out of the following five criteria: a high level of abdominal obesity along with visceral fat accumulation (measured by waist circumference), elevated triglyceride (TG) levels, low high-density lipoprotein cholesterol (HDL-C) levels, elevated blood pressure, and increased hyperglycemia and/or hyperinsulinemia [2]. MetS is primarily driven by increased consumption of high-calorie/low-fiber food and a decline in physical activity caused by mechanized transportation and sedentary lifestyles. Monitoring the prevalence of MetS across diverse populations is crucial due to its strong association with an increased risk of developing type 2 diabetes mellitus [2], cardiovascular disease (CVD) [3], and chronic kidney disease [4]. It is estimated that approximately 1.5 billion people (20% of the global population) have MetS [5], in line with the observations of a recent meta-analysis (ranging between 12.5 and 31.4%) [6]. From a financial perspective, the economic burden of MetS, encompassing healthcare expenses and the loss of potential economic productivity, amounts to trillions of dollars [7]. Interestingly, contrary to expectations, there is no significant association between the increase in MetS prevalence and a country's economic status. This trend is observable in African nations where rapid urbanization and the high cost of healthy foods promote unhealthy lifestyle choices, and the prevalence of MetS is increasing [5].

In the following review, we comprehensively examine the role of two key components of MetS, HDL and TG. We first overview the biogenesis of HDL and TG, discuss their role in the cardiovascular system, and explore the detrimental impact of cardiovascular risk factors. We also examine the dynamic connection between HDL and TG particles and their contribution to MetS progression to finally examine potential therapeutic strategies.

2. TG and HDL Biogenesis

Lipid metabolism is a complex and intricately regulated process that encompasses the synthesis, breakdown, and transport of lipids, which are essential for energy homeostasis, cellular signaling, and maintenance of membrane structure. These lipids can originate from dietary sources, referred to as the exogenous pathway, or can be synthesized by cells via the endogenous pathway [8].

The exogenous pathway begins in the small intestine where dietary lipids are absorbed and metabolized (Figure 1). During digestion, lipases hydrolyze the ester bonds in TG, leading to the production of free fatty acids (FFAA) and 2-monoacylglycerol. These digestive products are then emulsified by bile acids and phospholipids (PL) in the intestinal lumen, to form micelles [9]. Upon absorption into the enterocyte, FFAA and 2-monoacylglycerol are used by intestinal cells to synthesize TG, while cholesterol is converted into cholesterol esters (CE). These molecules, along with PLs and apolipoprotein (apo) B48, are subsequently assembled into nascent chylomicrons [10,11]. Nascent chylomicrons circulate through the bloodstream, acquiring apoC-II and apoE from HDL. As they travel to various tissues, they pass through capillaries, where apoC-II activates lipoprotein lipase (LPL), an enzyme also stimulated by insulin. LPL hydrolyzes the TG content of chylomicrons, producing glycerol and FFAA. The FFAA are then taken up by cells for either oxidation or re-esterification into TGs [12,13]. As TGs are depleted from chylomicrons, smaller chylomicron remnant particles are formed. ApoC-II is transferred back to HDL, while apoE is recognized by remnant receptors on hepatocytes. This interaction facilitates the uptake of chylomicron remnants by the liver, where they are further degraded [14].

The endogenous lipid transport pathway is activated during fasting, triggering de novo cholesterol and TG synthesis in the liver [15]. As such, lipids are packaged and secreted as nascent very low-density lipoproteins (VLDL) characterized by the presence of surface apoB-100. Like chylomicrons, VLDL particles acquire apoC-II and apoE from HDL. Upon reaching the vasculature, LPL activation in capillary beds leads to the hydrolysis of TG from VLDL and the subsequent release of FFAA and glycerol [16]. A portion of the TG, PLs, and apoC-II is transferred to HDL, which converts VLDL into denser intermediate-density lipoproteins (IDL). Low-density lipoproteins (LDL), chylomicron remnants, and some IDL can be taken up by the liver via LDL receptors (LDLR) that recognize apoB100 and apoE on the lipoprotein surface. Moreover, TGs contained in the remaining IDL fraction are hydrolyzed by hepatic lipase, generating LDLs, which are predominantly composed of CE. LDL binds to LDLRs, which are present in the cell membranes of most tissues and are internalized through receptor-mediated endocytosis. Once inside the cell, lysosomal enzymes hydrolyze LDL, releasing free cholesterol. In hepatocytes, LDL internalization promotes the inhibition of HMG-CoA reductase, resulting in a decrease in hepatic cholesterol synthesis (Figure 1). This process helps maintain overall cholesterol homeostasis in the body [17,18].

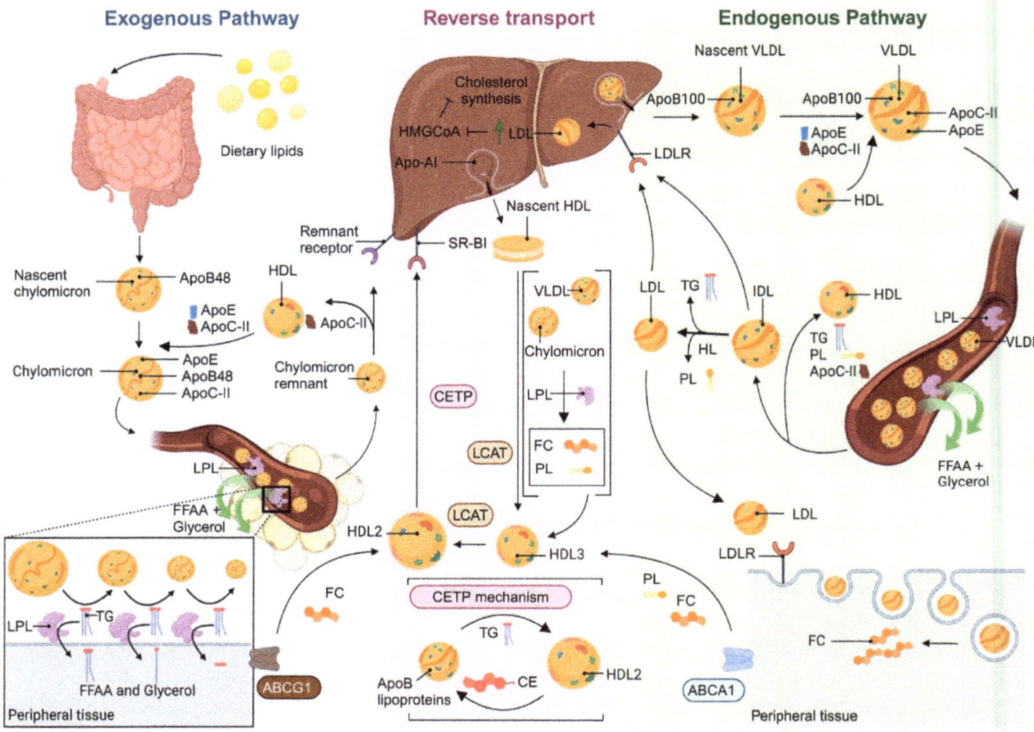

Figure 1. Overview of lipid metabolism pathways. The exogenous pathway starts in the small intestine, where dietary lipids are hydrolyzed, absorbed, and reassembled into nascent chylomicrons. These lipoproteins interact with HDL and acquire apoE and apoC-II. Mature chylomicrons transport TG and cholesterol to peripheral tissues, where LPL hydrolyses TG, releasing FFAA for energy or storage. The chylomicron remnants can interact with HDL and are taken up by the liver. The endogenous pathway is triggered during fasting, with the liver synthesizing VLDL to distribute TG and cholesterol. Nascent VLDL particles receive apoE and apoC-II from HDL's interactions. Mature VLDL is progressively metabolized into IDL and LDL, which return directly to the liver for degradation or deliver cholesterol to tissues by LDLR binding and endocytosis. HDL particles mediate reverse cholesterol transport, shuttling cholesterol from peripheral tissues to the liver for its excretion. ApoA-I is synthesized in the liver and acquires free cholesterol and PL as a result of LPL activity or via ABCA1 transporter from peripheral cells. LCAT esterifies free cholesterol on the HDL surface. As HDL matures, it engages with ABCG1 transporters from peripheral cells to acquire free cholesterol and interacts with CETP to transfer TG in exchange for CE with apoB-containing lipoproteins. Then, HDL can either deliver cholesterol directly to the liver via the SR-BI receptor or indirectly by via CETP apoB-containing lipoproteins, which are then cleared by the liver. Apo: apolipoprotein; TG: triglycerides; LPL: lipoprotein lipase; FFAA: free fatty acid; VLDL: very-low-density lipoproteins; IDL: intermediate-density lipoproteins; LDL: low-density lipoproteins; HDL: high-density lipoproteins; LDLR: LDL receptor; PL: phospholipids; LPL: lipoprotein lipase;

ABCA1: ATP-binding cassette protein A1; LCAT: lecithin–cholesterol acyltransferase; ABCG1: ATP-binding cassette protein G1; CETP: cholesteryl ester transfer protein; CE: cholesterol esters; SR-BI: scavenger receptor class B type I; Green arrow: increase. Created in BioRender.com.

HDL metabolism begins with the production of nascent HDL in the liver and intestine (Figure 1). These particles mature as they incorporate CE derived from cholesterol released by peripheral tissues, allowing HDL to play a central role in reverse cholesterol transport (RCT), shuttling cholesterol back to the liver [8]. The process starts with the synthesis of its main structural apolipoprotein, apoA-I, which acquires free cholesterol and PLs from chylomicrons and VLDL as a result of LPL activity, or via the ATP-binding cassette protein A1 (ABCA1) transporter, from peripheral tissues. ApoA-I acts as a cofactor for the enzyme lecithin–cholesterol acyltransferase (LCAT), which esterifies free cholesterol on the HDL surface, converting it into CE that is incorporated into the HDL core. As HDL matures, it engages with ATP-binding cassette protein G1 (ABCG1) transporters from peripheral cells to acquire free cholesterol and interacts with cholesteryl ester transfer protein (CETP), which facilitates the transfer of TG to HDL from apoB-containing lipoproteins [19]. Through this process, HDL can either deliver cholesterol directly to the liver via the scavenger receptor class B type I (SR-BI) or indirectly transfer CE to apoB-containing lipoproteins via CETP, which are then cleared by the liver [20]. HDL can perform a specific, rapid, and unidirectional cholesterol efflux via ABCA1 and ABCG1 receptors, whereas SR-B1 carries out a slower, passive, and bidirectional cholesterol efflux [21].

3. Understanding HDL: Insights into Functional and Dysfunctional Particles

The Framingham Heart study was the first large epidemiological trial to evidence an inverse association between HDL-C levels and ischemic heart disease [22]. As such, for every 1 mg/dL decrease in HDL-C, the risk of coronary heart disease increased by 2% in men and 3% in women. Several experimental and in vitro approaches have attributed HDL protective effects to its capacity to promote RCT (preventing atheroma plaque formation), exert antioxidant effects, enhance endothelial function, exert cardioprotection and prevent thrombus formation [23–25]. Recent epidemiological studies have also revealed a U-shaped association between HDL-C levels and all-cause mortality, with very high HDL-C levels potentially increasing coronary heart diseases risk [26–28]. Yet, more research is required to elucidate the mechanisms behind this phenomenon and to understand why extremely high HDL-C levels may be detrimental. Likewise, it has become increasingly apparent that the presence of cardiovascular risk factors or comorbid conditions remodel HDL particles into a dysfunctional state, causing them to lose their beneficial properties and potentially become harmful [29]. In the following sections, we explore the advantages of functional HDL particles and examine the potential risks associated with altered HDLs.

3.1. HDL Particles: Structure and Composition

HDL structure is characterized by a neutral lipid core composed mainly of CE and some TG, surrounded by a monolayer consisting of PLs and unesterified cholesterol that anchors various apolipoproteins [30,31]. HDLs have also been found to transport miRNAs that influence various cholesterol-related processes (Figure 2) [32,33] and other cardioprotective functions, such as inflammation regulation [34,35]. Of note, data also suggest that, beyond HDL particles, VLDL particles also carry miRNAs [36]. Over 200 different lipid species have been identified, which, together with protein variations, contribute to the high heterogeneity among HDL [30,31].

HDLs can be classified based on various characteristics; based on their shape and surface charge, they are categorized as pre-β particles or α-migrating; regarding their apolipoprotein content, particles containing only apoA-I are referred to as LpA-I, while those containing both apoA-I and apoA-II are classified as LpA-I:II; considering their size, subtypes range from the largest (HDL2a) to progressively smaller ones, including HDL2b, HDL3a, HDL3b, and HDL3c [20]; and by density, they are differentiated into dense HDL3, and less-dense HDL2 particles. Differences in composition exist within these latter HDL subfractions. As such, HDL3 particles contain lower sphingomyelin and free cholesterol levels, which enhance their fluidity and facilitate the incorporation of oxidized lipids [37], have a greater concentration of sphingosine-1-phosphate (S1P), and contain a higher proportion of proteins associated with cardiovascular protective functions (apoJ, PON1, PLTP, and PAF-AH) [38–40]. On the other hand, HDL2 particles are enriched with apoE and apoCs, suggesting a significant role in RCT due to their higher affinity for interacting with SR-BI and ABCG1 receptors [39]. HDL2 particles also exhibit a more pronounced vasodilatory effect, inducing greater secretion of prostacyclin (vasodilator) by endothelial cells and inhibiting the secretion of thromboxane A2 (a potent vasoconstrictor) [38]. However, excessively large HDL2 particles, with a very large diameter and high TG content, have been associated with an increased risk of coronary artery disease (CAD) [41].

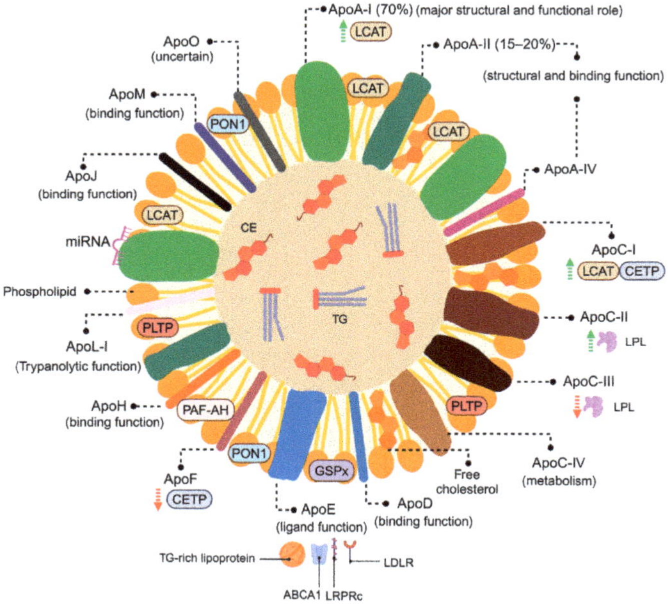

Figure 2. HDL structure and composition: ApoA-I constitutes 70% of the total protein content in HDL, activates LCAT, facilitates interactions with cell receptors, and has a major structural and functional role. ApoA-II represents 15–20% of the total protein and has structural and binding functions like apoA-IV. ApoC-I acts as modulator of CETP activity and as an LCAT activator. ApoC-II serves as an activator of LPL, while apoC-III inhibits its activity. ApoC-IV performs as a TG metabolism regulator. ApoD has been associated with the binding of small hydrophobic molecules. ApoE works as a ligand between TG-rich lipoproteins, ABCA1, LRPRc, and LDLR. Other apolipoproteins include apoF as a CETP inhibitor; apoH as a binder of negatively charged molecules; apoL-I as a trypanolytic factor of human serum; apoJ and apoM have been linked with the binding of small hydrophobic molecules. The function of apoO has yet to be fully elucidated [20]. The HDL lipidome is predominantly composed of PL (40–60%) and CE (30–40%), with the remainder consisting of TG (5–12%) and free cholesterol (5–10%). Moreover, HDL carries enzymes involved in lipid metabolism (LCAT and PLTP) and antioxidant activity (PON1, PAF-AH, and GSPx) [42]. HDLs have also been found to transport miRNAs that influence various cholesterol-related processes [33]. HDL: high-density lipoproteins;

Apo: Apolipoprotein; LCAT: lecithin–cholesterol acyltransferase; CETP: cholesteryl ester transfer protein; LPL: lipoprotein-lipase; TG: triglycerides; ABCA1: ATP-binding cassette protein A1; LRPRc: LDL receptor-related protein; LDLR: LDL receptor; PL: phospholipids; CE: cholesterol esters; LCAT: lecithin–cholesterol acyltransferase; PLTP: phospholipid transfer protein; PON1: paraxonase 1; PAF-AH: platelet-activating factor-acetyl hydrolase; GSPx: glutathione selenoperoxidase; Green arrow: activation; Red arrow: inhibition. Created in BioRender.com.

3.2. Functional HDL Particles

3.2.1 Antioxidant Properties

HDL displays antioxidant properties through apoA-I, PON1, and LCAT [43,44], which are involved in the reduction or hydrolyzation of oxidized lipids [43]. These antioxidative functions require SR-BI and ABCG1 activation [44]. HDL can remove oxidized lipids from lipoproteins and cellular membranes, avoiding endothelial cell apoptosis [45]. Additionally, HDL can prevent LDL oxidation by removing lipid hydroperoxides [43] and can inhibit LDL aggregation through interactions with hydrophobic domains, thus preventing their clustering [46].

PON1 has historically been described as an enzymatic protein capable of hydrolyzing lipid peroxides, thereby reducing the risk of atherosclerosis [47]. Conversely, other studies have shown that PON1 does not exhibit the capacity for phospholipid hydrolysis, thereby limiting its antioxidant capacity to an indirect role [48].

A direct function for apoA-I in reducing oxidative stress has also been demonstrated, along with its fundamental role in the activation of PON1 and LCAT [49]. Two methionine residues in apoA-I (Met112, Met148) are oxidized to sulfoxides during the reduction of lipid peroxides to redox-inactive hydroxides [50,51]. Additionally, CETP has been reported to facilitate the transfer of lipid peroxides from apoB-containing lipoproteins toward HDL [52], while apoM has been suggested to contribute to oxidized phospholipid binding [53].

3.2.2. Vasodilatory and Antithrombotic Properties

HDLs exert multiple beneficial effects on the cardiovascular system [54]. HDLs promote vasodilation by increasing nitric oxide (NO) [55] and prostacyclin [56] production. This process begins with HDL binding to SR-B1 receptors on endothelial cells, which triggers the activation of AMPK, subsequently activating eNOS via the Akt signaling pathway [57]. Additionally, ABCG1-mediated cholesterol efflux lowers the concentration of oxidized cholesterol molecules, facilitating the activation of eNOS dimers and increasing NO production [58]. Of note, through lipid removal, HDLs also exhibit antiapoptotic and anti-inflammatory effects in the endothelium and macrophages [25,59–61]. A third pathway for eNOS activation involves the HDL/apoM/S1P complex, which also leads to Akt signaling activation. This pathway primarily maintains vascular integrity and further promotes cell survival and endothelial cell migration [62]. Higher NO production, in turn, leads to the reduced transcriptional activation of NF-kB in endothelial cells, resulting in a decreased expression of adhesion molecules (VCAM-1, ICAM-1, and P-selectin), pro-inflammatory receptors (TLR-2), and cytokines (MCP-1 and IL-8). In addition, HDLs may exert antithrombotic effects [63] by interacting with endothelial SR-B1 and subsequent NO release (inhibits platelet activation) [64,65] or by inhibiting thrombin-induced tissue factor expression [66]. In fact, the increase in NO also influences oxidative stress, as it acts as an antioxidant by terminating radical chain reactions and inhibiting oxidases. Additionally, NO protects against NADPH oxidase-derived reactive oxygen species (ROS) production in the vascular endothelium [67].

3.2.3. Glucose Metabolism

HDLs also play a crucial role in glucose uptake and maintaining glucose homeostatic blood levels. The interaction of ApoA-I with ABCA1, ABCG1, and SR-B1 has been shown to activate the translocation of GLUT4 in skeletal muscle, endothelial cells, and adipocytes through the AMPK signaling pathway independently or synergistically with insulin [68]. This interaction induces an intracellular calcium increase and subsequent activation of CaMKK [68,69]. Several studies involving HDL infusions have reported increased GLUT4 transcript levels and a higher degree of GLUT4 translocation [70–72] regardless of HDL cholesterol efflux capacity [70,73]. Moreover, apoA-I binding to the β-cells membranes via ABCA1 has been described to exclude forkhead box protein O1 (FoxO1) from the nucleus and enhance the expression of *Pdx1*, a transcription factor that increases insulin secretion and regulates the expression of various genes associated with β-cell identity, functionality, and survival [74,75], besides increasing the number of insulin granules at the β-cell surface [76]. In addition, data suggest that HDLs may reduce glucagon secretion from α-cells [77].

3.2.4. Others

HDL intravenous infusion has also been shown to reduce infarct size and improve cardiac function post-myocardial infarction [78,79]. The mechanisms behind this involve a reduction in apoptosis execution through the activation of RISK and SAFE signaling. The RISK pathway, which encompasses the PI3K/AKT/eNOS axis, serves to protect endothelial cells from pro-inflammatory signaling induced by TNFα, whereas the SAFE pathway is believed to be activated by S1P bound to HDL [80].

In addition to their cardiovascular protective effects, HDLs have been suggested to inhibit LPS-induced cellular activation [81], to protect against certain parasitic species [82], to regulate neural tissue formation, and to contribute to β-amyloid clearance [83]. As such, low levels of apoA-I and HDL-C have been correlated with the early onset of Parkinson's disease [84,85] and the development of Alzheimer's disease [86,87].

3.3. HDL Adverse Remodelling: The Impact of Cardiovascular Risk Factors and Comorbid Conditions in HDL Functionality

The structure and composition of HDLs are essential for binding to key receptors, which enables their primary role in RCT as well as their anti-inflammatory, anti-platelet, antioxidant, anti-apoptotic, and glucose uptake functions. Consequently, any changes to HDL can disturb their homeostasis, leading to decreased functionality and potentially transforming HDL into a harmful entity. This is particularly evident in chronic and severe conditions such as CVD [88], obesity [89], chronic kidney disease [90], liver disease [91], and diabetes [92]. Consequently, the "HDL quality over quantity hypothesis" has gained popularity as a possible explanation for missing protective effects in secondary prevention [93].

Various cardiovascular risk factors, including aging, smoking, infections, pollutants, dietary imbalances, glycation, and oxidative stress, have been shown to negatively impact HDL functionality [94]. We have reported, in highly translatable animal models by means of cardiac magnetic resonance imaging, that diet-induced hypercholesterolemia disrupts HDL function, impairing its cardioprotective [79] and atheroprotective effects [95]. These functional changes were associated with alterations in their proteomic, lipidomic, and miRNA profile [96]. Interestingly, we found that adverse remodeling of HDL can be reversed by implementing a low-fat diet and reducing LDL-C levels to a normal physiological state [97].

Hyperglycemia, one of the main features of diabetes, results in non-enzymatic glycation of plasma protein and has also been shown to adversely affect HDL composition [92]. Structural alterations in apoA-I due to glycation disrupt critical regions, impairing the activation of LCAT [98], decreasing macrophage-mediated RCT, reducing the suppression of adhesion molecule expression, and promoting ROS generation [99]. Glycation also shortens the half-life of apoA-I, further compromising HDL functionality [100]. Additionally, glycated HDL induces mitochondrial dysfunction in endothelial cells, increasing ROS levels and enhancing apoptosis [101]. Furthermore, glycated HDL exhibits a reduced ability to counteract the harmful effects of oxLDL on endothelial vasorelaxation [101].

Hypertriglyceridemia increases TG-enriched HDL levels, which have been shown to enhance net cholesterol efflux from macrophages while reducing the esterification rate due to low LCAT activity. This leads to a redistribution of cholesterol within the HDL, due to the increased TG/CE ratio, which enhances core fluidity, altering HDL lipoprotein composition [102]. These changes alter the conformation of apoA-I domains, reducing their ability to act as lipid acceptors and decreasing their exposure to the aqueous phase, thereby impairing their binding function [103] and RCT [104]. On the other hand, HDL alterations have been detected before the onset of hypertriglyceridemia in patients with MetS, including a reduction of S1P levels and subsequent impairment of eNOS activation [105,106].

Moreover, hypertriglyceridemia enhances CETP activity and reduces LPL activity [107], promoting large cholesterol ester-core-depleted HDL particles, which become targets for hepatic lipase [108], or for endothelial lipases, which hydrolyze TG as well as PLs [109]. Consequently, these modifications result in a decreased affinity for apoA-I, which reduces its plasma residence time [110] and functionality [20].

Excessive ROS levels generated by cellular lipotoxicity or by myeloperoxidase during atherosclerosis can induce structural modifications in HDL through the oxidation of the tyrosine 192 residue of apoA-I, leading to the formation of oxidized amino acid species and impairing HDL's ability to mediate ABCA1-dependent cholesterol efflux [111,112]. Additionally, myeloperoxidase has been reported to reduce the anti-apoptotic effects of HDL, increase plaque instability [113], and diminish its antioxidant capacity by lowering PON1 activity [114]. Moreover, ROS can act on the polyunsaturated fatty acid tails of PLs or CE, generating a lipid radical that reacts with oxygen to form a lipid peroxyl radical. This oxidative molecule can propagate the reaction to adjacent PLs or polyunsaturated fatty acids, ultimately leading to HDL dysfunction [111,115].

On the other hand, genetic mutations affecting enzymes, proteins, and receptors have been shown to disrupt HDL metabolism, altering their plasma levels, modifying their composition, and impairing their beneficial properties [116]. As such, the reduction in LCAT activity, either derived from genetic mutations or exposure to pathological conditions [116], has been associated with lower HDL particle maturation and decreased HDL-C plasma levels. Likewise, genetic modifications that reduce CETP activity are associated with a decreased risk of CVD [117], resulting in increased HDL-C levels and reduced LDL-C levels. CETP-deficient individuals typically exhibit higher concentrations of HDL2a-C and enhanced SR-B1/ABCG1-mediated cholesterol efflux [118]. While these HDLs retain normal anti-inflammatory and antioxidant properties, they display reduced NO production, potentially due to lower content on S1P [119].

4. The Role of TG and FFAA in Metabolic and Cardiovascular Risk

According to the latest European guidelines, elevated fasting TG levels were defined as $\geq$150 mg/dL ($\geq$1.7 mmol/L), moderate hypertriglyceridemia as 150–880 mg/dL (1.7–10 mmol/L), and severe hypertriglyceridemia as >885 mg/dL (>10 mmol/L). Moreover, levels exceeding 440 mg/dL (5 mmol/L) may require action to prevent acute pancreatitis, with a higher risk at levels above 880 mg/dL (10 mmol/L) [120]. A study performed in 2020 showed hypertriglyceridemia prevalence (sex- and age-adjusted) of 27.0% in the Spanish global population, 34.6% in men, and 21.4% in women [121]. In the same year, the prevalence of hypertriglyceridemia was reported in the US as 25.9%; of which, 31.6% were receiving statin treatment [122]. There are extensive data regarding the causal association between TG and the increased risk of cardiovascular events, even in patients receiving effective LDL-lowering therapy [123]. It has been observed that, in a fasting state, each 88 mg/dL increase in TG levels raises the risk of coronary heart disease by 32% in men and 76% in women [124].

Elevated FFAA can adversely affect lipid metabolism, glucose control, and vascular function, highlighting the importance of maintaining balanced levels of TG levels for overall cardiovascular health. As described below and in Figure 3, FFAA can stimulate the liver's production of VLDL [125]. This process often results in elevated serum TG levels while concurrently decreasing HDL-C concentrations [126]. In addition, elevated FFAA can impair cellular metabolism and insulin action in skeletal muscle, adipose tissue, and the liver [68,127]. This impairment reduces the effectiveness of insulin in facilitating glucose uptake, which can lead to increased blood glucose concentrations. Lastly, increased FFAA can stimulate vasoconstriction and enhance sodium reabsorption in the kidneys, contributing to increased blood pressure [128].

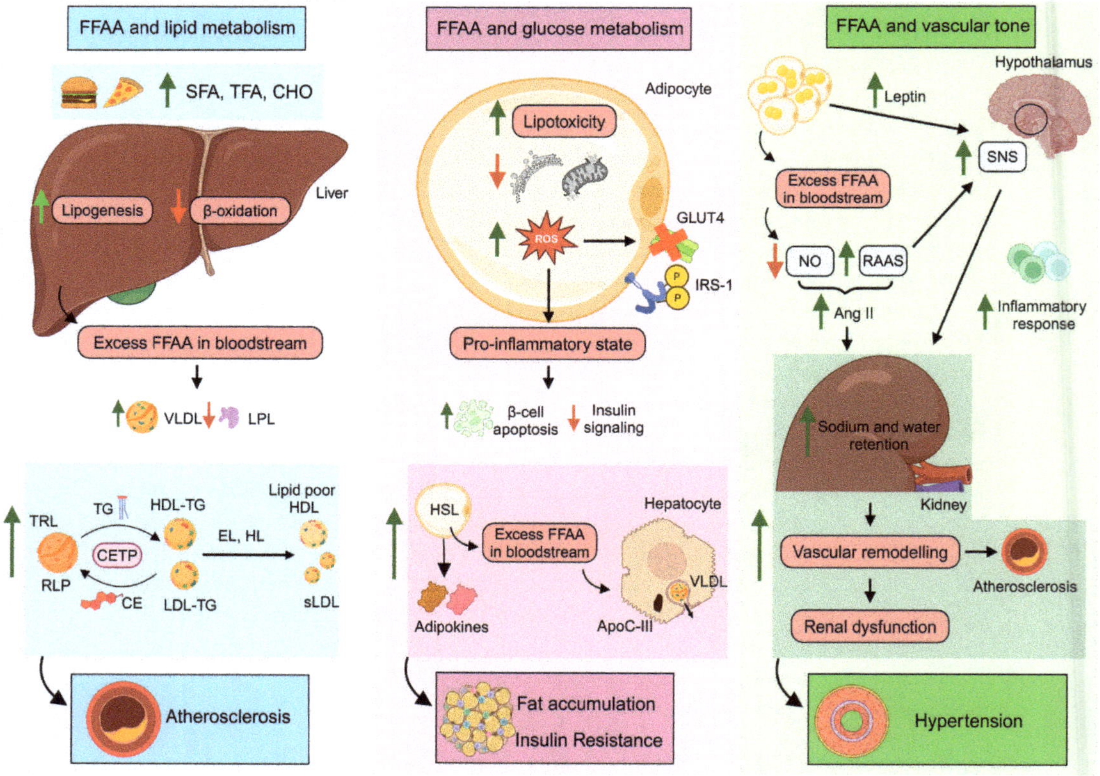

Figure 3. Adverse effects of high FFAA levels on lipid metabolism, glucose control, and vascular tone. (**Left**): The excessive consumption of foods rich in SFA, TFA, and carbohydrates disrupts hepatic

metabolic pathways, leading to enhanced VLDL production and decreased LPL activity. This results in elevated TRL and RLP levels because of the upregulation of CETP activity. Increased CETP activity, in turn, results in lipid poor HDL and small LDL, enhancing the risk of atherosclerosis progression. (**Center**): An excess of FFAA can promote cellular lipotoxicity and generate ROS, impairing the cell's glucose metabolism and contributing to an inflammatory state that may induce β-cell apoptosis and the development of IR. IR leads to increased secretion of FFAA and adipokines from adipocytes, stimulating VLDL and apoC-III synthesis in hepatocytes. This cascade results in further fat accumulation and exacerbates IR. (**Right**): In the case of vascular tone, an excessive release of leptin and FFAA stimulates the SNS, reduces endothelial NO production, and activates RAAS. RAAS further triggers SNS and Ang II synthesis, leading to an increase in renal sodium and water retention and promoting inflammatory cell infiltration. Collectively, these processes contribute to vascular remodeling and renal dysfunction, culminating in systemic vascular resistance and hypertension. FFAA: free fatty acids; SFA: saturated fatty acids; TFA: trans fatty acids; CHO: carbohydrates; VLDL: very low-density lipoproteins; LPL: lipoprotein lipase; TG: triglycerides; TRL: TG-rich lipoproteins; CETP: cholesteryl ester transfer protein; HDL: high-density lipoproteins; LDL: low-density lipoproteins; EL: endothelial lipase; HL: hepatic lipase; RLP: remnant lipoprotein particles; sLDL: small LDL; CE: cholesterol ester; GLUT4: glucose transporter type 4; IRS-1: Insulin receptor substrate 1; ROS: reactive oxygen species; HSL: hormone-sensitive lipase; IR: insulin resistance; ApoC-III: apolipoprotein C-III; SNS: sympathetic nervous activity; NO: nitric oxide; RAAS: renin–angiotensin–aldosterone system; Ang II: angiotensin II; Green arrow: increase; Red arrow: decrease. Created in BioRender.com.

4.1. FFAA and Lipid Metabolism: TG-Rich Lipoproteins and Remnant Lipoprotein Particles

A contributor to hypertriglyceridemia is a diet high in saturated fatty acids and refined sugars, among others [129]. The uptake of circulating FFAA by the liver, skeletal muscle, and other tissues is essential for lipid storage and mobilization [130]. Saturated fatty acids have been shown to reduce the expression, protein levels, and activity of hepatic LDLR, thereby decreasing LDL uptake and increasing blood LDL-C levels [131,132]. On the other hand, trans fatty acids contribute to an increase in LDL-C by reducing the catabolic rate of LDL-apoB without affecting its production levels. Trans fatty acids also increase the metabolic rate of apoA-I from HDL, without impacting its production rate [133,134]. Moreover, trans fatty acids elevate CETP activity, leading to greater TG/CE exchange between apoB-containing proteins and HDL, lowering HDL-C levels [135]. Furthermore, dietary carbohydrates serve as substrates in the liver for de novo FFAA synthesis, particularly during caloric excess. This process is amplified by glucose-induced insulin secretion, which also enhances hepatic FFAA production [136]. Excess in carbohydrate intake allows fructose to bypass the intestinal metabolism, enabling it to reach the liver directly, where it stimulates hepatic lipogenesis via SREBP1c and ChREBP. Unlike glucose, fructose metabolism does not have self-regulatory mechanisms, leading to an uncontrolled supply of substrates for lipogenesis. Additionally, fructose inhibits FFAA oxidation, contributing to higher TG hepatic levels. On top of this, fructose does not stimulate insulin production, avoiding LPL activation and reducing the clearance of TG-rich lipoproteins (TRL) [137,138].

The excess of FFAA in the bloodstream from the exogenous or/and endogenous pathway is absorbed and stored by the liver as TG [130]. This process leads to the overproduction and release of hepatic VLDL (particularly larger and TG-rich VLDL) [125], which hinders the lipolysis of chylomicrons by competing at the LPL level [139]. Additionally, hypertriglyceridemia has been shown to reduce the expression of LPL in muscle and adipose tissues [107], impairing the enzyme's ability to bind to the lipoprotein surface, disrupting lipolysis [140] and facilitating the transport of TRL back to the liver [139]. The rise in TRL heightens CETP activity. This excessive exchange yields TG-rich LDL and HDL particles, which are hydrolyzed by lipases, producing small, dense, and pro-atherogenic LDL particles and lipid-poor HDL particles that are rapidly catabolized. This process explains the observed association between high TG levels and low HDL-C plasma concentrations [136], which contribute to the development of atherosclerosis. Specifically, increased TG levels facilitate the intimal accumulation of LDL particles, while decreased HDL-C levels—particularly the loss of HDL's protective functions—hinder the removal of vascular cholesterol, as stated above.

On the other hand, there is an increase in the number and the half-life of TRL. The hydrolysis of TG from TRL within the endothelial lumen by LPL generates remnant lipoprotein particles (RLP). These particles are smaller than chylomicrons and VLDL, allowing them to penetrate the endothelium and reach the intimal layer. RLPs are also CE-rich molecules, as they remain a target for CETP [141]. Notably, they are considered even more pro-atherogenic than LDL-C, as they can be taken up directly by macrophages without oxidation, leading to foam cell formation and promoting the initial stages of atheroma plaque development [142]. Additionally, due to their size, RLPs can carry up to 40 times more cholesterol than LDL [143].

4.2. FFAA and Glucose Control

In healthy conditions, FFAA are taken up via specific membrane receptors, such as FA transport proteins 1–6 or CD36, depending on the cell type. Once inside the cell, FFAA are either stored as TG or utilized through β-oxidation as substrates for mitochondrial respiration. The binding of insulin to its membrane receptor in adipocyte cells triggers the inactivation of hormone-sensitive lipase, the enzyme responsible for hydrolyzing TG into glycerol and FFAA [144]. Moreover, insulin promotes glucose disposal in skeletal muscle cells by the translocation of GLUT4 through the activation of the IRβ/IRS-1/PI3K/Akt/AS160 pathway [145]. Under metabolic alterations, an excess of FFAA can disrupt these cellular pathways, promoting organ lipotoxicity mediated by the accumulation of TG, diacylglycerol, and ceramides [146,147]. Furthermore, it may induce endoplasmic reticulum stress and mitochondrial dysfunction, triggering the production of ROS. ROS, in turn, damages proteins involved in glucose uptake while also inducing changes in cellular homeostasis. These changes promote the activation of various intracellular pathways, including TNF-α, JNK, and PKC, among others, increasing serine over threonine phosphorylation of IRS-1, thereby impairing insulin signaling [147,148]. Moreover, oxidative stress stimulates pro-inflammatory cytokines, inflammasome activation, and macrophage tissue infiltration, resulting in cellular apoptosis. When this damage occurs in β-cells, it favors the onset of insulin resistance (IR) [127]. However, in a state of IR, hormone-sensitive lipase remains active, resulting in an increase in glycerol and FFAA and a subsequent increase in hepatic VLDL-TG secretion [149].

IR has been associated with enhanced apoC-III levels. ApoC-III hinders the binding of TRL to the cell surface, where LPL is situated. By doing so, apoC-III impairs the hydrolytic activity of LPL, as it displaces apoC-II, which is a crucial cofactor necessary for LPL to function on the lipoprotein surface. This displacement reduces the efficiency of LPL in hydrolyzing TG into FFAA, ultimately affecting lipid metabolism and leading to elevated levels of TG in the bloodstream [150]. *Apoc3* expression is partially regulated by the FoxO1 pathway, which plays a crucial role in controlling apoC-III production in the liver. Insulin facilitates the phosphorylation and subsequent inactivation of the FoxO1 pathway, resulting in the inhibition of *apoc3* gene expression and a decrease in apoC-III levels [151]. In contrast, glucose exerts an opposing effect by promoting increased apoC-III production [152]. Initially, elevated levels of apoC-III are a consequence of IR; however, as the condition advances, apoC-III itself contributes to impaired insulin signaling. This creates a feedback loop where sustained increases in circulating FFAA lead to heightened apoC-III concentrations in lipoproteins, which then remain in circulation for extended periods, exacerbating IR. On the other hand, fat accumulation in adipose tissue leads to an imbalance in TG turnover resulting in several described morpho-functional changes. These changes include alterations in adipocyte size and extracellular matrix reorganization, triggering the production of cytokines, known as adipokines (leptin, resistin, and visfatin), which have been associated with the development of IR [153,154].

4.3. FFAA Levels and the Vascular Tone

Recent studies have suggested that TG may act as an independent risk factor for the development of hypertension [155]. The accumulation of FFAA in renal tissues increases ROS production and impairs NO synthesis [156], which contributes to the activation of the renin–angiotensin–aldosterone system (RAAS) and, further, angiotensin II formation. Angiotensin II is a potent vasoconstrictor that stimulates the release of aldosterone and vasopressin, favoring sodium and water retention along the nephron [128,157]. Nevertheless, RAAS activates the hypothalamus, triggering sympathetic outflow towards the kidneys and promoting the activation of renal dendritic cells, which accumulate isoLG (isolevuglandins), enhancing the production of IL-6 and IL-1β [158]. This, in turn, facilitates inflammatory cell infiltration, exacerbating dysfunction and damage within renal tissue [159]. Inflammatory cells, along with cytokines and chemokines such as IL-1β, TNF-α, IFN-γ, and IL-17A, infiltrate the kidney and regulate the expression and activity of sodium transporters, leading to prolonged sodium and water retention, causing further renal damage. On top of this tissue damage, vascular remodeling occurs, characterized by the narrowing of the vascular lumen due to medial thickening and capillary loss (rarefaction) [160]. This reduction in cross-sectional area further increases systemic vascular resistance, perpetuating hypertension [161] and renal dysfunction [162].

5. The TG/HDL-C Ratio

Taking into consideration the key role of HDL and TG on lipid metabolism and cardiovascular risk, the TG/HDL-C ratio has emerged as a strong predictor of CAD and MetS [163,164]. The TG/HDL-C ratio has been shown to be an independent and more potent predictor of CAD than LDL-C and total-C/HDL-C or LDL-C/HDL-C ratios [164]. As such, high values of the TG/HDL-C ratio have been associated with a 2-fold increase in all-cause mortality and a 1.5- to 3-fold increase in cardiovascular events over a 5–6-year follow-up period, independent of traditional coronary risk factors and angiographic CAD severity [165,166]. Additionally, there has been an almost 2-fold increase in non-fatal myocardial infarction in intermediate-low risk patients with the highest TG/HDL-C ratio [167]. Likewise, the TG/HDL-C ratio has been considered to better identify MetS as compared to total-C/HDL-C and LDL-C/HDL-C ratios [168,169]. However, the TG/HDL-C ratio should not be used as an absolute value without considering age, ethnicity, genetics, and lifestyle [170].

6. Therapeutic Management to Target TG and HDL-C Levels

6.1. Lifestyle Changes

Exercise: The body prioritizes glucose or FFAA as the main source of energy production depending on the type, duration, and intensity of exercise. This workload is quantified in terms of VO_{2max}, which is defined as the maximum oxygen consumption a person can utilize per unit of time. During low-intensity exercise, with a VO_{2max} of around 25%, energy is predominantly derived from the β-oxidation of plasma FFAA [171]. As exercise intensity increases to a moderate level, nearing 65% VO_{2max}, energy demand is primarily met by FFAA released through the lipolysis of TG stored in adipose tissue. Beyond this level, classified as high-intensity exercise, there is a progressive shift toward glucose metabolism at the expense of FFAA utilization [172]. Some studies have observed that engaging in physical activity at 65–80% VO_{2max} is necessary to achieve a reduction in TG and an increase in HDL-C levels [173]. Interestingly, several studies with a large number of participants have demonstrated that prolonged intense exercise improves HDL-related cholesterol efflux [174,175]. Additionally, both acute [176] and chronic [177] exercise has been shown to enhance the antioxidant properties of HDL [174], and several studies involving patients with MetS have observed enhanced anti-inflammatory capacity associated with a decrease in TG and free cholesterol levels, alongside an increase in esterified cholesterol in HDL3b [178]. These changes correlated with greater protection against endothelial cell injury, evidenced by the reduced expression of V-CAM and decreased monocyte endothelial adhesion [179,180].

During exercise, muscle contraction leads to the release of peptides and cytokines (known as myokines) [181], including IL-6, IL-15, myostatin, irisin, and FNDCs. These myokines affect adipose tissue, particularly white adipose tissue, which serves as the primary energy storage site in the form of TG, predominantly located in intra-abdominal visceral depots [182]. Moreover, myokines activate a process known as browning, which involves the conversion of white adipose tissue into brown adipose tissue, a subtype of adipose tissue primarily responsible for energy expenditure and heat generation due to its high mitochondrial content and UCP-1 expression [182,183]. Effects on other organs have also been described, such as the pancreas, where several myokines protect β-cells from pro-inflammatory processes [184]. Furthermore, it has been reported that increased glucose uptake by the muscle is accompanied by an increase in hepatic glucose production [185], a reduction in appetite [185], the regulation of bone growth [186], and improvements in endothelial function and revascularization [187].

Diet: There is strong evidence from epidemiological studies indicating that increasing compliance with the Mediterranean diet is associated with reduced fatal and non-fatal CVD [188,189]. As such, experimental studies have proven that the intake of Mediterranean diet components preserves endothelial function [190,191], lessens platelet reactivity [192,193], reduces LDL oxidation [194], increases HDL-C levels [194], and protects against myocardial infarction damage [195–197]. The landmark PREDIMED trial reported a lower incidence of cardiovascular events in participants consuming a Mediterranean diet supplemented with extra virgin olive oil (EVOO) or nuts as compared to those who followed a low-fat diet [198]. Of note, participants recruited in the study presented diabetes or $\geq$3 risk factors (smoking, overweight or obesity, hypertension, dyslipidemia, and family history of early-onset CVD). Following these seminal findings, sub-studies were conducted to examine the effect of the Mediterranean diet on HDL functionality. An increase in cholesterol efflux was observed in those following the EVOO/nut supplementation, which was associated with an upregulation of HDL-related genes, changes in HDL-associated lipids, and improved antioxidant capacity [199]. No changes were noted in the levels of the major apolipoproteins [199]. Additionally, in the EVOO-supplemented group, an increase in LCAT activity and a decline in CETP activity were observed compared to pre-diet levels [199]. HDL also displayed enhanced antioxidant activity, which was found to be associated with an increase in PON1 content and a reduction in LDL oxidation, likely to protect LCAT from oxidative modifications [199,200]. On the other hand, HDL structural changes were also reported in the Mediterranean diet groups (particularly in the EVOO arm), showing a reduction in TG concentration and an increase in PL levels on the HDL surface. Overall, the benefits attributed to EVOO (omega-9 fatty acids) intake on HDL particles were associated with polyphenol content [201,202]. Positive effects for omega-3 fatty acids found in fish have also been described, including a reduction in TG levels [203] and an improvement in HDL beneficial effects [204].

Lycopene, a powerful antioxidant found in tomatoes, has also been associated with higher HDL-related PON1 and LCAT activity, as well as reduced serum amyloid A content and CETP activity [205]. Positive effects have also been observed with the consumption of walnuts and avocados, foods rich in polyphenols and MUFA. Walnut consumption has shown to improve HDL cholesterol removal and endothelial function [206], while avocado consumption has led to reductions in LDL-C and non-HDL-C levels, as well as a decrease in small and dense LDL particles [207]. Additionally, moderate alcohol intake (40 g of alcohol/day) has been associated with an increase in HDL-C levels, higher PON1, and reduced CETP activity [194,208–211]. Finally, beneficial effects have been observed from consuming whole grains, legumes, some vegetables, fruits, and seeds (all low-glycemic index carbohydrate) in overall CV health [212–215].

6.2. Drug Therapy

6.2.1. Effort to Improve Primary Cardiovascular Endpoints by Increasing HDL-C Levels or HDL-Mimetics

The efficacy of CETP inhibitors has been tested in multiple phase III clinical trials in combination with statin therapy, aiming to achieve a dual positive effect on atherosclerosis by limiting its progression with statins and favoring its regression via HDL. However, most of the trials failed to meet these expectations, as we recently reviewed in Schoch et al. [23].

On the other hand, although significant improvements have been achieved in the field of HDL mimetics at an experimental level, they have consistently failed to demonstrate benefits in the clinical setting [24]. As such, a recent clinical trial administering CSL112, a human apolipoprotein A-I derived from plasma, did not show a reduction in the risk of major adverse cardiovascular events over a 90-day period [216].

6.2.2. Others Therapeutic Strategies

Drug therapies for the management of TG and HDL-C levels are detailed in Table 1.

Table 1. Drug therapies for the management of TG and HDL-C level. CETP: cholesteryl ester transfer protein; HDL: high-density lipoproteins; TG: triglycerides; MetS: metabolic syndrome; IPE: icosapent ethyl; EPA: eicosapentaenoic acid; DHA: docosahexaenoic acid; ↑: increase; ↓: decrease; CV: cardiovascular; CVD: cardiovascular disease; T2DM: diabetes mellitus type II; MACE: major adverse cardiovascular events.

Drug Class	Example(s)	Doses (Oral)	Clinical Indications (Type of Patients)	Positive Outcomes	Clinical Outcomes	Reference
Vitamin B3	Niacin	500–2000 mg/d	CVD, MetS	↑HDL by ~15–30%, ↓TG by ~20–50%	No effect or ↓CV events	[217–219]
CETP Inhibitors	Dalcetrapib;	600 mg/d	Recent acute coronary syndrome;	↑HDL by ~31–40%; no significant ↓TG;	No significant ↓CV events;	[220]
	Evacetrapib;	130 mg/d	Acute coronary syndrome, cerebrovascular disease, T2DM with CVD;	↑HDL by ~130%, ↓TG by ~6%;	No significant ↓CV events;	[221]
	Torceratrip	60 mg/d	High CV risk;	↑HDL by ~72%, ↓TG by ~10%;	↑CV events, ↑death;	[222]
	Anacetrapib	100 mg/d	High CVD risk, low HDL levels	↑HDL by ~145%, ↓TG by ~9%	↓CV events (men)	[223]
Omega-3 Fatty Acids	IPE	4 g/d	High CV risk or T2DM	↑HDL by ~3%, ↓TG by ~20%	↓CV events	[224]
	EPA + DHA	4 g/d	High risk of CVD with low HDL, elevated TG	↑HDL by ~5%, ↓TG by ~19%	No significant ↓MACE	[225]
Fibrates	Fenofibrate	200 mg/d	T2DM	↑HDL by ~5%, ↓TG by ~29%	No significant ↓primary outcome	[226]
	Gemfibrozil	1200 mg/d	CVD, low HDL, elevated TG	↑HDL by ~6%, ↓TG by ~31%	↓MACE	[227]
Statin + Fibrate	Simvastatin + Fenofibrate	40 + 160 mg/d	Low HDL, high TG	↑HDL by ~8%, ↓TG by ~26%	No significant ↓primary outcome	[228]
Thiazolidinediones	Pioglitazone	15–45 mg/d,	T2DM with CVD	↑HDL by ~19%, ↓TG by ~11%	↓CV events, ↓death	[229]
Statins	Rosuvastatin	20 mg/d	High CV risk	No significant ↑HDL, ↓TG by ~19%	↓MACE	[230]

7. Future Perspectives and Directions

The HDL field still has several important areas that require further investigation. It is becoming increasingly accepted that HDL structure and function are better indicators of HDL's protective function than measuring the amount of cholesterol transported by the HDL particles. Yet, it remains to be determined which specific HDL features are most strongly associated with protection against CVD to tackle them from a therapeutic perspective. In addition, while some Mendelian randomization studies have shown a causal relationship between certain HDL traits and decreased CVD risk [41,231,232], more research is needed to fully understand the genetic components influencing HDL functionality and their impact on cardiovascular health, as well as the U-shaped HDL-related behavior.

Within the TG field, determining whether TGs themselves or other components of TRLs are the primary culprit in increasing cardiovascular risk is crucial. In addition, the efficacy and safety of the new TG-lowering therapies (i.e. inhibitors of angiopoietin-like 3 protein and apolipoprotein C-III) in reducing cardiovascular events remain to be assessed in robust clinical trials. In fact, whether targeting TG production, lipolysis, hepatic clearance, or a combination of these mechanisms yields the best outcomes deserves attention. Finally, a deeper understanding of the complex interactions between HDL particles and TG within the context of MetS is essential. Investigating the molecular mechanisms that govern their biogenesis and reciprocal relationship will provide crucial insights into how alterations in these lipid particles contribute to the metabolic disease beyond providing new therapeutic targets to effectively manage MetS patients.

Author Contributions: S.A. has contributed to the drafting of the manuscript and revising the figures. L.R.-E. and G.G. contributed to the design and development of the figures and the text. N.M.-G. revised the content of the paper. G.V. was key in the conception and design of the review, revising it critically for important intellectual content and for the final approval of the manuscript submitted. All authors have read and agreed to the published version of the manuscript.

Funding: This work was supported by Grant PID2021-128891OB-I00 (to G.V.), PLEC2021-007664—Unión Europea NextGenerationEU/PRTR (to G.V.), and Grant M-ERA-NET-3/PCI2023-143431—EU Horizon 2020 (to G.V.) funded by MCIN/AEI/10.13039/501100011033 and Fondo Europeo de Desarrollo Regional (FEDER) A way of making Europe; and the Generalitat of Catalunya-Secretaria d'Universitats i Recerca del Departament d'Economia i Coneixement de la Generalitat [2017SGR1480 to L.B.] and 2016PROD00043 (Agencia Gestión Ayudas Universitarias Investigación: AGAUR). This study is part of the studies of S.A. for the Doctorate in Biomedicine at the University of Barcelona.

Conflicts of Interest: The authors declare no conflicts of interest.

Abbreviations

The following abbreviations are used in this manuscript:

ABCA1	ATP-binding cassette protein A1
ABCG1	ATP-binding cassette protein G1
Apo	apolipoprotein
CAD	coronary artery disease
CE	cholesterol esters
CETP	cholesteryl ester transfer protein
CVD	cardiovascular disease
EVOO	extra virgin olive oil
FFAA	free fatty acids
FoxO1	forkhead box protein O1
HDL	high-density lipoproteins

IDL	intermediate-density lipoproteins
IR	insulin resistance
LCAT	lecithin–cholesterol acyltransferase
LDL	low-density lipoproteins
LDLR	LDL receptor
MetS	metabolic syndrome
MUFA	mono-saturated fatty acids
NO	nitric oxide
PL	phospholipids
RAAS	renin–angiotensin–aldosterone system
RCT	reverse cholesterol transport
RISK	reperfusion injury signaling kinase
RLP	remnant lipoprotein particles
ROS	reactive oxygen species
SAFE	survivor activating factor enhancement
S1P	sphingosine-1-phosphate
SR-BI	scavenger receptor class B type I
TG	triglycerides
TRL	TG-rich lipoprotein
VCAM-1	vascular cell adhesion molecule-1
VLDL	very low-density lipoproteins

References

1. Enzi, G.; Busetto, L.; Inelmen, E.M.; Coin, A.; Sergi, G. Historical Perspective: Visceral Obesity and Related Comorbidity in Joannes Baptista Morgagni's "De Sedibus et Causis Morborum per Anatomen Indagata". *Int. J. Obes. Relat. Metab. Disord.* **2003**, *27*, 534–535. [CrossRef] [PubMed]
2. Nilsson, P.M.; Tuomilehto, J.; Rydén, L. The Metabolic Syndrome—What Is It and How Should It Be Managed? *Eur. J. Prev. Cardiol.* **2019**, *26*, 33–46. [CrossRef]
3. Martínez-Larrad, M.T.; Corbatón-Anchuelo, A.; Fernández-Pérez, C.; Lazcano-Redondo, Y.; Escobar-Jiménez, F.; Serrano-Ríos, M. Metabolic Syndrome, Glucose Tolerance Categories and the Cardiovascular Risk in Spanish Population. *Diabetes Res. Clin. Pract.* **2016**, *114*, 23–31. [CrossRef] [PubMed]
4. Fwu, C.-W.; Schulman, I.H.; Lawrence, J.M.; Kimmel, P.L.; Eggers, P.; Norton, J.; Chan, K.; Mendley, S.R.; Barthold, J.S. Association of Obesity, Metabolic Syndrome, and Diabetes With Urinary Incontinence and Chronic Kidney Disease: Analysis of the National Health and Nutrition Examination Survey, 2003–2020. *J. Urol.* **2024**, *211*, 124–133. [CrossRef] [PubMed]
5. Ferrari, C.K.B. *Epidemiology of Metabolic Syndrome: Global Scenario*; Elsevier Inc.: Amsterdam, The Netherlands, 2024; ISBN 9780323857321.
6. Noubiap, J.J.; Nansseu, J.R.; Lontchi-Yimagou, E.; Nkeck, J.R.; Nyaga, U.F.; Ngouo, A.T.; Tounouga, D.N.; Tianyi, F.L.; Foka, A.J.; Ndoadoumgue, A.L.; et al. Geographic Distribution of Metabolic Syndrome and Its Components in the General Adult Population: A Meta-Analysis of Global Data from 28 Million Individuals. *Diabetes Res. Clin. Pract.* **2022**, *188*, 109924. [CrossRef]
7. Elabbassi, W.N.; Haddad, H.A. The Epidemic of the Metabolic Syndrome. *Saudi Med. J.* **2005**, *26*, 373–375.
8. Badimon, L.; Chiva-Blanch, G. Lipid Metabolism in Dyslipidemia and Familial Hypercholesterolemia. In *The Molecular Nutrition of Fats*; Academic Press: Cambridge, MA, USA, 2019; pp. 307–322. ISBN 9780128112977.
9. D'Aquila, T.; Hung, Y.H.; Carreiro, A.; Buhman, K.K. Recent Discoveries on Absorption of Dietary Fat: Presence, Synthesis, and Metabolism of Cytoplasmic Lipid Droplets within Enterocytes. *Biochim. Biophys. Acta Mol. Cell Biol. Lipids* **2016**, *1861*, 730–747.
10. Feingold, K.R. Lipid and Lipoprotein Metabolism. *Endocrinol. Metab. Clin. North. Am.* **2022**, *51*, 437–458.
11. Klop, B.; Elte, J.W.F.; Cabezas, M.C. Dyslipidemia in Obesity: Mechanisms and Potential Targets. *Nutrients* **2013**, *5*, 1218–1240. [CrossRef]
12. Orešič, M.; Vidal-Puig, A. *A Systems Biology Approach to Study Metabolic Syndrome*; Springer International Publishing: Berlin/Heidelberg, Germany, 2014; ISBN 9783319010076.
13. Moon, J.H.; Kim, K.; Choi, S.H. Lipoprotein Lipase: Is It a Magic Target for the Treatment of Hypertriglyceridemia. *Endocrinol. Metab.* **2022**, *37*, 575–586. [CrossRef]
14. Borén, J.; Taskinen, M.R.; Björnson, E.; Packard, C.J. Metabolism of Triglyceride-Rich Lipoproteins in Health and Dyslipidaemia. *Nat. Rev. Cardiol.* **2022**, *19*, 577–592. [PubMed]

15. Bahiru, E.; Hsiao, R.; Phillipson, D.; Watson, K.E. Mechanisms and Treatment of Dyslipidemia in Diabetes. *Curr. Cardiol. Rep.* **2021**, *23*, 26. [CrossRef]
16. Karam, I. Hyperlipidemia Background and Progress. *SM Atheroscler. J.* **2017**, *1*, 1003.
17. Feingold, K.R. *Introduction to Lipids and Lipoproteins*; Feingold, K.R., Ahmed, S.F., Anawalt, B., Blackman, M.R., Boyce, A., Chrousos, G., Corpas, E., de Herder, W.W., Dhatariya, K., Dungan, K., et al., Eds.; Endotext: South Dartmouth, MA, USA, 2000.
18. Heeren, J.; Scheja, L. Metabolic-Associated Fatty Liver Disease and Lipoprotein Metabolism. *Mol. Metab.* **2021**, *50*, 101238. [CrossRef]
19. Rohrer, L.; Ohnsorg, P.M.; Lehner, M.; Landolt, F.; Rinninger, F.; von Eckardstein, A. High-Density Lipoprotein Transport through Aortic Endothelial Cells Involves Scavenger Receptor BI and ATP-Binding Cassette Transporter G1. *Circ. Res.* **2009**, *104*, 1142–1150. [CrossRef]
20. Kontush, A.; Lindahl, M.; Lhomme, M.; Calabresi, L.; Chapman, M.J.; Davidson, W.S. Structure of HDL: Particle Subclasses and Molecular Components. In *Handbook of Experimental Pharmacology*; Springer: Cham, Switzerland, 2015; Volume 224, pp. 3–51. [CrossRef]
21. von Eckardstein, A.; Nofer, J.R.; Assmann, G. High Density Lipoproteins and Arteriosclerosis. Role of Cholesterol Efflux and Reverse Cholesterol Transport. *Arterioscler. Thromb. Vasc. Biol.* **2001**, *21*, 13–27. [CrossRef]
22. Miller, G.J.; Miller, N.E. Plasma-High-Density-Lipoprotein Concentration and Development of Ischaemic Heart-Disease. *Lancet* **1975**, *305*, 16–19. [CrossRef]
23. Schoch, L.; Alcover, S.; Padró, T.; Ben-Aicha, S.; Mendieta, G.; Badimon, L.; Vilahur, G. Update of HDL in Atherosclerotic Cardiovascular Disease. *Clin. Investig. Arterioscler.* **2023**, *35*, 297–314.
24. Ben-Aicha, S.; Badimon, L.; Vilahur, G. Advances in HDL: Much More than Lipid Transporters. *Int. J. Mol. Sci.* **2020**, *21*, 732. [CrossRef]
25. Vilahur, G. High-Density Lipoprotein Benefits beyond the Cardiovascular System: A Potential Key Role for Modulating Acquired Immunity through Cholesterol Efflux. *Cardiovasc. Res.* **2017**, *113*, e51–e53. [CrossRef]
26. Lu, J.; Han, G.; Liu, X.; Chen, B.; Peng, K.; Shi, Y.; Zhang, M.; Yang, Y.; Cui, J.; Song, L.; et al. Association of High-Density Lipoprotein Cholesterol with All-Cause and Cause-Specific Mortality in a Chinese Population of 3.3 Million Adults: A Prospective Cohort Study. *Lancet Reg. Health West. Pac.* **2024**, *42*, 100874. [CrossRef] [PubMed]
27. Mørland, J.G.; Magnus, P.; Vollset, S.E.; Leon, D.A.; Selmer, R.; Tverdal, A. Associations between Serum High-Density Lipoprotein Cholesterol Levels and Cause-Specific Mortality in a General Population of 345 000 Men and Women Aged 20–79 Years. *Int. J. Epidemiol.* **2023**, *52*, 1257–1267. [CrossRef] [PubMed]
28. Chen, J.-X.; Li, Y.; Zhang, Y.-B.; Wang, Y.; Zhou, Y.-F.; Geng, T.; Liu, G.; Pan, A.; Liao, Y.-F. Nonlinear Relationship between High-Density Lipoprotein Cholesterol and Cardiovascular Disease: An Observational and Mendelian Randomization Analysis. *Metabolism* **2024**, *154*, 155817. [CrossRef]
29. Badimon, L.; Vilahur, G. HDL Particles—More Complex than We Thought. *Thromb. Haemost.* **2014**, *112*, 857. [CrossRef] [PubMed]
30. Rohatgi, A.; Westerterp, M.; von Eckardstein, A.; Remaley, A.; Rye, K.A. HDL in the 21st Century. *Circulation* **2021**, *143*, 2293–2309. [CrossRef]
31. Silva, R.A.G.D.; Huang, R.; Morris, J.; Fang, J.; Gracheva, E.O.; Ren, G.; Kontush, A.; Jerome, W.G.; Rye, K.A.; Davidson, W.S. Structure of Apolipoprotein A-I in Spherical High Density Lipoproteins of Different Sizes. *Proc. Natl. Acad. Sci. USA* **2008**, *105*, 12176–12181. [CrossRef]
32. Rayner, K.J.; Moore, K.J. MicroRNA Control of High-Density Lipoprotein Metabolism and Function. *Circ. Res.* **2014**, *114*, 183–192. [CrossRef]
33. Ben-Aicha, S.; Escate, R.; Casani, L.; Padro, T.; Pena, E.; Arderiu, G.; Mendieta, G.; Badimon, L.; Vilahur, G. High-Density Lipoprotein Remodelled in Hypercholesterolaemic Blood Induce Epigenetically Driven down-Regulation of Endothelial HIF-1a Expression in a Preclinical Animal Model. *Cardiovasc. Res.* **2021**, *116*, 1288–1299. [CrossRef]
34. Wu, Q.; Sheng, Q.; Michell, D.; Ramirez-Solano, M.; Posey, O.; Phothisane, A.; Shaik, S.; Vickers, K.C.; Ormseth, M.J. Anti-Inflammatory Effect of High-Density Lipoprotein Blunted by Delivery of Altered MicroRNA Cargo in Patients With Rheumatoid Arthritis. *Arthritis Rheumatol.* **2024**, *76*, 684–695. [CrossRef]
35. Graham, A. Modulation of the Cellular MicroRNA Landscape: Contribution to the Protective Effects of High-Density Lipoproteins (HDL). *Biology* **2023**, *12*, 1232. [CrossRef]
36. Rossi-Herring, G.; Belmonte, T.; Rivas-Urbina, A.; Benítez, S.; Rotllan, N.; Crespo, J.; Llorente-Cortés, V.; Sánchez-Quesada, J.L.; de Gonzalo-Calvo, D. Circulating Lipoprotein-Carried MiRNome Analysis Reveals Novel VLDL-Enriched MicroRNAs That Strongly Correlate with the HDL-MicroRNA Profile. *Biomed. Pharmacother.* **2023**, *162*, 114623. [CrossRef]
37. Kontush, A.; Chapman, M.J. Antiatherogenic Function of HDL Particle Subpopulations: Focus on Antioxidative Activities. *Curr. Opin. Lipidol.* **2010**, *21*, 312–318. [CrossRef]
38. Oravec, S.; Demuth, K.; Myara, I.; Hornych, A. The Effect of High Density Lipoprotein Subfractions on Endothelial Eicosanoid Secretion. *Thromb. Res.* **1998**, *92*, 65–71. [CrossRef]

39. Pirillo, A.; Catapano, A.L.; Norata, G.D. Biological Consequences of Dysfunctional HDL. *Curr. Med. Chem.* **2018**, *26*, 1644–1664. [CrossRef]
40. Kontush, A.; Chapman, M. Antiatherogenic Small, Dense HDL—Guardian Angel of the Arterial Wall? *Nat. Clin. Pract. Cardiovasc. Med.* **2006**, *3*, 144–153. [CrossRef] [PubMed]
41. Prats-Uribe, A.; Sayols-Baixeras, S.; Fernández-Sanlés, A.; Subirana, I.; Carreras-Torres, R.; Vilahur, G.; Civeira, F.; Marrugat, J.; Fitó, M.; Hernáez, Á.; et al. High-Density Lipoprotein Characteristics and Coronary Artery Disease: A Mendelian Randomization Study. *Metabolism* **2020**, *112*, 154351. [CrossRef] [PubMed]
42. Kontush, A.; Lhomme, M.; Chapman, M.J. Unraveling the Complexities of the HDL Lipidome. *J. Lipid Res.* **2013**, *54*, 2950–2963. [CrossRef] [PubMed]
43. Zerrad-Saadi, A.; Therond, P.; Chantepie, S.; Couturier, M.; Rye, K.-A.; Chapman, M.J.; Kontush, A. HDL3-Mediated Inactivation of LDL-Associated Phospholipid Hydroperoxides Is Determined by the Redox Status of Apolipoprotein A-I and HDL Particle Surface Lipid Rigidity: Relevance to Inflammation and Atherogenesis. *Arterioscler. Thromb. Vasc. Biol.* **2009**, *29*, 2169–2175. [CrossRef]
44. de Souza, J.A.; Vindis, C.; Nègre-Salvayre, A.; Rye, K.-A.; Couturier, M.; Therond, P.; Chantepie, S.; Salvayre, R.; Chapman, M.J.; Kontush, A. Small, Dense HDL 3 Particles Attenuate Apoptosis in Endothelial Cells: Pivotal Role of Apolipoprotein A-I. *J. Cell Mol. Med.* **2010**, *14*, 608–620. [CrossRef]
45. Kontush, A.; Chantepie, S.; Chapman, M.J. Small, Dense HDL Particles Exert Potent Protection of Atherogenic LDL against Oxidative Stress. *Arterioscler. Thromb. Vasc. Biol.* **2003**, *23*, 1881–1888. [CrossRef]
46. Khoo, J.C.; Miller, E.; McLoughlin, P.; Steinberg, D. Prevention of Low Density Lipoprotein Aggregation by High Density Lipoprotein or Apolipoprotein A-I. *J. Lipid Res.* **1990**, *31*, 645–652. [CrossRef] [PubMed]
47. Durrington, P.N.; Bashir, B.; Soran, H. Paraoxonase 1 and Atherosclerosis. *Front. Cardiovasc. Med.* **2023**, *10*, 1065967. [CrossRef]
48. Jakubowski, H. The Molecular Bases of Anti-Oxidative and Anti-Inflammatory Properties of Paraoxonase 1. *Antioxidants* **2024**, *13*, 1292. [CrossRef]
49. Rye, K.-A.; Barter, P.J. Cardioprotective Functions of HDLs1. *J. Lipid Res.* **2014**, *55*, 168–179. [CrossRef] [PubMed]
50. Panzenböck, U.; Stocker, R. Formation of Methionine Sulfoxide-Containing Specific Forms of Oxidized High-Density Lipoproteins. *Biochim. Biophys. Acta (BBA)—Proteins Proteom.* **2005**, *1703*, 171–181. [CrossRef]
51. Brock, J.W.C.; Jenkins, A.J.; Lyons, T.J.; Klein, R.L.; Yim, E.; Lopes-Virella, M.; Carter, R.E.; Thorpe, S.R.; Baynes, J.W. Increased Methionine Sulfoxide Content of ApoA-I in Type 1 Diabetes. *J. Lipid Res.* **2008**, *49*, 847–855. [CrossRef]
52. Hine, D.; MacKness, B.; MacKness, M. Cholesteryl-Ester Transfer Protein Enhances the Ability of High-Density Lipoprotein to Inhibit Low-Density Lipoprotein Oxidation. *IUBMB Life* **2011**, *63*, 772–774. [CrossRef]
53. Elsøe, S.; Ahnström, J.; Christoffersen, C.; Hoofnagle, A.N.; Plomgaard, P.; Heinecke, J.W.; Binder, C.J.; Björkbacka, H.; Dahlbäck, B.; Nielsen, L.B. Apolipoprotein M Binds Oxidized Phospholipids and Increases the Antioxidant Effect of HDL. *Atherosclerosis* **2012**, *221*, 91–97. [CrossRef]
54. Choi, B.G.; Vilahur, G.; Viles-Gonzalez, J.F.; Badimon, J.J. The Role of High-Density Lipoprotein Cholesterol in Atherothrombosis. *Mt. Sinai J. Med.* **2006**, *73*, 690–701.
55. Drew, B.G.; Fidge, N.H.; Gallon-Beaumier, G.; Kemp, B.E.; Kingwell, B.A. High-Density Lipoprotein and Apolipoprotein AI Increase Endothelial NO Synthase Activity by Protein Association and Multisite Phosphorylation. *Proc. Natl. Acad. Sci. USA* **2004**, *101*, 6999–7004. [CrossRef]
56. Beitz, J.; Förster, W. Influence of Human Low Density and High Density Lipoprotein Cholesterol on the in Vitro Prostaglandin I2 Synthetase Activity. *Biochim. Biophys. Acta* **1980**, *620*, 352–355. [CrossRef] [PubMed]
57. Yuhanna, I.S.; Zhu, Y.; Cox, B.E.; Hahner, L.D.; Osborne-Lawrence, S.; Lu, P.; Marcel, Y.L.; Anderson, R.G.; Mendelsohn, M.E.; Hobbs, H.H.; et al. High-Density Lipoprotein Binding to Scavenger Receptor-BI Activates Endothelial Nitric Oxide Synthase. *Nat. Med.* **2001**, *7*, 853–857. [CrossRef] [PubMed]
58. Terasaka, N.; Yu, S.; Yvan-Charvet, L.; Wang, N.; Mzhavia, N.; Langlois, R.; Pagler, T.; Li, R.; Welch, C.L.; Goldberg, I.J.; et al. ABCG1 and HDL Protect against Endothelial Dysfunction in Mice Fed a High-Cholesterol Diet. *J. Clin. Investig.* **2008**, *118*, 3701–3713. [CrossRef] [PubMed]
59. Terasaka, N.; Wang, N.; Yvan-Charvet, L.; Tall, A.R. High-Density Lipoprotein Protects Macrophages from Oxidized Low-Density Lipoprotein-Induced Apoptosis by Promoting Efflux of 7-Ketocholesterol via ABCG1. *Proc. Natl. Acad. Sci. USA* **2007**, *104*, 15093–15098. [CrossRef]
60. Norata, G.D.; Pirillo, A.; Catapano, A.L. HDLs, Immunity, and Atherosclerosis. *Curr. Opin. Lipidol.* **2011**, *22*, 410–416. [CrossRef]
61. Norata, G.D.; Pirillo, A.; Ammirati, E.; Catapano, A.L. Emerging Role of High Density Lipoproteins as a Player in the Immune System. *Atherosclerosis* **2012**, *220*, 11–21. [CrossRef]
62. Kratzer, A.; Giral, H.; Landmesser, U. High-Density Lipoproteins as Modulators of Endothelial Cell Functions: Alterations in Patients with Coronary Artery Disease. *Cardiovasc. Res.* **2014**, *103*, 350–361. [CrossRef]

63. Badimon, L.; Vilahur, G. LDL-Cholesterol versus HDL-Cholesterol in the Atherosclerotic Plaque: Inflammatory Resolution versus Thrombotic Chaos. *Ann. N. Y. Acad. Sci.* **2012**, *1254*, 18–32. [CrossRef]
64. Calkin, A.C.; Drew, B.G.; Ono, A.; Duffy, S.J.; Gordon, M.V.; Schoenwaelder, S.M.; Sviridov, D.; Cooper, M.E.; Kingwell, B.A.; Jackson, S.P. Reconstituted High-Density Lipoprotein Attenuates Platelet Function in Individuals with Type 2 Diabetes Mellitus by Promoting Cholesterol Efflux. *Circulation* **2009**, *120*, 2095–2104. [CrossRef]
65. Chen, L.Y.; Mehta, J.L. Inhibitory Effect of High-Density Lipoprotein on Platelet Function Is Mediated by Increase in Nitric Oxide Synthase Activity in Platelets. *Life Sci.* **1994**, *55*, 1815–1821. [CrossRef]
66. Viswambharan, H.; Ming, X.-F.; Zhu, S.; Hubsch, A.; Lerch, P.; Vergères, G.; Rusconi, S.; Yang, Z. Reconstituted High-Density Lipoprotein Inhibits Thrombin-Induced Endothelial Tissue Factor Expression through Inhibition of RhoA and Stimulation of Phosphatidylinositol 3-Kinase but Not Akt/Endothelial Nitric Oxide Synthase. *Circ. Res.* **2004**, *94*, 918–925. [CrossRef] [PubMed]
67. Luo, M.; Tian, R.; Lu, N. Nitric Oxide Protected against NADPH Oxidase-Derived Superoxide Generation in Vascular Endothelium: Critical Role for Heme Oxygenase-1. *Int. J. Biol. Macromol.* **2019**, *126*, 549–554. [CrossRef]
68. Han, R.; Lai, R.; Ding, Q.; Wang, Z.; Luo, X.; Zhang, Y.; Cui, G.; He, J.; Liu, W.; Chen, Y. Apolipoprotein A-I Stimulates AMP-Activated Protein Kinase and Improves Glucose Metabolism. *Diabetologia* **2007**, *50*, 1960–1968. [CrossRef]
69. Drew, B.G.; Duffy, S.J.; Formosa, M.F.; Natoli, A.K.; Henstridge, D.C.; Penfold, S.A.; Thomas, W.G.; Mukhamedova, N.; de Courten, B.; Forbes, J.M.; et al. High-Density Lipoprotein Modulates Glucose Metabolism in Patients with Type 2 Diabetes Mellitus. *Circulation* **2009**, *119*, 2103–2111. [CrossRef] [PubMed]
70. Tang, S.; Tabet, F.; Cochran, B.J.; Cuesta Torres, L.F.; Wu, B.J.; Barter, P.J.; Rye, K.A. Apolipoprotein A-I Enhances Insulin-Dependent and Insulin-Independent Glucose Uptake by Skeletal Muscle. *Sci. Rep.* **2019**, *9*, 1350. [CrossRef]
71. Dugani, C.B.; Klip, A. Glucose Transporter 4: Cycling, Compartments and Controversies. *EMBO Rep.* **2005**, *6*, 1137–1142. [CrossRef]
72. Karlsson, H.K.R.; Chibalin, A.V.; Koistinen, H.A.; Yang, J.; Koumanov, F.; Wallberg-Henriksson, H.; Zierath, J.R.; Holman, G.D. Kinetics of GLUT4 Trafficking in Rat and Human Skeletal Muscle. *Diabetes* **2009**, *58*, 847–854. [CrossRef] [PubMed]
73. Drew, B.G.; Rye, K.A.; Duffy, S.J.; Barter, P.; Kingwell, B.A. The Emerging Role of HDL in Glucose Metabolism. *Nat. Rev. Endocrinol.* **2012**, *8*, 237–245. [CrossRef]
74. Gao, T.; McKenna, B.; Li, C.; Reichert, M.; Nguyen, J.; Singh, T.; Yang, C.; Pannikar, A.; Doliba, N.; Zhang, T.; et al. Pdx1 Maintains β Cell Identity and Function by Repressing an α Cell Program. *Cell Metab.* **2014**, *19*, 259–271. [CrossRef]
75. Cochran, B.J.; Bisoendial, R.J.; Hou, L.; Glaros, E.N.; Rossy, J.; Thomas, S.R.; Barter, P.J.; Rye, K.A. Apolipoprotein A-I Increases Insulin Secretion and Production from Pancreatic β-Cells via a G-Protein-CAMPPKA-FoxO1-Dependent Mechanism. *Arterioscler. Thromb. Vasc. Biol.* **2014**, *34*, 2261–2267. [CrossRef]
76. Nilsson, O.; Del Giudice, R.; Nagao, M.; Grönberg, C.; Eliasson, L.; Lagerstedt, J.O. Apolipoprotein A-I Primes Beta Cells to Increase Glucose Stimulated Insulin Secretion. *Biochim. Biophys. Acta Mol. Basis Dis.* **2020**, *1866*, 165613. [CrossRef]
77. Mancuso, E.; Mannino, G.C.; Fuoco, A.; Leo, A.; Citraro, R.; Averta, C.; Spiga, R.; Russo, E.; De Sarro, G.; Andreozzi, F.; et al. HDL (High-Density Lipoprotein) and ApoA-1 (Apolipoprotein A-1) Potentially Modulate Pancreatic α-Cell Glucagon Secretion. *Arterioscler. Thromb. Vasc. Biol.* **2020**, *40*, 2941–2952. [CrossRef]
78. Theilmeier, G.; Schmidt, C.; Herrmann, J.; Keul, P.; Schäfers, M.; Herrgott, I.; Mersmann, J.; Larmann, J.; Hermann, S.; Stypmann, J.; et al. High-Density Lipoproteins and Their Constituent, Sphingosine-1-Phosphate, Directly Protect the Heart against Ischemia/Reperfusion Injury in Vivo via the S1P3 Lysophospholipid Receptor. *Circulation* **2006**, *114*, 1403–1409. [CrossRef] [PubMed]
79. Vilahur, G.; Gutiérrez, M.; Casaní, L.; Cubedo, J.; Capdevila, A.; Pons-Llado, G.; Carreras, F.; Hidalgo, A.; Badimon, L. Hypercholesterolemia Abolishes High-Density Lipoprotein-Related Cardioprotective Effects in the Setting of Myocardial Infarction. *J. Am. Coll. Cardiol.* **2015**, *66*, 2469–2470.
80. Sposito, A.C.; De Lima-Junior, J.C.; Moura, F.A.; Barreto, J.; Bonilha, I.; Santana, M.; Virginio, V.W.; Sun, L.; Carvalho, L.S.F.; Soares, A.A.S.; et al. Reciprocal Multifaceted Interaction between HDL (High-Density Lipoprotein) and Myocardial Infarction. *Arterioscler. Thromb. Vasc. Biol.* **2019**, *39*, 1550–1564.
81. Pajkrt, D.; Doran, J.E.; Koster, F.; Lerch, P.G.; Arnet, B.; van der Poll, T.; ten Cate, J.W.; van Deventer, S.J. Antiinflammatory Effects of Reconstituted High-Density Lipoprotein during Human Endotoxemia. *J. Exp. Med.* **1996**, *184*, 1601–1608. [CrossRef] [PubMed]
82. Hajduk, S.L.; Moore, D.R.; Vasudevacharya, J.; Siqueira, H.; Torri, A.F.; Tytler, E.M.; Esko, J.D. Lysis of Trypanosoma Brucei by a Toxic Subspecies of Human High Density Lipoprotein. *J. Biol. Chem.* **1989**, *264*, 5210–5217. [CrossRef]
83. Cho, K.-H. Structural and Functional Impairments of Reconstituted High-Density Lipoprotein by Incorporation of Recombinant β-Amyloid42. *Molecules* **2021**, *26*, 4317. [CrossRef] [PubMed]
84. Polymeropoulos, M.H.; Lavedan, C.; Leroy, E.; Ide, S.E.; Dehejia, A.; Dutra, A.; Pike, B.; Root, H.; Rubenstein, J.; Boyer, R.; et al. Mutation in the α-Synuclein Gene Identified in Families with Parkinson's Disease. *Science* **1997**, *276*, 2045–2047. [CrossRef]
85. Hsiao, J.-H.T.; Halliday, G.M.; Kim, W.S. α-Synuclein Regulates Neuronal Cholesterol Efflux. *Molecules* **2017**, *22*, 1769. [CrossRef]

86. Stukas, S.; Robert, J.; Wellington, C.L. High-Density Lipoproteins and Cerebrovascular Integrity in Alzheimer's Disease. *Cell Metab.* **2014**, *19*, 574–591. [CrossRef]
87. Shih, Y.-H.; Tsai, K.-J.; Lee, C.-W.; Shiesh, S.-C.; Chen, W.-T.; Pai, M.-C.; Kuo, Y.-M. Apolipoprotein C-III Is an Amyloid-β-Binding Protein and an Early Marker for Alzheimer's Disease. *J. Alzheimer's Dis.* **2014**, *41*, 855–865. [CrossRef]
88. Rader, D.J.; Hovingh, G.K. HDL and Cardiovascular Disease. *Lancet* **2014**, *384*, 618–625. [CrossRef] [PubMed]
89. Stadler, J.T.; Lackner, S.; Mörkl, S.; Trakaki, A.; Scharnagl, H.; Borenich, A.; Wonisch, W.; Mangge, H.; Zelzer, S.; Meier-Allard, N.; et al. Obesity Affects HDL Metabolism, Composition and Subclass Distribution. *Biomedicines* **2021**, *9*, 242. [CrossRef] [PubMed]
90. Holzer, M.; Schilcher, G.; Curcic, S.; Trieb, M.; Ljubojevic, S.; Stojakovic, T.; Scharnagl, H.; Kopecky, C.M.; Rosenkranz, A.R.; Heinemann, A.; et al. Dialysis Modalities and HDL Composition and Function. *J. Am. Soc. Nephrol.* **2015**, *26*, 2267–2276. [CrossRef]
91. Trieb, M.; Horvath, A.; Birner-Gruenberger, R.; Spindelboeck, W.; Stadlbauer, V.; Taschler, U.; Curcic, S.; Stauber, R.E.; Holzer, M.; Pasterk, L.; et al. Liver Disease Alters High-Density Lipoprotein Composition, Metabolism and Function. *Biochim. Biophys. Acta* **2016**, *1861*, 630–638. [CrossRef]
92. Srivastava, R.A.K. Dysfunctional HDL in Diabetes Mellitus and Its Role in the Pathogenesis of Cardiovascular Disease. *Mol. Cell Biochem.* **2018**, *440*, 167–187. [CrossRef]
93. Ahmed, T.; Bowden, R.G. Assessing High-Density Lipoprotein: Shifting Focus from Quantity to Quality in Cardiovascular Disease Risk Assessment. *Int. J. Transl. Med.* **2024**, *4*, 369–380. [CrossRef]
94. Cho, K.H. The Current Status of Research on High-Density Lipoproteins (HDL): A Paradigm Shift from HDL Quantity to HDL Quality and HDL Functionality. *Int. J. Mol. Sci.* **2022**, *23*, 3967. [CrossRef]
95. Ben-Aicha, S.; Casaní, L.; Muñoz-García, N.; Joan-Babot, O.; Peña, E.; Aržanauskaitė, M.; Gutierrez, M.; Mendieta, G.; Padró, T.; Badimon, L.; et al. HDL (High-Density Lipoprotein) Remodeling and Magnetic Resonance Imaging-Assessed Atherosclerotic Plaque Burden: Study in a Preclinical Experimental Model. *Arterioscler. Thromb. Vasc. Biol.* **2020**, *40*, 2481–2493. [CrossRef]
96. Padró, T.; Cubedo, J.; Camino, S.; Béjar, M.T.; Ben-Aicha, S.; Mendieta, G.; Escolà-Gil, J.C.; Escate, R.; Gutiérrez, M.; Casani, L.; et al. Detrimental Effect of Hypercholesterolemia on High-Density Lipoprotein Particle Remodeling in Pigs. *J. Am. Coll. Cardiol.* **2017**, *70*, 165–178. [CrossRef] [PubMed]
97. Schoch, L.; Sutelman, P.; Suades, R.; Casani, L.; Padro, T.; Badimon, L.; Vilahur, G. Hypercholesterolemia-Induced HDL Dysfunction Can Be Reversed: The Impact of Diet and Statin Treatment in a Preclinical Animal Model. *Int. J. Mol. Sci.* **2022**, *23*, 8596. [CrossRef]
98. Nobecourt, E.; Davies, M.J.; Brown, B.E.; Curtiss, L.K.; Bonnet, D.J.; Charlton, F.; Januszewski, A.S.; Jenkins, A.J.; Barter, P.J.; Rye, K.-A. The Impact of Glycation on Apolipoprotein A-I Structure and Its Ability to Activate Lecithin:Cholesterol Acyltransferase. *Diabetologia* **2007**, *50*, 643–653. [CrossRef]
99. Hoang, A.; Murphy, A.J.; Coughlan, M.T.; Thomas, M.C.; Forbes, J.M.; O'Brien, R.; Cooper, M.E.; Chin-Dusting, J.P.F.; Sviridov, D. Advanced Glycation of Apolipoprotein A-I Impairs Its Anti-Atherogenic Properties. *Diabetologia* **2007**, *50*, 1770–1779. [CrossRef] [PubMed]
100. Kashyap, S.R.; Osme, A.; Ilchenko, S.; Golizeh, M.; Lee, K.; Wang, S.; Bena, J.; Previs, S.F.; Smith, J.D.; Kasumov, T. Glycation Reduces the Stability of ApoAI and Increases HDL Dysfunction in Diet-Controlled Type 2 Diabetes. *J. Clin. Endocrinol. Metab.* **2018**, *103*, 388–396. [CrossRef]
101. Matsunaga, T.; Nakajima, T.; Miyazaki, T.; Koyama, I.; Hokari, S.; Inoue, I.; Kawai, S.; Shimomura, H.; Katayama, S.; Hara, A.; et al. Glycated High-Density Lipoprotein Regulates Reactive Oxygen Species and Reactive Nitrogen Species in Endothelial Cells. *Metabolism* **2003**, *52*, 42–49. [CrossRef]
102. Skeggs, J.W.; Morton, R.E. LDL and HDL Enriched in Triglyceride Promote Abnormal Cholesterol Transport. *J. Lipid Res.* **2002**, *43*, 1264–1274. [CrossRef]
103. Kontush, A.; De Faria, E.C.; Chantepie, S.; Chapman, M.J. A Normotriglyceridemic, Low HDL-Cholesterol Phenotype Is Characterised by Elevated Oxidative Stress and HDL Particles with Attenuated Antioxidative Activity. *Atherosclerosis* **2005**, *182*, 277–285. [CrossRef] [PubMed]
104. Lagrost, L. Regulation of Cholesteryl Ester Transfer Protein (CETP) Activity: Review of in Vitro and in Vivo Studies. *Biochim. Biophys. Acta* **1994**, *1215*, 209–236. [CrossRef]
105. Denimal, D.; Nguyen, A.; Pais de Barros, J.P.; Bouillet, B.; Petit, J.M.; Vergès, B.; Duvillard, L. Major Changes in the Sphingophospholipidome of HDL in Non-Diabetic Patients with Metabolic Syndrome. *Atherosclerosis* **2016**, *246*, 106–114. [CrossRef]
106. Denimal, D.; Monier, S.; Brindisi, M.C.; Petit, J.M.; Bouillet, B.; Nguyen, A.; Demizieux, L.; Simoneau, I.; Pais De Barros, J.P.; Vergès, B.; et al. Impairment of the Ability of Hdl from Patients with Metabolic Syndrome but without Diabetes Mellitus to Activate ENOS: Correction by S1P Enrichment. *Arterioscler. Thromb. Vasc. Biol.* **2017**, *37*, 804–811. [CrossRef]
107. Clemente-Postigo, M.; Queipo-Ortuño, M.I.; Fernandez-Garcia, D.; Gomez-Huelgas, R.; Tinahones, F.J.; Cardona, F. Adipose Tissue Gene Expression of Factors Related to Lipid Processing in Obesity. *PLoS ONE* **2011**, *6*, e24783. [CrossRef]

108. Verwer, B.J.; Scheffer, P.G.; Vermue, R.P.; Pouwels, P.J.; Diamant, M.; Tushuizen, M.E. NAFLD Is Related to Post-Prandial Triglyceride-Enrichment of HDL Particles in Association with Endothelial and HDL Dysfunction. *Liver Int.* **2020**, *40*, 2439–2444. [CrossRef] [PubMed]
109. Annema, W.; Tietge, U.J.F. Role of Hepatic Lipase and Endothelial Lipase in High-Density Lipoprotein-Mediated Reverse Cholesterol Transport. *Curr. Atheroscler. Rep.* **2011**, *13*, 257–265. [CrossRef]
110. Brites, F.D.; Bonavita, C.D.; De Geitere, C.; Cloës, M.; Delfly, B.; Yael, M.J.; Fruchart, J.; Wikinski, R.W.; Castro, G.R. Alterations in the Main Steps of Reverse Cholesterol Transport in Male Patients with Primary Hypertriglyceridemia and Low HDL-Cholesterol Levels. *Atherosclerosis* **2000**, *152*, 181–192. [CrossRef] [PubMed]
111. Davies, S.S. HDL Function and Atherosclerosis: Reactive Dicarbonyls as Promising Targets of Therapy. *Circ. Res.* **2023**, *132*, 1521–1545. [CrossRef]
112. Bergt, C.; Pennathur, S.; Fu, X.; Byun, J.; O'Brien, K.; McDonald, T.O.; Singh, P.; Anantharamaiah, G.M.; Chait, A.; Brunzell, J.; et al. The Myeloperoxidase Product Hypochlorous Acid Oxidizes HDL in the Human Artery Wall and Impairs ABCA1-Dependent Cholesterol Transport. *Proc. Natl. Acad. Sci. USA* **2004**, *101*, 13032–13037. [CrossRef]
113. Lu, N.; Xie, S.; Li, J.; Tian, R.; Peng, Y.-Y. Myeloperoxidase-Mediated Oxidation Targets Serum Apolipoprotein A-I in Diabetic Patients and Represents a Potential Mechanism Leading to Impaired Anti-Apoptotic Activity of High Density Lipoprotein. *Clin. Chim. Acta* **2015**, *441*, 163–170. [CrossRef]
114. Nathan, D.M.; Genuth, S.; Lachin, J.; Cleary, P.; Crofford, O.; Davis, M.; Rand, L.; Siebert, C. The Effect of Intensive Treatment of Diabetes on the Development and Progression of Long-Term Complications in Insulin-Dependent Diabetes Mellitus. *N. Engl. J. Med.* **1993**, *329*, 977–986. [CrossRef]
115. Brame, C.J.; Boutaud, O.; Davies, S.S.; Yang, T.; Oates, J.A.; Roden, D.; Roberts, L.J. Modification of Proteins by Isoketal-Containing Oxidized Phospholipids*. *J. Biol. Chem.* **2004**, *279*, 13447–13451. [CrossRef]
116. Norata, G.D.; Pirillo, A.; Catapano, A.L. Modified HDL: Biological and Physiopathological Consequences. *Nutr. Metab. Cardiovasc. Dis.* **2006**, *16*, 371–386. [CrossRef] [PubMed]
117. Johannsen, T.H.; Frikke-Schmidt, R.; Schou, J.; Nordestgaard, B.G.; Tybjærg-Hansen, A. Genetic Inhibition of CETP, Ischemic Vascular Disease and Mortality, and Possible Adverse Effects. *J. Am. Coll. Cardiol.* **2012**, *60*, 2041–2048. [CrossRef] [PubMed]
118. Chantepie, S.; Bochem, A.E.; Chapman, M.J.; Hovingh, G.K.; Kontush, A. High-Density Lipoprotein (HDL) Particle Subpopulations in Heterozygous Cholesteryl Ester Transfer Protein (CETP) Deficiency: Maintenance of Antioxidative Activity. *PLoS ONE* **2012**, *7*, e49336.
119. Gomaraschi, M.; Ossoli, A.; Pozzi, S.; Nilsson, P.; Cefalù, A.B.; Averna, M.; Kuivenhoven, J.A.; Hovingh, G.K.; Veglia, F.; Franceschini, G.; et al. ENOS Activation by HDL Is Impaired in Genetic CETP Deficiency. *PLoS ONE* **2014**, *9*, e95925.
120. Mach, F.; Baigent, C.; Catapano, A.L.; Koskinas, K.C.; Casula, M.; Badimon, L.; Chapman, M.J.; De Backer, G.G.; Delgado, V.; Ference, B.A.; et al. 2019 ESC/EAS Guidelines for the Management of Dyslipidaemias: Lipid Modification to Reduce Cardiovascular Risk: The Task Force for the Management of Dyslipidaemias of the European Society of Cardiology (ESC) and European Atherosclerosis Society (EAS). *Eur. Heart J.* **2020**, *41*, 111–188. [CrossRef]
121. Ruiz-García, A.; Arranz-Martínez, E.; López-Uriarte, B.; Rivera-Teijido, M.; Palacios-Martínez, D.; Dávila-Blázquez, G.M.; Rosillo-González, A.; González-Posada Delgado, J.A.; Mariño-Suárez, J.E.; Revilla-Pascual, E.; et al. Prevalence of Hypertriglyceridemia in Adults and Related Cardiometabolic Factors. SIMETAP-HTG Study. *Clin. Investig. Arterioscler.* **2020**, *32*, 242–255. [CrossRef] [PubMed]
122. Fan, W.; Philip, S.; Granowitz, C.; Toth, P.P.; Wong, N.D. Prevalence of US Adults with Triglycerides $\geq$ 150 Mg/Dl: NHANES 2007–2014. *Cardiol. Ther.* **2020**, *9*, 207–213. [CrossRef]
123. Nordestgaard, B.G.; Chapman, M.J.; Ray, K.; Borén, J.; Andreotti, F.; Watts, G.F.; Ginsberg, H.; Amarenco, P.; Catapano, A.; Descamps, O.S.; et al. Lipoprotein(a) as a Cardiovascular Risk Factor: Current Status. *Eur. Heart J.* **2010**, *31*, 2844–2853. [CrossRef]
124. Ildefonso Arocha Rodulfo, J.; Ponte Negretti, C.I.; Candia, F.A. Triglicéridos En Ayunas y Pospradiales, y Su Contribución al Estudio Del Riesgo Cardiometabólico. *Clínica Investig. Arterioscler.* **2009**, *21*, 290–297. [CrossRef]
125. Koutsari, C.; Mundi, M.S.; Ali, A.H.; Patterson, B.W.; Jensen, M.D. Systemic Free Fatty Acid Disposal into Very Low-Density Lipoprotein Triglycerides. *Diabetes* **2013**, *62*, 2386–2395. [CrossRef]
126. Capell, W.H.; Zambon, A.; Austin, M.A.; Brunzell, J.D.; Hokanson, J.E. Compositional Differences of LDL Particles in Normal Subjects with LDL Subclass Phenotype A and LDL Subclass Phenotype B. *Arterioscler. Thromb. Vasc. Biol.* **1996**, *16*, 1040–1046. [CrossRef] [PubMed]
127. Lupi, R.; Dotta, F.; Marselli, L.; Del Guerra, S.; Masini, M.; Santangelo, C.; Patané, G.; Boggi, U.; Piro, S.; Anello, M.; et al. Prolonged Exposure to Free Fatty Acids Has Cytostatic and Pro-Apoptotic Effects on Human Pancreatic Islets: Evidence That β-Cell Death Is Caspase Mediated, Partially Dependent on Ceramide Pathway, and Bcl-2 Regulated. *Diabetes* **2002**, *51*, 1437–1442. [CrossRef] [PubMed]
128. Kambham, N.; Markowitz, G.S.; Valeri, A.M.; Lin, J.; D'Agati, V.D. Obesity-Related Glomerulopathy: An Emerging Epidemic. *Kidney Int.* **2001**, *59*, 1498–1509. [CrossRef]

129. Simha, V. Management of Hypertriglyceridemia. *BMJ* **2020**, *371*, m3109. [CrossRef] [PubMed]
130. Parafati, M.; Lascala, A.; Morittu, V.M.; Trimboli, F.; Rizzuto, A.; Brunelli, E.; Coscarelli, F.; Costa, N.; Britti, D.; Ehrlich, J.; et al. Bergamot Polyphenol Fraction Prevents Nonalcoholic Fatty Liver Disease via Stimulation of Lipophagy in Cafeteria Diet-Induced Rat Model of Metabolic Syndrome. *J. Nutr. Biochem.* **2015**, *26*, 938–948. [CrossRef]
131. Dietschy, J.M. Dietary Fatty Acids and the Regulation of Plasma Low Density Lipoprotein Cholesterol Concentrations. *J. Nutr.* **1998**, *128*, 444S–448S. [CrossRef]
132. Horton, J.D.; Goldstein, J.L.; Brown, M.S. SREBPs: Activators of the Complete Program of Cholesterol and Fatty Acid Synthesis in the Liver. *J. Clin. Investig.* **2002**, *109*, 1125–1131. [CrossRef]
133. Lichtenstein, A.H. Dietary Trans Fatty Acids and Cardiovascular Disease Risk: Past and Present. *Curr. Atheroscler. Rep.* **2014**, *16*, 433. [CrossRef]
134. Matthan, N.R.; Welty, F.K.; Barrett, P.H.R.; Harausz, C.; Dolnikowski, G.G.; Parks, J.S.; Eckel, R.H.; Schaefer, E.J.; Lichtenstein, A.H. Dietary Hydrogenated Fat Increases High-Density Lipoprotein ApoA-I Catabolism and Decreases Low-Density Lipoprotein ApoB-100 Catabolism in Hypercholesterolemic Women. *Arterioscler. Thromb. Vasc. Biol.* **2004**, *24*, 1092–1097. [CrossRef]
135. van Tol, A.; Zock, P.L.; van Gent, T.; Scheek, L.M.; Katan, M.B. Dietary Trans Fatty Acids Increase Serum Cholesterylester Transfer Protein Activity in Man. *Atherosclerosis* **1995**, *115*, 129–134. [CrossRef]
136. Feingold, K.R. *The Effect of Diet on Cardiovascular Disease and Lipid and Lipoprotein Levels*; Feingold, K.R., Anawalt, B., Blackman, M.R., Boyce, A., Chrousos, G., Corpas, E., de Herder, W.W., Dhatariya, K., Dungan, K., Hofland, J., et al., Eds.; Endotext: South Dartmouth, MA, USA, 2024.
137. Softic, S.; Meyer, J.G.; Wang, G.-X.; Gupta, M.K.; Batista, T.M.; Lauritzen, H.P.M.M.; Fujisaka, S.; Serra, D.; Herrero, L.; Willoughby, J.; et al. Dietary Sugars Alter Hepatic Fatty Acid Oxidation via Transcriptional and Post-Translational Modifications of Mitochondrial Proteins. *Cell Metab.* **2019**, *30*, 735–753.e4. [CrossRef] [PubMed]
138. Kroemer, G.; López-Otín, C.; Madeo, F.; de Cabo, R. Carbotoxicity—Noxious Effects of Carbohydrates. *Cell* **2018**, *175*, 605–614. [CrossRef]
139. Brunzell, J.D.; Hazzard, W.R.; Porte, D.J.; Bierman, E.L. Evidence for a Common, Saturable, Triglyceride Removal Mechanism for Chylomicrons and Very Low Density Lipoproteins in Man. *J. Clin. Investig.* **1973**, *52*, 1578–1585. [CrossRef] [PubMed]
140. Karpe, F.; Olivecrona, T.; Walldius, G.; Hamsten, A. Lipoprotein Lipase in Plasma after an Oral Fat Load: Relation to Free Fatty Acids. *J. Lipid Res.* **1992**, *33*, 975–984. [CrossRef]
141. Padro, T.; Muñoz-Garcia, N.; Badimon, L. The Role of Triglycerides in the Origin and Progression of Atherosclerosis. *Clin. Investig. Arterioscler.* **2021**, *33*, 20–28. [CrossRef] [PubMed]
142. Varbo, A.; Nordestgaard, B.G. Remnant Cholesterol and Triglyceride-Rich Lipoproteins in Atherosclerosis Progression and Cardiovascular Disease. *Arterioscler. Thromb. Vasc. Biol.* **2016**, *36*, 2133–2135.
143. Nakajima, K.; Nakano, T.; Tanaka, A. The Oxidative Modification Hypothesis of Atherosclerosis: The Comparison of Atherogenic Effects on Oxidized LDL and Remnant Lipoproteins in Plasma. *Clin. Chim. Acta* **2006**, *367*, 36–47. [CrossRef]
144. Meijssen, S.; Castro Cabezas, M.; Ballieux, C.G.M.; Derksen, R.J.; Bilecen, S.; Erkelens, D.W. Insulin Mediated Inhibition of Hormone Sensitive Lipase Activity in Vivo in Relation to Endogenous Catecholamines in Healthy Subjects. *J. Clin. Endocrinol. Metab.* **2001**, *86*, 4193–4197. [CrossRef]
145. Sun, X.J.; Miralpeix, M.; Myers, M.G.; Glasheen, E.M.; Backer, J.M.; Kahn, C.R.; White, M.F. Expression and Function of IRS-1 in Insulin Signal Transmission. *J. Biol. Chem.* **1992**, *267*, 22662–22672. [CrossRef]
146. Koves, T.R.; Ussher, J.R.; Noland, R.C.; Slentz, D.; Mosedale, M.; Ilkayeva, O.; Bain, J.; Stevens, R.; Dyck, J.R.B.; Newgard, C.B.; et al. Mitochondrial Overload and Incomplete Fatty Acid Oxidation Contribute to Skeletal Muscle Insulin Resistance. *Cell Metab.* **2008**, *7*, 45–56. [CrossRef]
147. Yu, C.; Chen, Y.; Cline, G.W.; Zhang, D.; Zong, H.; Wang, Y.; Bergeron, R.; Kim, J.K.; Cushman, S.W.; Cooney, G.J.; et al. Mechanism by Which Fatty Acids Inhibit Insulin Activation of Insulin Receptor Substrate-1 (IRS-1)-Associated Phosphatidylinositol 3-Kinase Activity in Muscle. *J. Biol. Chem.* **2002**, *277*, 50230–50236. [CrossRef] [PubMed]
148. Kruszynska, Y.T.; Worrall, D.S.; Ofrecio, J.; Frias, J.P.; Macaraeg, G.; Olefsky, J.M. Fatty Acid-Induced Insulin Resistance: Decreased Muscle PI3K Activation but Unchanged Akt Phosphorylation. *J. Clin. Endocrinol. Metab.* **2002**, *87*, 226–234. [CrossRef] [PubMed]
149. Qu, S.; Zhang, T.; Dong, H.H. Effect of Hepatic Insulin Expression on Lipid Metabolism in Diabetic Mice. *J. Diabetes* **2016**, *8*, 314–323. [CrossRef]
150. Taskinen, M.R.; Packard, C.J.; Borén, J. Emerging Evidence That ApoC-III Inhibitors Provide Novel Options to Reduce the Residual CVD. *Curr. Atheroscler. Rep.* **2019**, *21*, 27. [CrossRef]
151. Goyal, S.; Tanigawa, Y.; Zhang, W.; Chai, J.-F.; Almeida, M.; Sim, X.; Lerner, M.; Chainakul, J.; Ramiu, J.G.; Seraphin, C.; et al. APOC3 Genetic Variation, Serum Triglycerides, and Risk of Coronary Artery Disease in Asian Indians, Europeans, and Other Ethnic Groups. *Lipids Health Dis.* **2021**, *20*, 113. [CrossRef]

152. Caron, S.; Verrijken, A.; Mertens, I.; Samanez, C.H.; Mautino, G.; Haas, J.T.; Duran-Sandoval, D.; Prawitt, J.; Francque, S.; Vallez, E.; et al. Transcriptional Activation of Apolipoprotein CIII Expression by Glucose May Contribute to Diabetic Dyslipidemia. *Arterioscler. Thromb. Vasc. Biol.* **2011**, *31*, 513–519. [CrossRef] [PubMed]
153. Arner, E.; Westermark, P.O.; Spalding, K.L.; Britton, T.; Rydén, M.; Frisén, J.; Bernard, S.; Arner, P. Adipocyte Turnover: Relevance to Human Adipose Tissue Morphology. *Diabetes* **2010**, *59*, 105–109. [CrossRef]
154. Chen, C.; Jiang, J.; Lü, J.-M.; Chai, H.; Wang, X.; Lin, P.H.; Yao, Q. Resistin Decreases Expression of Endothelial Nitric Oxide Synthase through Oxidative Stress in Human Coronary Artery Endothelial Cells. *Am. J. Physiol. Heart Circ. Physiol.* **2010**, *299*, H193–H201. [CrossRef]
155. Tomita, Y.; Sakata, S.; Arima, H.; Yamato, I.; Ibaraki, A.; Ohtsubo, T.; Matsumura, K.; Fukuhara, M.; Goto, K.; Kitazono, T. Relationship between Casual Serum Triglyceride Levels and the Development of Hypertension in Japanese. *J. Hypertens.* **2021**, *39*, 677–682. [CrossRef]
156. Oishi, K.; Zheng, B.; Kuo, J.F. Inhibition of Na,K-ATPase and Sodium Pump by Protein Kinase C Regulators Sphingosine, Lysophosphatidylcholine, and Oleic Acid. *J. Biol. Chem.* **1990**, *265*, 70–75. [CrossRef]
157. Norlander, A.E.; Madhur, M.S.; Harrison, D.G. The Immunology of Hypertension. *J. Exp. Med.* **2018**, *215*, 21–33, Erratum in *J. Exp. Med.* **2018**, *215*, 719. [CrossRef] [PubMed]
158. Kirabo, A.; Fontana, V.; de Faria, A.P.C.; Loperena, R.; Galindo, C.L.; Wu, J.; Bikineyeva, A.T.; Dikalov, S.; Xiao, L.; Chen, W.; et al. DC Isoketal-Modified Proteins Activate T Cells and Promote Hypertension. *J. Clin. Investig.* **2014**, *124*, 4642–4656. [CrossRef] [PubMed]
159. Xiao, L.; Kirabo, A.; Wu, J.; Saleh, M.A.; Zhu, L.; Wang, F.; Takahashi, T.; Loperena, R.; Foss, J.D.; Mernaugh, R.L.; et al. Renal Denervation Prevents Immune Cell Activation and Renal Inflammation in Angiotensin II–Induced Hypertension. *Circ. Res.* **2015**, *117*, 547–557. [CrossRef] [PubMed]
160. Folkow, B. Physiological Aspects of Primary Hypertension. *Physiol. Rev.* **1982**, *62*, 347–504. [CrossRef]
161. Bobik, A. The Structural Basis of Hypertension: Vascular Remodelling, Rarefaction and Angiogenesis/Arteriogenesis. *J. Hypertens.* **2005**, *23*, 1473–1475. [CrossRef]
162. Norlander, A.E.; Madhur, M.S. Inflammatory Cytokines Regulate Renal Sodium Transporters: How, Where, and Why? *Am. J. Physiol.-Ren. Physiol.* **2017**, *313*, F141–F144. [CrossRef]
163. Criqui, M.H.; Heiss, G.; Cohn, R.; Cowan, L.D.; Suchindran, C.M.; Bangdiwala, S.; Kritchevsky, S.; Jacobs, D.R.J.; O'Grady, H.K.; Davis, C.E. Plasma Triglyceride Level and Mortality from Coronary Heart Disease. *N. Engl. J. Med.* **1993**, *328*, 1220–1225. [CrossRef]
164. Gaziano, J.M.; Hennekens, C.H.; O'Donnell, C.J.; Breslow, J.L.; Buring, J.E. Fasting Triglycerides, High-Density Lipoprotein, and Risk of Myocardial Infarction. *Circulation* **1997**, *96*, 2520–2525. [CrossRef]
165. Sultani, R.; Tong, D.C.; Peverelle, M.; Lee, Y.S.; Baradi, A.; Wilson, A.M. Elevated Triglycerides to High-Density Lipoprotein Cholesterol (TG/HDL-C) Ratio Predicts Long-Term Mortality in High-Risk Patients. *Heart Lung Circ.* **2020**, *29*, 414–421. [CrossRef]
166. Bittner, V.; Johnson, B.D.; Zineh, I.; Rogers, W.J.; Vido, D.; Marroquin, O.C.; Bairey-Merz, C.N.; Sopko, G. The Triglyceride/High-Density Lipoprotein Cholesterol Ratio Predicts All-Cause Mortality in Women with Suspected Myocardial Ischemia: A Report from the Women's Ischemia Syndrome Evaluation (WISE). *Am. Heart J.* **2009**, *157*, 548–555. [CrossRef]
167. Caselli, C.; De Caterina, R.; Smit, J.M.; Campolo, J.; El Mahdiui, M.; Ragusa, R.; Clemente, A.; Sampietro, T.; Clerico, A.; Liga, R.; et al. Triglycerides and Low HDL Cholesterol Predict Coronary Heart Disease Risk in Patients with Stable Angina. *Sci. Rep.* **2021**, *11*, 20714. [CrossRef]
168. Rezapour, M.; Shahesmaeili, A.; Hossinzadeh, A.; Zahedi, R.; Najafipour, H.; Gozashti, M.H. Comparison of Lipid Ratios to Identify Metabolic Syndrome. *Arch. Iran. Med.* **2018**, *21*, 572–577. [PubMed]
169. Shin, H.-G.; Kim, Y.-K.; Kim, Y.-H.; Jung, Y.-H.; Kang, H.-C. The Relationship between the Triglyceride to High-Density Lipoprotein Cholesterol Ratio and Metabolic Syndrome. *Korean J. Fam. Med.* **2017**, *38*, 352–357. [CrossRef]
170. Wakabayashi, I.; Daimon, T. Comparison of Discrimination for Cardio-Metabolic Risk by Different Cut-off Values of the Ratio of Triglycerides to HDL Cholesterol. *Lipids Health Dis.* **2019**, *18*, 156. [CrossRef] [PubMed]
171. Achten, J.; Gleeson, M.; Jeukendrup, A.E. Determination of the Exercise Intensity That Elicits Maximal Fat Oxidation. *Med. Sci. Sports Exerc.* **2002**, *34*, 92–97. [CrossRef] [PubMed]
172. Romijn, J.A.; Coyle, E.F.; Sidossis, L.S.; Gastaldelli, A.; Horowitz, J.F.; Endert, E.; Wolfe, R.R. Regulation of Endogenous Fat and Carbohydrate Metabolism in Relation to Exercise Intensity and Duration. *Am. J. Physiol. Endocrinol. Metab.* **1993**, *265*, 380–391. [CrossRef]
173. Fikenzer, K.; Fikenzer, S.; Laufs, U.; Werner, C. Effects of Endurance Training on Serum Lipids. *Vasc. Pharmacol.* **2018**, *101*, 9–20. [CrossRef]
174. Ruiz-Ramie, J.J.; Barber, J.L.; Sarzynski, M.A. Effects of Exercise on HDL Functionality. *Curr. Opin. Lipidol.* **2019**, *30*, 16–23. [CrossRef]

175. Sarzynski, M.A.; Ruiz-Ramie, J.J.; Barber, J.L.; Slentz, C.A.; Apolzan, J.W.; McGarrah, R.W.; Harris, M.N.; Church, T.S.; Borja, M.S.; He, Y.; et al. Effects of Increasing Exercise Intensity and Dose on Multiple Measures of HDL (High-Density Lipoprotein) Function. *Arterioscler. Thromb. Vasc. Biol.* **2018**, *38*, 943–952. [CrossRef]
176. Välimäki, I.A.; Vuorimaa, T.; Ahotupa, M.; Vasankari, T.J. Strenuous Physical Exercise Accelerates the Lipid Peroxide Clearing Transport by HDL. *Eur. J. Appl. Physiol.* **2016**, *116*, 1683–1691. [CrossRef]
177. Tiainen, S.; Luoto, R.; Ahotupa, M.; Raitanen, J.; Vasankari, T. 6-Mo Aerobic Exercise Intervention Enhances the Lipid Peroxide Transport Function of HDL. *Free Radic. Res.* **2016**, *50*, 1279–1285. [CrossRef] [PubMed]
178. Casella-Filho, A.; Chagas, A.C.P.; Maranhão, R.C.; Trombetta, I.C.; Cesena, F.H.Y.; Silva, V.M.; Tanus-Santos, J.E.; Negrão, C.E.; da Luz, P.L. Effect of Exercise Training on Plasma Levels and Functional Properties of High-Density Lipoprotein Cholesterol in the Metabolic Syndrome. *Am. J. Cardiol.* **2011**, *107*, 1168–1172. [CrossRef] [PubMed]
179. Sang, H.; Yao, S.; Zhang, L.; Li, X.; Yang, N.; Zhao, J.; Zhao, L.; Si, Y.; Zhang, Y.; Lv, X.; et al. Walk-Run Training Improves the Anti-Inflammation Properties of High-Density Lipoprotein in Patients with Metabolic Syndrome. *J. Clin. Endocrinol. Metab.* **2015**, *100*, 870–879. [CrossRef]
180. Roberts, C.K.; Ng, C.; Hama, S.; Eliseo, A.J.; Barnard, R.J. Effect of a Short-Term Diet and Exercise Intervention on Inflammatory/Anti-Inflammatory Properties of HDL in Overweight/Obese Men with Cardiovascular Risk Factors. *J. Appl. Physiol. (1985)* **2006**, *101*, 1727–1732. [CrossRef] [PubMed]
181. Petersen, A.M.W.; Pedersen, B.K. The Anti-Inflammatory Effect of Exercise. *J. Appl. Physiol.* **2005**, *98*, 1154–1162. [CrossRef]
182. Kajimura, S.; Spiegelman, B.M.; Seale, P. Brown and Beige Fat: Physiological Roles beyond Heat Generation. *Cell Metab.* **2015**, *22*, 546–559. [CrossRef]
183. Garritson, J.D.; Boudina, S. The Effects of Exercise on White and Brown Adipose Tissue Cellularity, Metabolic Activity and Remodeling. *Front. Physiol.* **2021**, *12*, 772894.
184. Rutti, S.; Dusaulcy, R.; Hansen, J.S.; Howald, C.; Dermitzakis, E.T.; Pedersen, B.K.; Pinget, M.; Plomgaard, P.; Bouzakri, K. Angiogenin and Osteoprotegerin Are Type II Muscle Specific Myokines Protecting Pancreatic Beta-Cells against Proinflammatory Cytokines. *Sci. Rep.* **2018**, *8*, 10072. [CrossRef]
185. Wasserman, D.H.; Lacy, D.B.; Colburn, C.A.; Bracy, D.; Cherrington, A.D. Efficiency of Compensation for Absence of Fall in Insulin during Exercise. *Am. J. Physiol.* **1991**, *261*, E587–E597. [CrossRef]
186. Gomarasca, M.; Banfi, G.; Lombardi, G. Myokines: The Endocrine Coupling of Skeletal Muscle and Bone. *Adv. Clin. Chem.* **2020**, *94*, 155–218. [CrossRef]
187. Ouchi, N.; Oshima, Y.; Ohashi, K.; Higuchi, A.; Ikegami, C.; Izumiya, Y.; Walsh, K. Follistatin-like 1, a Secreted Muscle Protein, Promotes Endothelial Cell Function and Revascularization in Ischemic Tissue through a Nitric-Oxide Synthase-Dependent Mechanism. *J. Biol. Chem.* **2008**, *283*, 32802–32811. [CrossRef]
188. Sofi, F.; Abbate, R.; Gensini, G.F.; Casini, A. Accruing Evidence on Benefits of Adherence to the Mediterranean Diet on Health: An Updated Systematic Review and Meta-Analysis. *Am. J. Clin. Nutr.* **2010**, *92*, 1189–1196. [PubMed]
189. Badimon, L.; Vilahur, G.; Padro, T. Nutraceuticals and Atherosclerosis: Human Trials. *Cardiovasc. Ther.* **2010**, *28*, 202–215. [PubMed]
190. Vilahur, G.; Cubedo, J.; Padró, T.; Casaní, L.; Mendieta, G.; González, A.; Badimon, L. Intake of Cooked Tomato Sauce Preserves Coronary Endothelial Function and Improves Apolipoprotein A-I and Apolipoprotein J Protein Profile in High-Density Lipoproteins. *Transl. Res.* **2015**, *166*, 44–56. [CrossRef] [PubMed]
191. Vilahur, G.; Padró, T.; Casaní, L.; Mendieta, G.; López, J.A.; Streitenberger, S.; Badimon, L. Polyphenol-Enriched Diet Prevents Coronary Endothelial Dysfunction by Activating the Akt/ENOS Pathway. *Rev. Española Cardiol. (Engl. Ed.)* **2015**, *68*, 216–225. [CrossRef]
192. Vilahur, G.; Badimon, L. Antiplatelet Properties of Natural Products. *Vascul Pharmacol.* **2013**, *59*, 67–75.
193. López-Yerena, A.; Padro, T.; de Santisteban Villaplana, V.; Muñoz-García, N.; Pérez, A.; Vilahur, G.; Badimon, L. Vascular and Platelet Effects of Tomato Soffritto Intake in Overweight and Obese Subjects. *Nutrients* **2023**, *15*, 5084. [CrossRef]
194. Padro, T.; Muñoz-García, N.; Vilahur, G.; Chagas, P.; Deyà, A.; Antonijoan, R.M.; Badimon, L. Moderate Beer Intake and Cardiovascular Health in Overweight Individuals. *Nutrients* **2018**, *10*, 1237. [CrossRef]
195. Vilahur, G.; Casaní, L.; Peña, E.; Crespo, J.; Juan-Babot, O.; Ben-Aicha, S.; Mendieta, G.; Béjar, M.T.; Borrell, M.; Badimon, L. Silybum Marianum Provides Cardioprotection and Limits Adverse Remodeling Post-Myocardial Infarction by Mitigating Oxidative Stress and Reactive Fibrosis. *Int. J. Cardiol.* **2018**, *270*, 28–35. [CrossRef]
196. Vilahur, G.; Sutelman, P.; Mendieta, G.; Ben-Aicha, S.; Borrell-Pages, M.; Peña, E.; Crespo, J.; Casaní, L.; Badimon, L. Triglyceride-Induced Cardiac Lipotoxicity Is Mitigated by Silybum Marianum. *Atherosclerosis* **2021**, *324*, 91–101. [CrossRef]
197. Vilahur, G.; Casani, L.; Guerra, J.M.; Badimon, L. Intake of Fermented Beverages Protect against Acute Myocardial Injury: Target Organ Cardiac Effects and Vasculoprotective Effects. *Basic. Res. Cardiol.* **2012**, *107*, 291. [CrossRef] [PubMed]

198. Ramón, E.; Emilio, R.; Jordi, S.-S.; Maria-Isabel, C.; Dolores, C.; Fernando, A.; Enrique, G.-G.; Valentina, R.-G.; Miquel, F.; José, L.; et al. Primary Prevention of Cardiovascular Disease with a Mediterranean Diet Supplemented with Extra-Virgin Olive Oil or Nuts. *N. Engl. J. Med.* **2018**, *378*, e34. [CrossRef]
199. Hernáez, Á.; Castañer, O.; Elosua, R.; Pintó, X.; Estruch, R.; Salas-Salvadó, J.; Corella, D.; Arós, F.; Serra-Majem, L.; Fiol, M.; et al. Mediterranean Diet Improves High-Density Lipoprotein Function in High-Cardiovascular-Risk Individuals. *Circulation* **2017**, *135*, 633–643. [CrossRef]
200. Wang, K.; Subbaiah, P.V. Importance of the Free Sulfhydryl Groups of Lecithin-Cholesterol Acyltransferase for Its Sensitivity to Oxidative Inactivation1The Results of These Studies Were Partly Presented at the American Heart Association Meeting in Dallas, TX, November 1998.1. *Biochim. Biophys. Acta (BBA)—Mol. Cell Biol. Lipids* **2000**, *1488*, 268–277. [CrossRef]
201. Hernáez, A.; Farràs, M.; Fitó, M. Olive Oil Phenolic Compounds and High-Density Lipoprotein Function. *Curr. Opin. Lipidol.* **2016**, *27*, 47–53. [CrossRef]
202. Hernáez, Á.; Fernández-Castillejo, S.; Farràs, M.; Catalán, Ú.; Subirana, I.; Montes, R.; Solà, R.; Muñoz-Aguayo, D.; Gelabert-Gorgues, A.; Díaz-Gil, Ó.; et al. Olive Oil Polyphenols Enhance High-Density Lipoprotein Function in Humans. *Arterioscler. Thromb. Vasc. Biol.* **2014**, *34*, 2115–2119. [CrossRef]
203. Skulas-Ray, A.C.; Wilson, P.W.F.; Harris, W.S.; Brinton, E.A.; Kris-Etherton, P.M.; Richter, C.K.; Jacobson, T.A.; Engler, M.B.; Miller, M.; Robinson, J.G.; et al. Omega-3 Fatty Acids for the Management of Hypertriglyceridemia: A Science Advisory from the American Heart Association. *Circulation* **2019**, *140*, E673–E691. [PubMed]
204. Tanaka, N.; Ishida, T.; Nagao, M.; Mori, T.; Monguchi, T.; Sasaki, M.; Mori, K.; Kondo, K.; Nakajima, H.; Honjo, T.; et al. Administration of High Dose Eicosapentaenoic Acid Enhances Anti-Inflammatory Properties of High-Density Lipoprotein in Japanese Patients with Dyslipidemia. *Atherosclerosis* **2014**, *237*, 577–583. [CrossRef]
205. McEneny, J.; Wade, L.; Young, I.S.; Masson, L.; Duthie, G.; McGinty, A.; McMaster, C.; Thies, F. Lycopene Intervention Reduces Inflammation and Improves HDL Functionality in Moderately Overweight Middle-Aged Individuals. *J. Nutr. Biochem.* **2013**, *24*, 163–168. [CrossRef]
206. Berryman, C.E.; Grieger, J.A.; West, S.G.; Chen, C.-Y.O.; Blumberg, J.B.; Rothblat, G.H.; Sankaranarayanan, S.; Kris-Etherton, P.M. Acute Consumption of Walnuts and Walnut Components Differentially Affect Postprandial Lipemia, Endothelial Function, Oxidative Stress, and Cholesterol Efflux in Humans with Mild Hypercholesterolemia. *J. Nutr.* **2013**, *143*, 788–794. [CrossRef]
207. Wang, L.; Bordi, P.L.; Fleming, J.A.; Hill, A.M.; Kris-Etherton, P.M. Effect of a Moderate Fat Diet With and Without Avocados on Lipoprotein Particle Number, Size and Subclasses in Overweight and Obese Adults: A Randomized, Controlled Trial. *J. Am. Heart Assoc.* **2024**, *4*, e001355. [CrossRef]
208. Beulens, J.W.J.; Sierksma, A.; van Tol, A.; Fournier, N.; van Gent, T.; Paul, J.-L.; Hendriks, H.F.J. Moderate Alcohol Consumption Increases Cholesterol Efflux Mediated by ABCA1. *J. Lipid Res.* **2004**, *45*, 1716–1723. [CrossRef] [PubMed]
209. van der Gaag, M.S.; van Tol, A.; Vermunt, S.H.F.; Scheek, L.M.; Schaafsma, G.; Hendriks, H.F.J. Alcohol Consumption Stimulates Early Steps in Reverse Cholesterol Transport. *J. Lipid Res.* **2001**, *42*, 2077–2083. [CrossRef] [PubMed]
210. Mäkelä, S.M.; Jauhiainen, M.; Ala-Korpela, M.; Metso, J.; Lehto, T.M.; Savolainen, M.J.; Hannuksela, M.L. HDL2 of Heavy Alcohol Drinkers Enhances Cholesterol Efflux from Raw Macrophages via Phospholipid-Rich HDL2b Particles. *Alcohol. Clin. Exp. Res.* **2008**, *32*, 991–1000. [CrossRef]
211. Casani, L.; Segales, E.; Vilahur, G.; Bayes De Luna, A.; Badimon, L. Moderate Daily Intake of Red Wine Inhibits Mural Thrombosis and Monocyte Tissue Factor Expression in an Experimental Porcine Model. *Circulation* **2004**, *110*, 460–465. [CrossRef]
212. Giacco, R.; Costabile, G.; Della Pepa, G.; Anniballi, G.; Griffo, E.; Mangione, A.; Cipriano, P.; Viscovo, D.; Clemente, G.; Landberg, R.; et al. A Whole-Grain Cereal-Based Diet Lowers Postprandial Plasma Insulin and Triglyceride Levels in Individuals with Metabolic Syndrome. *Nutr. Metab. Cardiovasc. Dis.* **2014**, *24*, 837–844. [CrossRef]
213. Bozzetto, L.; Annuzzi, G.; Costabile, G.; Costagliola, L.; Giorgini, M.; Alderisio, A.; Strazzullo, A.; Patti, L.; Cipriano, P.; Mangione, A.; et al. A CHO/Fibre Diet Reduces and a MUFA Diet Increases Postprandial Lipaemia in Type 2 Diabetes: No Supplementary Effects of Low-Volume Physical Training. *Acta Diabetol.* **2014**, *51*, 385–393. [CrossRef]
214. Lambert, C.; Cubedo, J.; Padró, T.; Vilahur, G.; López-Bernal, S.; Rocha, M.; Hernández-Mijares, A.; Badimon, L. Effects of a Carob-Pod-Derived Sweetener on Glucose Metabolism. *Nutrients* **2018**, *10*, 271. [CrossRef]
215. Reynolds, A.; Mann, J.; Cummings, J.; Winter, N.; Mete, E.; Te Morenga, L. Carbohydrate Quality and Human Health: A Series of Systematic Reviews and Meta-Analyses. *Lancet* **2019**, *393*, 434–445. [CrossRef]
216. Gibson, C.M.; Duffy, D.; Korjian, S.; Bahit, M.C.; Chi, G.; Alexander, J.H.; Lincoff, A.M.; Heise, M.; Tricoci, P.; Deckelbaum, L.I.; et al. Apolipoprotein A1 Infusions and Cardiovascular Outcomes after Acute Myocardial Infarction. *N. Engl. J. Med.* **2024**, *390*, 1560–1571. [CrossRef]
217. Guyton, J.R.; Slee, A.E.; Anderson, T.; Fleg, J.L.; Goldberg, R.B.; Kashyap, M.L.; Marcovina, S.M.; Nash, S.D.; O'Brien, K.D.; Weintraub, W.S.; et al. Relationship of Lipoproteins to Cardiovascular Events: The AIM-HIGH Trial (Atherothrombosis Intervention in Metabolic Syndrome with Low HDL/High Triglycerides and Impact on Global Health Outcomes). *J. Am. Coll. Cardiol.* **2013**, *62*, 1580–1584. [CrossRef] [PubMed]

218. Brown, B.G.; Zhao, X.Q.; Chait, A.; Fisher, L.D.; Cheung, M.C.; Morse, J.S.; Dowdy, A.A.; Marino, E.K.; Bolson, E.L.; Alaupovic, P.; et al. Simvastatin and Niacin, Antioxidant Vitamins, or the Combination for the Prevention of Coronary Disease. *N. Engl. J. Med.* **2001**, *345*, 1583–1592. [CrossRef]
219. Fu, Y.; Xu, C.; Wu, G. Dietary Niacin Intake and Its Association with All-Cause and Cardiovascular Mortality Rates in Individuals with Metabolic Syndrome. *Nutr. J.* **2024**, *23*, 90. [CrossRef] [PubMed]
220. Schwartz, G.G.; Olsson, A.G.; Abt, M.; Ballantyne, C.M.; Barter, P.J.; Brumm, J.; Chaitman, B.R.; Holme, I.M.; Kallend, D.; Leiter, L.A.; et al. Effects of Dalcetrapib in Patients with a Recent Acute Coronary Syndrome. *N. Engl. J. Med.* **2012**, *367*, 2089–2099. [CrossRef]
221. Lincoff, A.M.; Nicholls, S.J.; Riesmeyer, J.S.; Barter, P.J.; Brewer, H.B.; Fox, K.A.A.; Gibson, C.M.; Granger, C.; Menon, V.; Montalescot, G.; et al. Evacetrapib and Cardiovascular Outcomes in High-Risk Vascular Disease. *N. Engl. J. Med.* **2017**, *376*, 1933–1942. [CrossRef]
222. Barter, P.J.; Caulfield, M.; Eriksson, M.; Grundy, S.M.; Kastelein, J.J.P.; Komajda, M.; Lopez-Sendon, J.; Mosca, L.; Tardif, J.-C.; Waters, D.D.; et al. Effects of Torcetrapib in Patients at High Risk for Coronary Events. *N. Engl. J. Med.* **2007**, *357*, 2109–2122. [CrossRef] [PubMed]
223. Metzinger, M.P.; Saldanha, S.; Gulati, J.; Patel, K.V.; El-Ghazali, A.; Deodhar, S.; Joshi, P.H.; Ayers, C.; Rohatgi, A. Effect of Anacetrapib on Cholesterol Efflux Capacity: A Substudy of the DEFINE Trial. *J. Am. Heart Assoc.* **2020**, *9*, e018136. [CrossRef]
224. Bhatt, D.L.; Steg, P.G.; Miller, M.; Brinton, E.A.; Jacobson, T.A.; Ketchum, S.B.; Doyle, R.T.J.; Juliano, R.A.; Jiao, L.; Granowitz, C.; et al. Cardiovascular Risk Reduction with Icosapent Ethyl for Hypertriglyceridemia. *N. Engl. J. Med.* **2019**, *380*, 11–22. [CrossRef]
225. Nicholls, S.J.; Lincoff, A.M.; Garcia, M.; Bash, D.; Ballantyne, C.M.; Barter, P.J.; Davidson, M.H.; Kastelein, J.J.P.; Koenig, W.; McGuire, D.K.; et al. Effect of High-Dose Omega-3 Fatty Acids vs Corn Oil on Major Adverse Cardiovascular Events in Patients at High Cardiovascular Risk: The STRENGTH Randomized Clinical Trial. *JAMA* **2020**, *324*, 2268–2280. [CrossRef]
226. Keech, A.; Simes, R.J.; Barter, P.; Best, J.; Scott, R.; Taskinen, M.R.; Forder, P.; Pillai, A.; Davis, T.; Glasziou, P.; et al. Effects of Long-Term Fenofibrate Therapy on Cardiovascular Events in 9795 People with Type 2 Diabetes Mellitus (the FIELD Study): Randomised Controlled Trial. *Lancet* **2005**, *366*, 1849–1861. [CrossRef]
227. Rubins, H.B.; Robins, S.J.; Collins, D.; Fye, C.L.; Anderson, J.W.; Elam, M.B.; Faas, F.H.; Linares, E.; Schaefer, E.J.; Schectman, G.; et al. Gemfibrozil for the Secondary Prevention of Coronary Heart Disease in Men with Low Levels of High-Density Lipoprotein Cholesterol. Veterans Affairs High-Density Lipoprotein Cholesterol Intervention Trial Study Group. *N. Engl. J. Med.* **1999**, *341*, 410–418. [CrossRef] [PubMed]
228. Ginsberg, H.N.; Elam, M.B.; Lovato, L.C.; Crouse, J.R., 3rd; Leiter, L.A.; Linz, P.; Friedewald, W.T.; Buse, J.B.; Gerstein, H.C.; Probstfield, J.; et al. Effects of Combination Lipid Therapy in Type 2 Diabetes Mellitus. *N. Engl. J. Med.* **2010**, *362*, 1563–1574. [CrossRef] [PubMed]
229. Dormandy, J.A.; Charbonnel, B.; Eckland, D.J.A.; Erdmann, E.; Massi-Benedetti, M.; Moules, I.K.; Skene, A.M.; Tan, M.H.; Lefèbvre, P.J.; Murray, G.D.; et al. Secondary Prevention of Macrovascular Events in Patients with Type 2 Diabetes in the PROactive Study (PROspective PioglitAzone Clinical Trial In MacroVascular Events): A Randomised Controlled Trial. *Lancet* **2005**, *366*, 1279–1289. [CrossRef] [PubMed]
230. Ridker, P.M.; Danielson, E.; Fonseca, F.A.H.; Genest, J.; Gotto, A.M.J.; Kastelein, J.J.P.; Koenig, W.; Libby, P.; Lorenzatti, A.J.; MacFadyen, J.G.; et al. Rosuvastatin to Prevent Vascular Events in Men and Women with Elevated C-Reactive Protein. *N. Engl. J. Med.* **2008**, *359*, 2195–2207. [CrossRef]
231. Zheng, R.; Lind, L. A Combined Observational and Mendelian Randomization Investigation Reveals NMR-Measured Analytes to Be Risk Factors of Major Cardiovascular Diseases. *Sci. Rep.* **2024**, *14*, 10645. [CrossRef]
232. Zhao, Q.; Wang, J.; Miao, Z.; Zhang, N.R.; Hennessy, S.; Small, D.S.; Rader, D.J. A Mendelian Randomization Study of the Role of Lipoprotein Subfractions in Coronary Artery Disease. *eLife* **2021**, *10*, e58361. [CrossRef]

antioxidants

MDPI

Review

How Does HDL Participate in Atherogenesis? Antioxidant Activity Versus Role in Reverse Cholesterol Transport

Paul N. Durrington [1,*], Bilal Bashir [1,2] and Handrean Soran [1,2]

1 Faculty of Biology, Medicine and Health, Cardiovascular Research Group, University of Manchester, Manchester M13 9NT, UK; bilal.bashir2@mft.nhs.uk (B.B.); Handrean.Soran@mft.nhs.uk (H.S.)

2 Department of Diabetes, Endocrinology and Metabolism, Peter Mount Building, Manchester University NHS Foundation Trust, Manchester M13 9WL, UK

* Correspondence: pdurrington@manchester.ac.uk; Tel.: +44-161-275-1201; Fax: +44-161-275-1183

Abstract: Low-density lipoprotein (LDL) chemically modified by reactive oxygen species (ROS), for example, leaking from red blood cells in the vascular compartment, more readily crosses the vascular endothelium than does nonoxidatively modified LDL to enter tissue fluid. Oxidatively modified LDL (oxLDL) may also be created in the tissue fluid by ROS leaking from cells by design, for example, by inflammatory white cells, or simply leaking from other cells as a consequence of oxygen metabolism. As well as oxLDL, glycatively modified LDL (glycLDL) is formed in the circulation. High-density lipoprotein (HDL) appears capable of decreasing the burden of lipid peroxides formed on LDL exposed to ROS or to glucose and its metabolites. The mechanism for this that has received the most attention is the antioxidant activity of HDL, which is due in large part to the presence of paraoxonase 1 (PON1). PON1 is intimately associated with its apolipoprotein A1 component and with HDL's lipid domains into which lipid peroxides from LDL or cell membranes can be transferred. It is frequently overlooked that for PON1 to hydrolyze lipid substrates, it is essential that it remain by virtue of its hydrophobic amino acid sequences within a lipid micellar environment, for example, during its isolation from serum or genetically modified cells in tissue culture. Otherwise, it may retain its capacity to hydrolyze water-soluble substrates, such as phenyl acetate, whilst failing to hydrolyze more lipid-soluble molecules. OxLDL and probably glycLDL, once they have crossed the arterial endothelium by receptor-mediated transcytosis, are rapidly taken up by monocytes in a process that also involves scavenger receptors, leading to subendothelial foam cell formation. These are the precursors of atheroma, inducing more monocytes to cross the endothelium into the lesion and the proliferation and migration of myocytes present in the arterial wall into the developing lesion, where they transform into foam cells and fibroblasts. The atheroma progresses to have a central extracellular lake of cholesteryl ester following necrosis and apoptosis of foam cells with an overlying fibrous cap whilst continuing to grow concentrically around the arterial wall by a process involving oxLDL and glycLDL. Within the arterial wall, additional oxLDL is generated by ROS secreted by inflammatory cells and leakage from cells generally when couplet oxygen is reduced. PON1 is important for the mechanism by which HDL opposes atherogenesis, which may provide a better avenue of inquiry in the identification of vulnerable individuals and the provision of new therapies than have emerged from the emphasis placed on its role in RCT.

Keywords: antioxidant; LDL; paroxonase1; cardiovascular disease; high density lipoprotein; lipid peroxidation; atherosclerosis

1. Introduction

Fundamental questions about the role of lipoproteins in the pathogenesis of atheromatous diseases remain topics of active discussion. In this review, we shall focus particularly on our knowledge, or lack of it, concerning the mechanisms by which high-density lipoprotein (HDL) components by opposing oxidative modification and glycation can impede atherogenesis, firstly by preventing the passage of atherogenic lipoproteins from the circulating blood across the arterial endothelium into the subintima and secondly by decreasing the likelihood that, once there, they will cause the formation of foam cells and thence the growth of atheromatous plaques and their subsequent rupture. Because of the ubiquitous presence of HDL in tissue fluids, the antioxidative activities of HDL may also prevent the modification of other proteins, such as those of outer cell membranes, involved in the pathogenesis of many diseases other than atherosclerosis, which are the subject of other reviews and reports in this collection.

2. The Oxidant Theory of Atherosclerosis

The oxidant theory of atherosclerosis has recently been the subject of an excellent review from the group at La Jolla, University of California San Diego [1], where much of the concept underwent development under the leadership of the late Daniel Steinberg [2]. However, randomized clinical trials of antioxidant vitamins have yielded at best marginal benefit in the prevention of ASCVD incidents [3–5]. This has been widely interpreted as denying the hypothesis that oxidatively modified low-density lipoprotein (oxLDL) is a potent cause of atherogenesis. Nevertheless, whilst antioxidant vitamins can be shown to decrease the initial phase of lipid peroxidation (conjugated diene formation) on low-density lipoprotein (LDL), they may not be the best approach to prevent the later stages of LDL lipid peroxidative damage [6]. They, themselves, undergo oxidation, after which they are pro-oxidant, and they may increase potentially proatherogenic pathways, such as cholesteryl ester transfer [7].

The conversion of native LDL to oxLDL involves several stages. Antioxidants, such as vitamin E or ascorbate, prevent oxidation by themselves undergoing oxidation in preference to other substances. It was hoped that by intervening with pharmacological quantities of antioxidants of this type to prevent the earliest stage of LDL oxidation (the oxygen-free radical attack on its long-chain unsaturated fatty acyl groups of phospholipids and cholesteryl esters leading to conjugated diene formation), it would prevent atherosclerotic cardiovascular disease (ASCVD). However, they may not be the most effective or even physiological approach to prevent the subsequent generation of oxLDL. On the other hand, the hydrolysis of the breakdown products of oxygen-free radical attack, such as 9-hydroperoxy-10,12-octodecadienoic acid (9HPODE), to harmless carboxylic acids rather than allowing their breakdown into aldehydes (e.g., propanediol, hexanal, nonanal), unsaturated aldehydes (e.g., hexenal, nonenal), and their various hydroperoxy derivatives, which are damaging to the apolipoprotein B (apoB) of LDL, might be a better option. By just such a process, HDL may protect LDL from the accumulation of these breakdown products, which might otherwise adduct to the side chains of proline and arginine residues of apoB, leading to its fragmentation, following which it becomes a ligand for endothelial, macrophage, and transformed smooth muscle cell scavenger receptors [1,6]. This review will summarize some of the evidence for this supposition.

3. How HDL Protects Against Atherosclerosis

3.1. Participation in Reverse Cholesterol Transport

For many years, the inverse relationship between HDL cholesterol and ASCVD incidence has been considered to be because HDL metabolism protects against atherogenesis by being somehow rate-limiting for reverse cholesterol transport (RCT). RCT must occur because, for no known reason, the human liver secretes more cholesterol into the blood circulation than is required to fulfill the requirements of the tissues [8,9]. Therefore, if it is not to accumulate peripherally, the excess must be returned to the liver by a process that is termed RCT. It was proposed that HDL is the route by which RCT is accomplished [10]. Despite the zeal with which this idea has been pursued, evidence for a critical role for HDL in RCT has been hard to find, at least until the relatively recent finding that HDL can act as an acceptor for cholesterol exiting cells by the ATP-binding cassette transporter A1 (ABCA1 (also known as the cholesterol efflux regulatory protein)) [11,12]. Just how rate-limiting is this property of HDL in the process of RCT? Probably, the most convincing evidence that it is comes from epidemiological studies reporting that the capacity of serum to acquire cholesterol from laboratory-grown cells after removal of apoB-containing lipoproteins correlates inversely with ASCVD risk [12]. This is termed cholesterol efflux capacity (CEC). Almost certainly in the human, however, the greater part of the cholesterol acquired by HDL in this manner is rapidly esterified by lecithin: cholesterol acyltransferase (LCAT) located on HDL and then transferred to LDL by cholesteryl ester transfer protein (CETP) [13]. From LDL, any cholesteryl ester not redelivered to the peripheral tissues is returned to the liver by the LDL receptor (LDLR) and LDL-like receptor protein (LRP) [13]. Thus, LDL as well as HDL contributes substantially to RCT [14]. The balance between LDL production and catabolism, not HDL, are the major forces governing the concentration of circulating cholesterol in humans [15,16]. Evidence that the involvement of HDL in RCT is not the only nor even a major explanation for its apparent protection against ASCVD is provided by inborn errors in its metabolism [17–25]. In loss-of-function mutations of ABCA1 (Tangier disease), cholesteryl ester laden foam cells (macrophages) are present in many tissues, including the tonsils, spleen, and liver, accompanied by profoundly diminished HDL. A defect in HDL metabolism, so severe as to wipe out circulating HDL almost entirely, might be expected to cause remarkably premature atherosclerosis if defective RCT was critical to the process. However, atheroma is not nearly as aggressive as in heterozygous familial hypercholesterolaemia or familial dysbetalipoproteinaemia [8,9,18–20]. Tissues other than the arteries accumulate cholesterol earlier than the arteries. Similarly, in LCAT deficiency, despite deposition of cholesterol in the kidney often severe enough to require renal transplantation and low circulating HDL, atherosclerosis is not a prominent feature [21]. Mutations affecting specifically the apoA1 gene, whilst associated with atherosclerosis, may be because they also affect chylomicron metabolism [22,23]. Genetic CETP deficiency produces high HDL cholesterol concentrations, but any protection it affords against ASCVD is disputed [24]. The small decrease in ASCVD incidence provided by pharmacological inhibition of CETP derives more from its modest LDL-lowering action rather than from its effect in raising HDL cholesterol concentration [25]. In summary, extreme disorders of HDL metabolism, which profoundly influence its involvement in RCT, are not associated with atherosclerosis of the severity expected. It is thus reasonable to consider other mechanisms by which HDL might protect against ASCVD.

3.2. *Impeding the Structural Modification of LDL by Oxidation and Glycation*

3.2.1. Source of Reactive Oxygen Species (ROS) in the Circulation

Aerobic respiration became possible as the atmosphere accumulated oxygen following the evolution of photosynthetic plants. This in turn permitted the advent of organisms with much faster metabolic rates than had hitherto been possible with simple anaerobic respiration. Oxidative metabolism, however, is not without its hazards. Until it participates in chemical reactions (oxidation), atmospheric oxygen (and thus most dissolved oxygen) exists as a couplet in which two oxygen molecules, each having six electrons in their outermost shell, share with each other two of these electrons to completely fill their outermost shells, creating stability. When oxygen (O_2) combines by sharing electrons with other atoms, the first stage must inevitably be the creation of superoxide in which the couplet has gained a single electron, but has yet to acquire an additional electron to complete its outer shell. It is thus highly reactive, having at that stage a similar outer shell to fluorine and thus a similar predilection for combining with carbon at alkene bonds, such as those in linoleate and arachidonate [18]. A typical human consumes nearly 400 L of oxygen every day, a substantial proportion of which enters the blood circulation, where it combines reversibly with hemoglobin in erythrocytes. For this to occur, the iron in hemoglobin must remain in the Fe^{II} state (ferrous). If only a small proportion of Fe^{II} is oxidized irreversibly to Fe^{III} (ferric) (methemoglobin), significant quantities of superoxide can be generated (as follows) with the potential to damage other vital molecules [26,27].

$$\mathbf{Hb\text{-}Fe^{II} + O_2 \rightarrow Hb\text{-}Fe^{III} + O_2^{\bullet -}}$$

Superoxide rapidly combines with hydrogen ions to form hydrogen peroxide.

$$\mathbf{2\,O_2^{\bullet -} + 2H^+ \rightarrow H_2O_2 + O_2}$$

Technically, hydrogen peroxide is not an oxygen-free radical, but it is water soluble and highly reactive. The term reactive oxygen species (ROS) is used to encompass true free radicals, such as superoxide, and their often more reactive and ubiquitous derivatives, such as hydrogen peroxide [28]. To overcome damaging ROS, the red cell contains an active pentose phosphate pathway (PPP) producing the reducing agent, NADPH, which maintains glutathione in a reduced state to neutralize superoxide [29]. Nevertheless, some must inevitably escape glutathione to react with protons to become hydrogen peroxide, which can readily diffuse from red cells to react, for example, with the alkene groups in phosphatidyl choline and cholesteryl esters of LDL to generate oxidatively modified LDL (oxLDL). HDL may provide an alternative pathway for the harmless removal of these lipid peroxides escaping across the erythrocyte outer cell membrane [30]. The PPP itself, despite its generally protective role, may also contribute to the chemical modification of proteins, such as apoB, because it produces metabolites linked to glycation (see later).

3.2.2. Oxidative Modification of LDL in the Circulation

There appears to be no disagreement about the notion that HDL ameliorates the biological effects of LDL oxidation that was observed in the earliest reports that LDL could damage cells in tissue culture [1]. Figure 1 shows an experiment where the oxidation of LDL by Cu^{II} ions has been prevented when HDL is also present [31]. OxLDL was detected by the method of el-Saadani, which makes use of the color reagent of a commercially available test kit for cholesterol [32]. This method measures the accumulation of the products of lipid peroxidation. In the presence of HDL, these largely disappear. They are fatty acyl hydroperoxides typically derived from linoleate and arachidonate, which rapidly break down to form ketones and aldehydes capable of adducting to the side chains of proline and arginine residues of apoB, leading to fragmentation of the apoB molecule, which thereby becomes a ligand for scavenger receptors, such as scavenger receptor class B type 1 (SR-B1 aka SCARB1; lectin-like oxidized LDL receptor1, LOX-1) [1]. The earlier phase of lipid peroxidation, namely conjugated diene formation detectable by ultraviolet (UV) absorbance, which is delayed by oral administration of antioxidant vitamins [6,7,33], is unaffected by HDL, whereas it is by oral administration of antioxidant vitamins [6,7,33]. This effect of antioxidant vitamins on conjugated diene formation is, however, short-lived compared to that of HDL on the later phases of lipid peroxide breakdown.

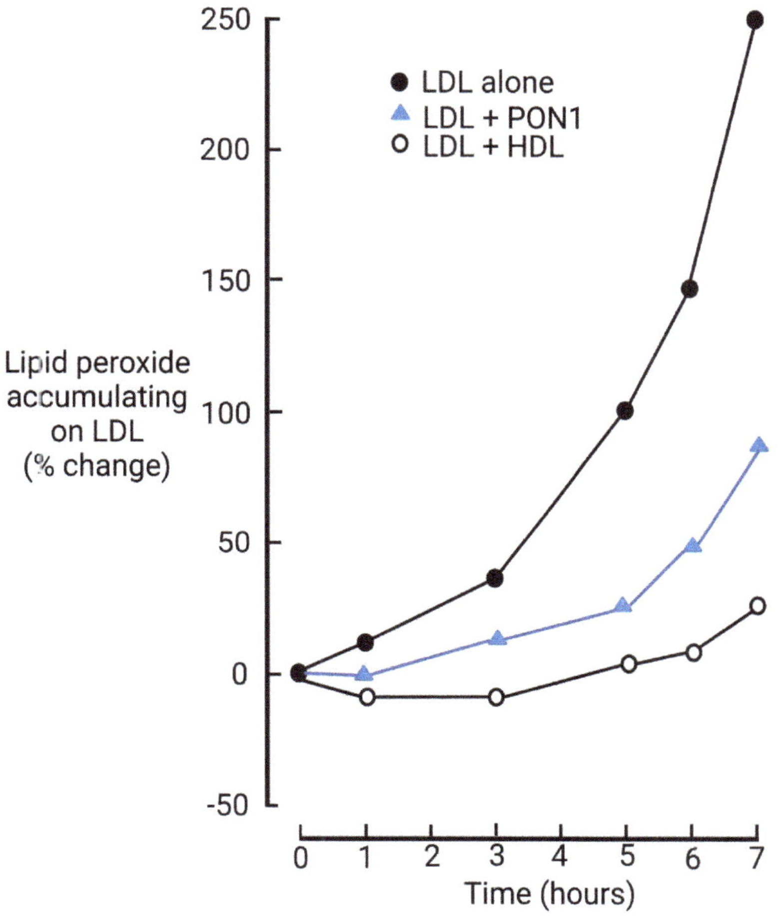

Figure 1. The generation of lipid peroxides over time when LDL is incubated with $CuSo_4$ 5 μM alone, with HDL and in the presence of paraoxonase 1 (PON1). Data from reference [31].

Probably, in the presence of HDL, phospholipid hydroperoxides are hydrolyzed to carbonic acids, and thus ketones and aldehydes do not accumulate [34–36]. Whatever the mechanism by which oxidative modification of LDL is impeded when HDL is present, it is likely to require transfer of phospholipid hydroperoxides from LDL to HDL presumably by phospholipid transfer protein and/or CETP [37]. This is extremely important, because, were a peroxidized phospholipid, for example, phosphatidylcholine (lecithin), to remain on LDL, its hydrolysis by phospholipase A2 (aka platelet activating factor acetylhydrolase) present on LDL would release the peroxidized fatty acyl group at Sn2 to breakdown into aldehydes and ketones on LDL and moreover leave behind lysophosphatidylcholine (lysolecithin) which is itself intensely damaging to LDL and tissues [38]. HDL is, however, also known to possess phospholipase A2 activity [39]. Thus, what can be the advantage of transferring phospholipid hydroperoxides to it from LDL? One important answer is that HDL, with its intensely hydrophobic environment maintained by the strongly detergent apolipoprotein A1 (apoA1) provides a safe environment for the release of toxic lipids, such as lysophatidylcholine. This must be the case because cholesterol secreted by the liver, mostly in VLDL, is free (unesterified), yet most of that in the circulation is esterified [8]. This is accomplished by LCAT present on HDL in the following reaction:

Cholesterol + Phosphatidylcholine → Cholesteryl ester + Lysophosphatidylcholine.

LCAT on HDL also esterifies free cholesterol effluxing from peripheral cells, which is initially taken up by small HDL particles (preβ-HDL) where it is esterified so that it can be packed into the intensely hydrophobic core of these particles to allow more free cholesterol to join their surface layer [40,41]. Thus, the particles enlarge to become HDL_3. Substantial gram-range quantities of cholesterol are esterified on HDL in this way every day and thus the stoichemical production of potentially toxic lysophosphatidylcholine is similarly great [8]. The production of lysophosphatidyl choline on HDL by LCAT, is a physiological process, which presumably does no damage to tissues. Thus, HDL must be a safe environment in which to hold lysophosphatidylcholine until it can be released to hepatocytes during the passage of HDL through the liver. Additionally, there is no apoB located on HDL to damage. Interestingly, much of the phospholipase A2 activity on HDL often attributed to the enzyme, phospholipase A2, may be due to paraoxonase 1 (PON1) [39]. Partially purified PON1 maintained in a lipid environment was reported by us to be highly effective in impeding Cu-induced oxidation of LDL lipids (Figure 1) (see [6] for discussion). LCAT, apoA1, and a hydrophobic, lipid environment are likely to be essential for the hydrolytic activity of PON1 towards lipid peroxides.

The composition of HDL varies greatly both within and between individuals. Proteomic investigations have revealed at least a hundred potential HDL components. Its antioxidant activity reflects the balance between PON1 activity, LCAT, and apoAI on the one hand and on the other the presence of pro-oxidant myeloperoxidase and of serum amyloid A (SAA) and apoAII, both of which displace PON1 from HDL [6]. HDL, deficient in PON1, rich in both SAA and myeloperoxidase with a low ratio of apoAI to AII, has been called proinflammatory HDL because of its association with acute and chronic inflammatory states, such as infection, rheumatoid arthritis, and autoimmune diseases. This type of HDL may also have a limited capacity to impede LDL oxidation and glycation or to promote cholesterol efflux, say from macrophage foam cells (see later).

3.2.3. Oxidative Modification of LDL in the Tissues

Cells in tissue culture oxidatively modify LDL [1,42,43]. In the case of endothelial and smooth muscle cells in tissue culture, this may simply be due to leakage of ROS from their cytoplasm. On the assumption that ROS also escape from cells in vivo, this would account for the generation of oxidatively modified LDL in the tissue fluid. Added to this, neutrophils and macrophages actively produce ROS to shower on invading pathogens and probably macromolecules recognized as misplaced or effete as a component of the host defense mechanism [44].

3.2.4. Lipoprotein (a)

Although there is a positive association between ASCVD incidence and lipoprotein(a) (Lp(a)), the mechanism remains elusive. Oxidized phospholipids have been reported to accumulate preferentially on Lp(a) in comparison to other LDL subclasses (apoB-containing lipoproteins) [1]. The rate at which LDL isolated from different individuals accumulates lipid peroxides in the presence of Cu^{II} differs greatly [33]. One factor that may contribute to this variation, which has never been explored, is the proportion of Lp(a) present in LDL used in these experiments. Lp(a), once it has crossed the arterial endothelial barrier, is retained there longer than more buoyant LDL [45], which may increase the extent to which it undergoes lipid peroxidation there.

3.2.5. Small, Dense LDL

In terms of hydrated density, small dense LDL (SD-LDL) is similar to Lp(a). Additionally, in common with Lp(a), SD-LDL is not cleared by the LDL receptor, spending more time in the blood and lymphatic circulation than more buoyant LDL [46]. SD-LDL is more susceptible to oxidative modification [47] and to glycation [48–50], which may be two sides of the same coin (see later). Circulating SD-LDL is increased in parallel with more buoyant LDL concentration in, for example, familial hypercholesterolemia, and as a proportion of LDL as a whole is increased in metabolic syndrome and diabetes. It contributes to serum apoB100 concentration, but not greatly to LDL cholesterol. Unless a method for measuring SD-LDL is available, its presence in increased concentrations can generally be expected when triglycerides are increased (perhaps only modestly) and HDL cholesterol is low [46,51,52].

3.2.6. LDL Glycation

In health approximately 3–4% of plasma LDL is glycated when the concentration is determined by boron affinity chromatography and apoB immunoassay [53]. The concentration is thus normally approximately 3 mg/dL. The percentage of serum LDL, which is glycated and its concentration rise as glycated hemoglobin increases; both are thus raised in diabetes [53]. In untreated familial hypercholesterolemia, whilst the percentage of LDL that is glycated, is relatively normal, the concentration of glycated LDL (glycLDL) is frequently as high as in diabetes because of the raised LDL levels [53]. Glycated LDL can cause foam cell formation and binds to the same receptors as oxidatively modified LDL (oxLDL) [54]. It may thus have similar atherogenicity. Allowing for methodological differences and definitions of how irreversibly glucose is bound to LDL, glycLDL concentration in serum is similar to or may even exceed that of oxLDL. It is thus likely to be a major player in atherogenesis and one that has been neglected. Just as SD-LDL undergoes oxidative modification more readily than more buoyant LDL, SD-LDL is more susceptible to glycation [48–50]. Moreover, HDL ex vivo has been reported to protect LDL against glycation [55]. Furthermore, HDL from people in the upper half of the PON1 activity distribution impedes glycation more effectively than HDL from the lower half of its population distribution [55].

Glycation is itself a process that generates ROS [56,57]. Thus, even when incubation of LDL with glucose occurs under nitrogen, not only glycLDL, but also oxLDL may be produced [58,59]. The explanation for this might be mechanistically similar to the effect of PON1 in decreasing LDL oxidative modification, because during glycation of LDL by glucose and its metabolites, the same nucleophilic side chains of lysine and arginine in apoB are attacked as are by aldehydes and ketones generated by lipid peroxidation. Both the generation of oxLDL and glycLDL may be accelerated when both ROS and glucose and its metabolites are present [59–68].

Despite employing higher glucose concentrations than are likely to occur in vivo, glycation of LDL ex vivo in the absence of oxygen is a slow process [48–55]: too slow to account for the proportion of LDL that is glycated in serum and that must be formed in the few days between hepatic VLDL secretion, conversion to LDL, and its catabolism [8]. Ex vivo, LDL glycation experiments have generally been performed under nitrogen in the absence of atmospheric oxygen, and thus ROS may not be present to the same extent as in vivo. In the presence of Cu^{II}, glycation of LDL is accelerated [58]. Glycation may also proceed more rapidly in vivo because more reactive metabolites of glucose are present. These can accelerate glycation of LDL. Interestingly, the erythrocyte PPP and glycolytic pathways are likely to be significant sources of ROS in the circulation. Gluconolactone has been shown to rapidly glycate proteins [60], and phosphogluconolactone generation is the first step in the PPP [61]. In this context, the lactonase activity of PON1 should not be overlooked in contemplating the mechanism by which HDL protects LDL against glycation. Methylglyoxal another potent glycating agent, is produced in the glycolysis pathway by nonenzymatic phosphate removal from two of its intermediates, glyceraldehyde 3-phosphate and dihydroxyacetone phosphate [62–68]. It is also a product of the PPP. Both the PPP and glycolysis are located in the erythrocyte cytoplasm, increasing the likelihood of the escape of their intermediates across the outer cell membrane of red blood cells coming into contact with LDL in the circulation [69]. They might explain the high proportion of glycLDL circulating even in nondiabetic people, despite the slow rate of LDL glycation in experiments with glucose itself. Such experiments, however, suggest that HDL, particularly PON1—rich HDL, is likely to impede apoB glycation [55].

3.3. Mechanism by Which the Antioxidative Action of HDL Protects Against Atherogenesis

3.3.1. Impeding the Passage of Atherogenic Lipoproteins Across the Arterial Endothelium

The arterial endothelium is not fenestrated, unlike endothelia in the reticuloendothelial system, which certainly do allow the passage of lipoproteins up to chylomicron dimensions. When chylomicrons circulate in excess, the smaller ones not only cross the fenestrated endothelia of liver, spleen, and bone marrow, but can be taken up by macrophages there, leading to foam cell formation and hepatosplenomegaly due to engorgement with lipid. Figure 2 shows a macrophage foam cell in the bone marrow in familial lipoprotein lipase deficiency [70].

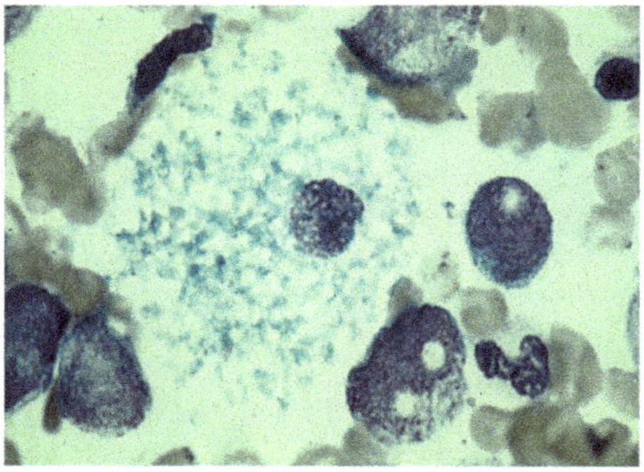

Figure 2. Foam cell in bone marrow aspirate from a patient with severe hypertriglyceridemia [70].

For many years, lipoproteins and other macromolecules were believed to cross the vascular endothelium by a simple process of filtration. It was reported that lipoproteins with a diameter exceeding 12 nm were excluded from crossing intact, healthy vascular endothelial membranes (Figure 3) [71]. This explained why HDL, with its molecular diameter of 7–13 nm and components of HDL, such as apoA1, are detectable in tissue fluid and lymph at concentrations at approximately one-fifth those in plasma [72]. Some other components, such as PON 1, are decreased proportionately more than apoA1, because of sequestration by cell membranes [73]. However, LDL, theoretically too large to cross intact vascular endothelia, is also present in tissue fluid, albeit at only about one tenth of its plasma concentration [72,74]. Indeed, if LDL is to fulfill its role in supplying cholesterol to tissues, its presence in tissue fluid is essential. Furthermore, the cholesterol present in atheromatous plaques is derived from LDL cholesterol [1,2]. Both apoB100 and apoB48 have been identified in atheromatous lesions, suggesting that not only LDL, but also small remnants of gut-derived lipoproteins can participate in atherogenesis [75–77]. Chylomicrons (Sf > 400) have a diameter of 100–10^5 nm. Chylomicron remnants, which in health are briefly present in the blood circulation as a small component of VLDL (Sf20–400), vary in diameter from 30–90 nm. To explain the presence of lipoproteins larger than HDL in tissue fluid, it was postulated that damage to the endothelial junctions or loss of endothelial cells was required to permit LDL and even larger lipoproteins to cross [78,79]. Such a situation might occur in established (mature) lesions, but is unsatisfactory to account for LDL as the cause of the precursor fatty streak and earlier atheromatous lesions occurring when the endothelium is intact. The theory that the passage of LDL across the arterial endothelium, leading to atherogenesis, is the result of mechanical or chemical damage to the endothelial junctions or loss of endothelial cells, particularly occurring at sites in the arterial tree where atherosclerosis frequently occurs, whilst undoubtedly true in established atheroma [78–80], is unlikely to explain initial lesion formation when the endothelium is intact. Another theory proposes that inflammation is the initiating event, increasing endothelial permeability to permit the passage of monocytes and lipoproteins across the arterial endothelium [81–83]. Many authors have written about endothelial dysfunction defined as a deficiency of nitric oxide (NO) [84,85]. NO bioavailability is decreased when superoxide or hydrogen peroxide reacts with it to form peroxynitrous acid (ONOOH), toxic to cellular structures.

$$O_2\bullet + NO \rightarrow ONOO^-$$

$$2\,H_2O_2 + NO \rightarrow ONOO^- + H_2O$$

Decreased NO bioavailability will undoubtedly affect the inflammatory responses of the arterial wall, particularly at sites prone to the development of atherosclerosis [84,85]. The essential question, however, is at what stage in the disease process? There is a vast literature on the inflammatory cytokine responses that occur during the development of atheromatous lesions [83]. Leucocyte chemoattractant chemokines followed by interleukin-1β (IL-1β) produced by monocytes recruited from the blood circulation and tissue macrophages within the lesion are heavily implicated [83]. The simple fact remains, however, that entry of LDL into tissues physiologically cannot depend on inflammation. LDL can cross the arterial endothelium without the need for inflammation; indeed, it has to do so if it is to perform its physiological function of delivering cholesterol to the tissues. Furthermore, there is no animal model of atherosclerosis in which the inflammatory response or individual inflammatory cytokines can be tested as a cause that does not involve an animal that has been rendered hypercholesterolemic [86]. As Anitschkov wrote, 'there can be no atheroma without cholesterol' [87].

Certainly, in the early stages of atherogenesis, there must be another explanation for how LDL crosses the arterial endothelium besides increased porosity due to damage or as a response to inflammation. The earliest lesion in atherosclerosis is the fatty streak, and by this stage, LDL has already crossed the arterial endothelium in quantities sufficient to produce cholesterol deposits. The location of these subendothelial deposits at junctions, at sites where arteries are tethered and not cushioned, and the very fact that the streaks are parallel with the direction of blood flow suggests that hemodynamics plays some part in their pathogenesis [88–90]. However, fatty streaks are uncommon in young people in populations in which cholesterol levels are low and where later atherosclerotic complications are few [91,92]. This makes it highly likely that LDL, (in particular, oxLDL—see later) initiates fatty streaks by penetrating or at least interacting with the arterial intima before it expresses adhesion molecules and secretes chemokines, leading to the recruitment of circulating leukocytes [93]. When monocytes-macrophages subsequently, of course, do infiltrate atherosclerotic plaques, they take up oxLDL and form "foam cells" that in turn release inflammatory mediators (tumor necrosis factor, interleukin-6, soluble intercellular adhesion molecule 1 and circulating vascular cell adhesion molecule 1), reinforcing the process. Nonetheless, the importance of oxLDL penetrating intact arterial endothelium is that it is likely to initiate the whole process. Furthermore, the importance of oxLDL from the circulation crossing the arterial endothelium is not confined to fatty streak generation in the initial stage of atherogenesis. It may also be essential for the mature atheroma to grow concentrically along the arterial wall. Inflammatory (monocyte recruitment and subsequent foam cell formation), maladaptive wound-healing responses (smooth muscle cell recruitment and subsequent fibrosis), and antibodies to oxLDL [1,81,83] are clearly essential, but the growth of the lesion occurs at its edges (shoulders on 2-dimensional microscopy) by a similar mechanism to the initiation of fatty streaks; the passage of oxLDL across relatively normally functioning arterial endothelium.

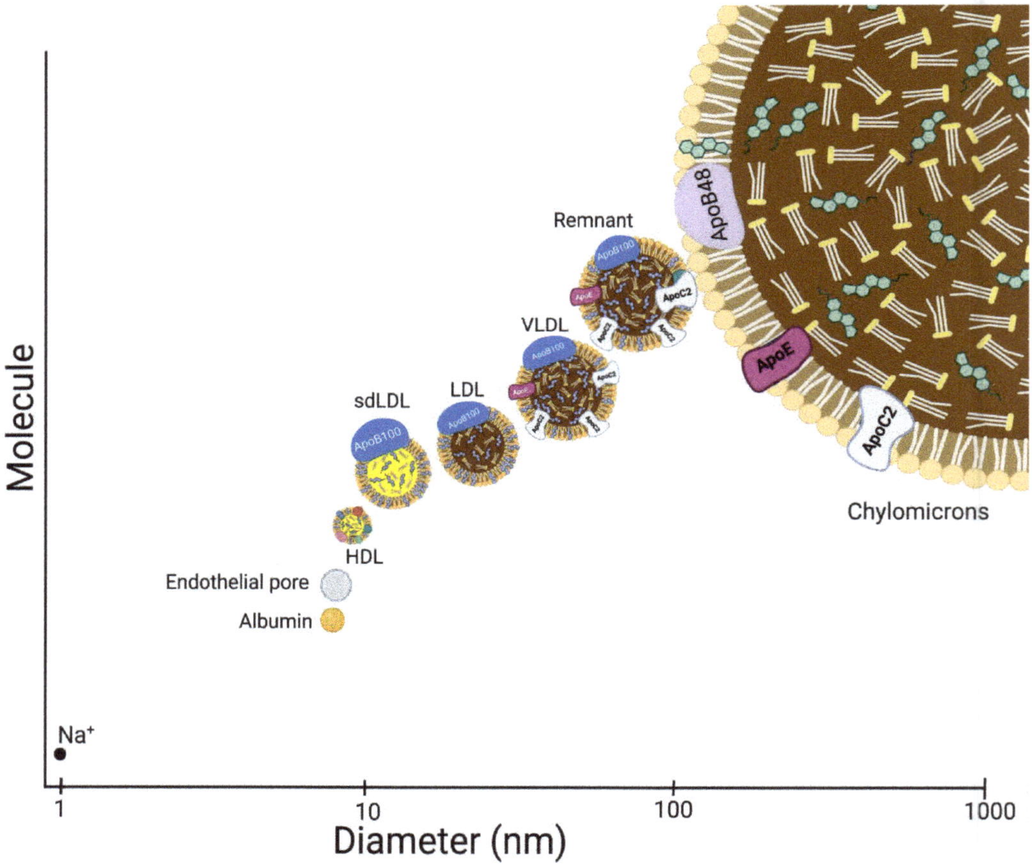

Figure 3. The molecular dimensions of lipoproteins, albumin, and sodium. The pore size of arterial endothelium was considered to be <12 nm, but the existence of anatomical pores in healthy, intact, noninflamed arterial (as opposed to capillary) endothelium now seems unlikely. HDL and LDL (particularly oxLDL and glycLDL) cross by receptor-mediated transcytosis. See text for references.

Thus, key to the initiation and expansion of atheroma is the subintimal influx and accumulation of LDL leading to the recruitment of blood monocytes. Both are encouraged in the presence of hyperlipidemia when the quantity of intimal LDL and the oxidative potential of the intima exceed the capacity of macrophages to remove it.

As undoubtedly HDL and LDL constitute a system for delivery and removal of cholesterol to and from tissues, they must be capable of transport across vascular endothelia into tissue fluid, and clearly this can no longer be considered to rely on simple filtration across the vascular endothelium. Furthermore, much of what has been written about the filtration of macromolecules relates to their passage across capillary endothelia, but there is greater resistance to the passive transfer of macromolecules across the arterial endothelium where atherogenesis occurs. Transfer is therefore now believed to occur by transcytosis and pinocytosis [94–108]. In transcytosis, molecules bind to receptors on, the apical surface of endothelial cells and are transported in endosomes through the cytoplasm to be released at their basal surface. Receptors proposed for transcytosis include the LDL receptor [94,95]. Because this receptor binds both apoB100 and apoE [9], both LDL (via apoB100) and chylomicron remnants (via apoE) could cross by this mechanism. However, the importance of this route for atherogenesis is questionable, firstly because it is saturable and thus only likely to operate when LDL cholesterol levels are lower than in adults. At typical adult concentrations of serum LDL cholesterol, the LDL receptor will be downregulated. Furthermore, in familial hypercholesterolemia, LDL receptor expression is impaired, whilst atherogenesis is rife [9].

Another receptor-mediated route proposed for endothelial transcytosis, proposed soon after the LDL receptor fell out of favor to serve this purpose, is the scavenger receptor class B1 (SR-B1 aka SCARB1) (Figure 4) [94–102]. This potentially allows the passage of both LDL and HDL into the arterial subintima. Mice overexpressing endothelial SRB1 (as opposed to hepatic or macrophage SR-B1) were protected against atherosclerosis. The SR-B1 is not saturable, and thus it permits LDL and HDL to cross the arterial endothelium to an increasingly greater extent as their serum levels increase. Passage of LDL across the arterial endothelium can also be mediated by direct pinocytosis via caveolae [102], by the actin receptor-like kinase 1 (ALK1), and by LOX-1 [102–105]. Of all these mechanisms, LOX-1 has recently been proposed to be responsible for the largest proportion of the LDL that crosses the arterial endothelium [102–105]. OxLDL is the preferred ligand for both SR-B1 and LOX-1, and its passage through the arterial endothelium by these routes is critical to the initiation of atheroma. GlycLDL also crosses from the arterial lumen by transcytosis [106,107], thus contributing to atherogenesis. HDL is transcytosed across the arterial endothelium not only by the SR-B1 receptor, but also by the ATP-binding cassette transporters A1 and G1 (ABCA1 and ABCG1) [94,98].

All these receptors can permit the passage of LDL and HDL across the arterial endothelium in either direction and could thus mediate the return of LDL or HDL cholesterol to the circulation. Whether transcytosis of LDL adequately explains why atheroma develops under intact, uninjured endothelium has been questioned [108]. It is argued that the source of the LDL cholesterol may be from the blood vessels (vasa vasorum) in the artery wall rather than the arterial lumen. Atherogenesis may thus occur when this cholesterol accumulates because its clearance rate by transcytosis into the arterial lumen lags behind its rate of arrival from vasa vasorum.

Does transcytosis explain why there is more HDL than LDL in tissue fluid? Size must play some part. Presumably, the smaller HDL particles undergo pinocytosis and receptor-mediated endocytosis more readily than the larger LDL. Whether lipoproteins larger than LDL can cross the intact arterial endothelium is unresolved, but is probably unlikely, except perhaps in the case of smaller VLDL and chylomicron remnant particles. More certain is that the relation between triglyceride-rich lipoproteins and atherosclerosis is due to the generation of cholesterol-depleted SD-LDL, which goes unobserved in epidemiological studies linking triglyceride levels to ASCVD incidence. SD-LDL is generated by CETP and the action of lipases during the circulation of triglyceride-rich lipoproteins [46,51]. Critical for atherogenesis is likely to be that the receptors involved in endothelial transcytosis, apart from the LDL receptor, which is generally down-regulated (see back), favor ox LDL and glyc LDL over native LDL [94–108].

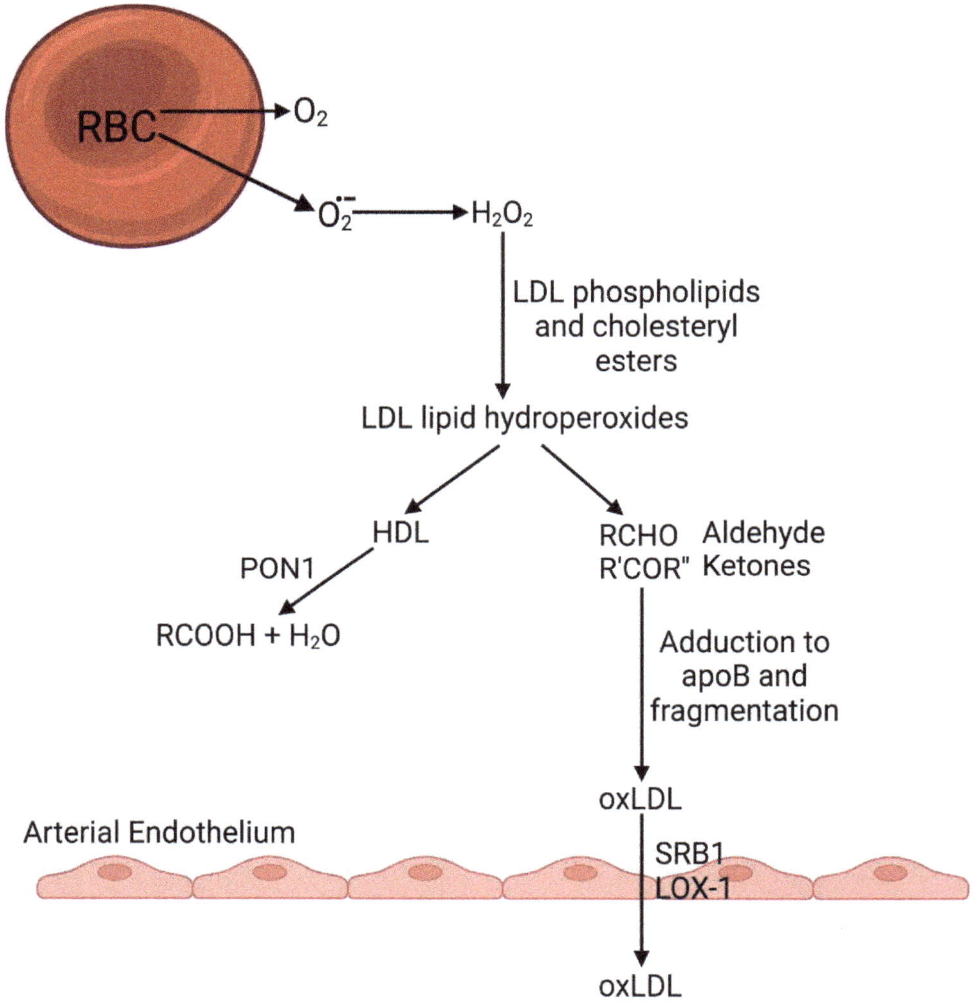

Figure 4. Events leading to the passage of LDL across the arterial endothelium. ROS are released into the circulation, for example, from red blood cells. There they react with the unsaturated acyl groups of lipoprotein phospholipids and cholesteryl esters on LDL to form lipid peroxides. The apolipoprotein B of LDL adducts to the ketones and aldehydes produced by the breakdown of lipid peroxides and then undergoes fragmentation. The resultant oxidatively modified LDL (oxLDL) undergoes endothelial transcytosis as the result of binding to scavenger receptors (SR-B1 and LOX-1). HDL can protect LDL against oxLDL formation.

Several studies have reported that transcytosis of LDL mediated by mechanisms other than the LDL receptor is impeded by HDL. This was first observed in fibroblasts [109], but applies also to arterial endothelial cells [110]. The mechanism is highly likely to involve the prevention of LDL oxidation by HDL, reducing the likelihood of LDL binding to SR-B1 and other receptors, showing a preference for binding to oxLDL over native LDL [94–108].

It represents a potential mechanism preventing atherogenesis. Just as the role of HDL in encouraging the efflux of cholesterol from cells is enhanced by HDL with higher PON1 content (see next section), so also may be the flux of ox LDL and glyc LDL across the arterial endothelium into the subintima. The inhibition by HDL and purified PON1 of the ox LDL-induced transmigration of monocytes across aortic endothelial cell monolayers was first demonstrated in cocultures by workers from Los Angeles [36].

3.3.2. Impeding Foam Cell Formation in the Arterial Wall

Foam cells are present throughout the atheromatous process from its origin in fatty streaks to the mature lesion with its fibrous cap overlying a lake of cholesterol [78,79,111,112]. Foam cells appear to orchestrate through the elaboration of cytokines and chemokines much of the growth of the plaque, attracting into it the monocytes and undifferentiated smooth muscle cells, both of which transform themselves into foam cells, swelling their numbers in the developing lesion. Foam cells are phagocytic macrophage-type cells that have within their cytoplasm abundant droplets of cholesteryl ester. As their numbers increase, they undergo apoptosis and necrosis to form the extracellular deposits of cholesteryl ester within the atheroma. Growth of the lesion is believed to take place at its edges where foam cell formation is most active, allowing the plaque to extend itself around the circumference of the artery very much as the original fatty streak had progressed. Smooth muscle cells entering the lesion not only swell the ranks of the foam cells, but also themselves transform into fibroblasts. Fibrosis, which may represent an aberrant wound-healing response, leads to the development of the fibrous cap overlying the lesion. However, the coup de grace, the rupture of the fibrous cap, leading to thrombosis and acute clinical events, is frequently in its shoulder region, where foam cells are abundant and may be mediated by metalloproteinases secreted by these foam cells, weakening fibrous tissue in that region.

Our understanding of how foam cells form has undergone a similar evolution to that of how receptors were recognized to be necessary for the transcytosis of LDL by arterial endothelial cells. In the case of monocyte-macrophages, it was found that the uptake of LDL by the LDL receptor was too slow to cause foam cell formation. Chemically modified LDL was, however, rapidly taken up, leading to foam cell generation (Figure 5). Naturally occurring chemical modifications of LDL that cause foam cell formation are oxLDL, glycLDL, and malondialdehyde-modified LDL. These are ligands for cluster differentiation 36 (CD36 aka scavenger receptor class B Type 3 (SCARB3)), SRA-1 and LOX-1 [111,112].

Because rapid uptake of LDL by monocyte-macrophages depends on the chemical modification of LDL, it might be expected that limiting the chemical modification of LDL would reduce the likelihood of its uptake, and both HDL and PON1 have been reported to diminish LDL-induced foam cell formation [2,36]. PON1-rich HDL can decrease the generation of both oxLDL and glycLDL [34,36,55].

The formation of foam cells, whether from monocyte-macrophages or smooth muscle cells, represents the balance between LDL uptake and the egress of cholesterol from the cells [113]. As discussed earlier, this cholesterol efflux may be through ABCA1 to small HDL and even smaller prebeta HDL particles, where it is packed into a central core after undergoing esterification by LCAT. It can also be accomplished by macrophage secretion of apolipoprotein E (apoE) [114]. HDL and paraoxonase have been reported to increase the efflux of cholesterol from macrophages [115]. The authors of the report concluded that the generation of lysophosphatidyl choline by paraoxonase, together with its effect in protecting against peroxidation of HDL and cellular membranes, increased the probability of HDL binding to and receiving cholesterol effluxing from macrophages. PON1 is known to redistribute from HDL to cell membranes [116]. As with arterial endothelial uptake of oxLDL, physical forces may contribute to the likelihood of foam cell formation within the arterial wall. Evidence suggests that macrophage cell types cultured under pressure take up oxLDL more readily to become foam cells [117].

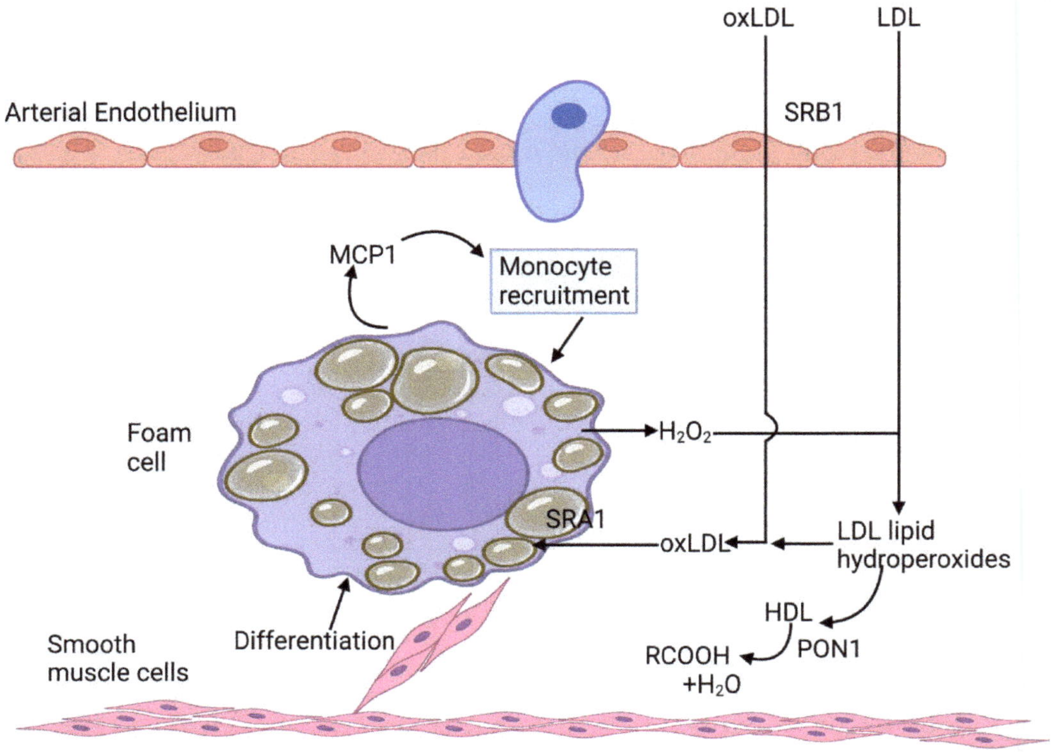

Figure 5. OxLDL arriving beneath the arterial wall attracts monocytes to enter from the blood circulation. These transform into monocyte-macrophages. More oxLDL is created by the generation of ROS by these monocyte-macrophages, which take up oxLDL via scavenger receptors (CD36 and SR-A1) to become foam cells. These permit the growth of the atheromatous lesion at its edges, whilst centrally the chemokines and cytokines they secrete attract increasing numbers of monocytes and other inflammatory cells into the lesion, stimulate smooth muscle proliferation, and transform into either fibroblasts secreting collagen or more foam cells. Foam cells eventually undergo necrosis or apoptosis, leaving behind the central lake of cholesteryl ester with its overlying fibrous cap.

3.4. Antioxidant Components of HDL

From the foregoing, HDL, by virtue of its capacity to hydrolyze lipid peroxides to harmless carboxylic acids before their breakdown into aldehydes and ketones, can decrease the formation of oxLDL both in the circulation and within the arterial wall. Foremost amongst the components of HDL likely to be important for the protection of LDL against oxidative modification appears to be PON1 [6,118]. Essential for its activity against hydrophobic substrates is the hydrophobic environment provided by the powerful detergent activity of apoA1 and by the enzyme LCAT, which creates the hydrophobic core of HDL.

PON1 was discovered in serum in 1953 and originally classified as 'A' esterase to distinguish it from esterases that were blocked by organophosphates, such as paraoxon (then used extensively in agriculture as a pesticide as its precursor, parathion) [119]. There followed extensive studies of its role in toxicology, which revealed the wide range of organic substrates it could hydrolyze and its location on HDL [6,120–124]. PON1 was found to be increasingly present in atheromatous lesions as they progressed [125]. PON1 activity is decreased in coronary heart disease [126–129], familial hypercholesterolemia [130], type1 and 2 diabetes mellitus [131,132], familial dysbetalipoproteinemia [133] (Figure 6), metabolic syndrome [134–140], polycystic ovary syndrome [141], and chronic renal disease [142]. PON1 is one of a family of paraoxonases, the other members of which are PON2, an intracellular enzyme, and PON3, a minor component of HDL. In 1991, PON1 partially purified from HDL was reported to prevent the accumulation of lipid peroxides on LDL under oxidizing conditions [34]. It was subsequently found that PON1 prevented minimally oxidized LDL-induced migration of human blood monocytes through a layer of cultured endothelial cells and decreased oxidation products of phosphatidyl choline [36].

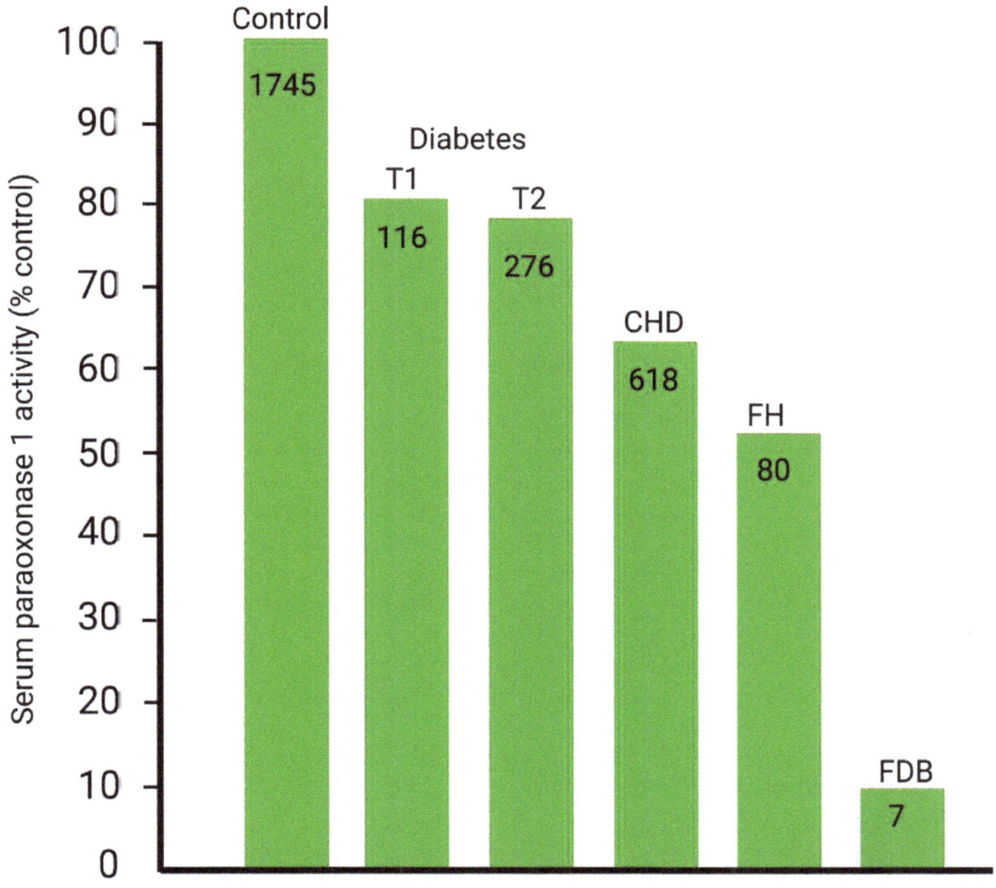

Figure 6. Median serum PON1 activity measured in our laboratory expressed as a percentage of control in Type 1 and Type 2 diabetes, coronary heart disease, familial hypercholesterolemia (FH), and familial dysbetalipoproteinemia (FDB). The number of individuals studied is shown. The controls were men recruited from the general population who did not experience acute myocardial infarction during follow-up. In 555 controls who were considered healthy at the time of venipuncture, median serum PON1 activity was higher at 184.4 U/L. Data from references [50,127–133].

PON1 has several polymorphisms, of which one has been frequently shown to be associated with ASCVD. This occurs as the result of whether glycine(Q) or arginine (R) is present in position 192 of its amino acid sequence. This polymorphism is also designated rs662. The 192R isoenzyme of PON1 is less active in protecting LDL against oxidative modification [6,143] and is more closely associated with ASCVD [6,144,145]. However, the 192Q enzyme confers protection too. It is thus the combined serum concentration of both isoenzymes, which in epidemiological studies is at least as predictive of ASCVD incidence as HDL cholesterol, particularly in diabetes and established ASCVD [6,146]. Activity assays that employ substrates to which PON1 does not display substrate specificity have high activity, and are nontoxic, such as phenyl acetate, have the most clinical utility [6,147]. One extreme example of nondiscordance between HDL cholesterol and PON1 activity is Tangier disease (see back), where serum HDL cholesterol is almost entirely absent, but PON1 activity is present within the normal range [148].

PON1 not only displays esterase activity, but has even greater lactonase activity and may have its evolutionary origin as a lactonase [149]. Its antiatherosclerotic role could thus be as an antioxidative enzyme, as a lactonase or both [118].

4. PON1 and ASCVD Causality

Epidemiological studies report that ASCVD cases have lower PON1 activity measured with paraoxon or phenyl acetate as a substrate compared to controls [6]. Activity of PON1 has generally been found to be a better discriminator than concentration. Most important amongst these are the prospective studies revealing that the association between lower PON1 activity and ASCVD is not the consequence of the ASCVD event or its treatment or due to lower levels being associated with survival, but that it predates the clinical event [6, 128,129,146,150,151]. Furthermore, low PON1 activity may explain cases of ASCVD when HDL cholesterol is high, which were previously thought anomalous [152]. However, epidemiology cannot prove causation. In theory, Mendelian randomization studies come closer to revealing causation, and the Q192R gene variant presents an opportunity for this type of investigation. There have been more than 100 reports, which have, with considerable consistency, demonstrated an association between the 192R (which is less effective than 192Q in decreasing LDL oxidation) and the likelihood of ASCVD [144,145]. However, 192R (even though less active than Q in hydrolyzing lipid peroxides) does still protects against oxidative modification of LDL, albeit less effectively than 192Q. Thus, higher concentrations can overcome its potentially adverse genotype effect [128]. Thus, the effect is smaller than might be expected from in vitro experiments in which similar concentrations were compared. Many other factors, including dyslipidemias and diabetes, are involved in determining PON1 activity, and these may be more influential than any gene so far discovered that modifies PON1 activity or concentration [153,154].

Animal experiments provide the strongest evidence that the epidemiologically observed inverse relationship between serum PON1 concentration and ASCVD is causal.

1. Serum PON1 activity varies greatly throughout the animal kingdom. Birds lack serum paraoxonase activity, whereas humans have substantial amounts, and rabbits, for example, even more. Human HDL protects LDL against oxidative modification, avian HDL fails to do so [155].
2. PON1 knockout mice are prone to atherosclerosis both induced by diet and apoE deficiency [156,157].
3. Over-expression of PON1 in mouse, rat, and rabbit models protects against atherosclerosis [135,158–161].

5. Objections to PON1 Being Essential for the Antioxidative, Antiglycative Role of HDL

There have, however, been reports critical of the proposal that a substantial component of the protection that HDL affords LDL against oxidative modification is due to its component PON1. These are as follows:

1. There are those that focus on the role of HDL in RCT in which so much research has been invested. They tend to dismiss the effect of HDL in decreasing LDL oxidation as due to the hydrolytic activity of PAFAH present on HDL [14,162–164]. Undoubtedly, HDL has PAFAH activity, and proteomic studies show PAFAH itself to be present in HDL. However, the majority of the PAFAH activity of HDL (not so LDL) is due to PON1. Furthermore, the effect of both whole HDL and partially purified PON1 in protecting LDL against oxidative modification is unaffected by inhibitors of PAFAH [39].
2. PON1 when highly purified loses its capacity to protect LDL against oxidation, therefore the effect of less highly purified PON1 is due to contamination by another enzyme truly responsible [165]. PON1 has hydrophobic domains and requires a lipid environment for its activity towards lipophilic substrates. It is difficult to maintain this lipid environment whilst achieving the final stage of purification, whether of PON1 from serum or of rPON1 from the culture media of genetically engineered cells [166–170].
3. There are numerous commercially available rPON1 preparations. Most, if not all, do not protect LDL against oxidation. Methods used to isolate the rPON1 have been optimized to maximize the yield with the aim of organophosphate hydrolysis. Initial screening is usually by phenyl acetate hydrolysis and then by testing potency as potential antidotes to organophosphate toxicity. The rPON1 thus produced may be lacking its hydrophobic environment depending on its method of isolation and may have structural modifications and tagging to enhance ease of isolation and potency as an organophosphate detoxicating enzyme. The antioxidant, antiatherogenic properties of PON1 were, however, reported to persist in rPON1 [171] prepared by one published method [172].
4. HDL can still protect LDL against oxidation in the absence of Ca^{2+} when paraoxon hydrolysis has thus been abolished [173]. However, soon after this report, it was revealed that Ca^{2+} is much less critical for phospholipid peroxide hydrolysis than for its aryl esterase and paraoxonase hydrolytic activities [174].
5. Mendelian randomization epidemiology based on the 192 polymorphism shows that the PON1 isoform is more active in promoting paraoxon hydrolysis. However, although this polymorphism is associated with ASCVD, in one report the association was not so strong as to rule out publication bias [175]. As has been earlier discussed, the impact of the R isoform on serum PON1 activity is not as strong as the authors of this report supposed. More recent meta-analyses have largely discounted publication bias as the explanation.
6 PON1 is the most active as a lactonase [149]. Although PON1 may have evolved as a lactonase, this does not mean that it is not involved in preventing a disease, such as atheroma, the clinical manifestations of which have only become apparent as a major epidemic in the last century [176]. If we allow that the protective effect of PON1 against ASCVD is not by protecting LDL against oxidative modification, then we must entertain that the discovery of its antiatherogenic role was serendipitous. Certainly, the possibility that its lactonase activity might be important, for example, against homocysteine thiolactone [177], should not be discounted, and further research should be directed in that area. However, the current evidence for an antioxidative role is compelling.

6. Conclusions

There is no doubt that HDL can protect LDL against oxidative modification. The extent to which HDL displays its antioxidative capacity is dependent on the balance between its pro- and antioxidant components, which varies between individuals, and on the propensity to develop certain diseases, such as ASCVD. Although primarily a lactonase, PON1 is the component of HDL that contributes most to its antioxidant activity. Epidemiology has revealed an inverse relationship between serum PON1 activity and ASCVD incidence. Experiments with genetically modified animals show convincingly that PON1 can prevent the development of atheroma. Furthermore, evidence suggests that in the circulation PON1 may protect LDL against oxidative modification, occurring, for example, as a consequence of hem metabolism, and against glycation due to glucose and its metabolites generated in the PPP and glycolysis pathway. OxLDL (and probably glycLDL) preferentially cross the arterial endothelium by receptor-mediated transcytosis, where their attempted removal by monocyte-macrophages creates foam cells. Within the arterial wall, additional oxLDL is generated by ROS secreted by inflammatory cells and leakage from cells generally when couplet oxygen is reduced. PON1 is important for the antioxidative mechanism by which HDL opposes atherogenesis, which may provide a better avenue of inquiry in the prevention and treatment of ASCVD [118] than has emerged from the emphasis on its role in RCT.

Author Contributions: P.N.D. was invited to contribute this editorial review in which he has been joined by B.B. and H.S. as joint authors. All three participated in its conception and design to ensure that its scope extended to areas of its topic not previously reviewed. P.N.D. prepared the original draft. All three authors contributed to later versions. B.B. and H.S. prepared the Figures. All authors have read and agreed to the published version of the manuscript.

Funding: This research review received no external funding.

Conflicts of Interest: The authors declare no conflict of interest in relation to this article.

References

1. Tsimikas, S.; Witztum, J.L. Oxidized phospholipids in cardiovascular disease. *Nat. Rev. Cardiol.* **2024**, *21*, 170–191. [CrossRef] [PubMed]
2. Steinberg, D.; Witztum, J.L. Oxidized low-density lipoprotein and atherosclerosis. *Arterioscler. Thromb. Vasc. Biol.* **2010**, *30*, 2311–2316. [CrossRef]
3. Heart Protection Study Collaborative Group. MRC/BHF Heart Protection Study of antioxidant vitamin supplementation in 20,536 high-risk individuals: A randomised placebo-controlled trial. *Lancet* **2002**, *360*, 23–33. [CrossRef] [PubMed]
4. Loffredo, L.; Perri, L.; Di Castelnuovo, A.; Iacoviello, L.; De Gaetano, G.; Violi, F. Supplementation with vitamin E alone is associated with reduced myocardial infarction: A meta-analysis. *Nutr. Metab. Cardiovasc. Dis.* **2015**, *25*, 354–363. [CrossRef]
5. Maggio, E.; Bocchini, V.P.; Carnevale, R.; Pignatelli, P.; Violi, F.; Loffredo, L. Vitamin E supplementation (alone or with other antioxidants) and stroke: A meta-analysis. *Nutr. Rev.* **2024**, *82*, 1069–1078. [CrossRef] [PubMed]
6. Durrington, P.N.; Bashir, B.; Soran, H. Paraoxonase 1 and atherosclerosis. *Front. Cardiovasc. Med.* **2023**, *10*, 1065967. [CrossRef]
7. Arrol, S.; Mackness, M.I.; Durrington, P.N. Vitamin E supplementation increases the resistance of both LDL and HDL to oxidation and increases cholesteryl ester transfer activity. *Atherosclerosis* **2000**, *150*, 129–134. [CrossRef]
8. Myant, N.B. *The Biology of Cholesterol and Related Steroids*; Elsevier: Amsterdam, The Netherlands, 1981. [CrossRef]
9. Brown, M.S.; Goldstein, J.L. How LDL receptors influence cholesterol and atherosclerosis. *Sci. Am.* **1984**, *251*, 58–66. [CrossRef]
10. Miller, G.J.; Miller, N.E. Plasma-high-density-lipoprotein concentration and development of ischaemic heart-disease. *Lancet* **1975**, *1*, 16–19. [CrossRef]
11. Ouimet, M.; Barrett, T.J.; Fisher, E.A. HDL and Reverse Cholesterol Transport. *Circ. Res.* **2019**, *124*, 1505–1518. [CrossRef]
12. Qiu, C.; Zhao, X.; Zhou, Q.; Zhang, Z. High-density lipoprotein cholesterol efflux capacity is inversely associated with cardiovascular risk: A systematic review and meta-analysis. *Lipids Health Dis.* **2017**, *16*, 212. [CrossRef] [PubMed]
13. Vitali, C.; Remaley, A.T.; Cuchel, M. Is Low-Density Lipoprotein Cholesterol the Key to Interpret the Role of Lecithin: Cholesterol Acyltransferase in Atherosclerosis? *Circulation* **2018**, *138*, 1008–1011. [CrossRef] [PubMed]

14. von Eckardstein, A.; Nordestgaard, B.G.; Remaley, A.T.; Catapano, A.L. High-density lipoprotein revisited: Biological functions and clinical relevance. *Eur. Heart J.* **2023**, *44*, 1394–1407. [CrossRef] [PubMed]
15. Durrington, P. HDL in risk prediction and its direct and indirect involvement in atherogenesis. *Atheroscler. Suppl.* **2002**, *3*, 3–12. [CrossRef]
16. Cedó, L.; Metso, J.; Santos, D.; García-León, A.; Plana, N.; Sabate-Soler, S.; Rotllan, N.; Rivas-Urbina, A.; Méndez-Lara, K.A.; Tondo, M.; et al. LDL Receptor Regulates the Reverse Transport of Macrophage-Derived Unesterified Cholesterol via Concerted Action of the HDL-LDL Axis: Insight From Mouse Models. *Circ. Res.* **2020**, *127*, 778–792. [CrossRef]
17. Assmann, G.; von Eckardstein, A.; Funke, H. High density lipoproteins, reverse transport of cholesterol, and coronary artery disease. Insights from mutations. *Circulation* **1993**, *87*, III28–III34.
18. Durrington, P.N. *Hyperlipidaemia: Diagnosis and Management*, 3rd ed.; Hodder Arnold: London, UK, 2007.
19. Tall, A.R.; Wang, N. Tangier disease as a test of the reverse cholesterol transport hypothesis. *J. Clin. Investig.* **2000**, *106*, 1205–1207. [CrossRef]
20. Koseki, M.; Yamashita, S.; Ogura, M.; Ishigaki, Y.; Ono, K.; Tsukamoto, K.; Hori, M.; Matsuki, K.; Yokoyama, S.; Harada-Shiba, M. Current Diagnosis and Management of Tangier Disease. *J. Atheroscler. Thromb.* **2021**, *28*, 802–810. [CrossRef]
21. Rousset, X.; Vaisman, B.; Amar, M.; Sethi, A.A.; Remaley, A.T. Lecithin: Cholesterol acyltransferase--from biochemistry to role in cardiovascular disease. *Curr. Opin. Endocrinol. Diabetes Obes.* **2009**, *16*, 163–171. [CrossRef]
22. Zanoni, P.; von Eckardstein, A. Inborn errors of apolipoprotein A-I metabolism: Implications for disease, research and development. *Curr. Opin. Lipidol.* **2020**, *31*, 62–70. [CrossRef]
23. Hancock-Cerutti, W.; Lhomme, M.; Dauteuille, C.; Lecocq, S.; Chapman, M.J.; Rader, D.J.; Kontush, A.; Cuchel, M. Paradoxical coronary artery disease in humans with hyperalphalipoproteinemia is associated with distinct differences in the high-density lipoprotein phosphosphingolipidome. *J. Clin. Lipidol.* **2017**, *11*, 1192–1200.e3. [CrossRef] [PubMed]
24. Hirano, K.I.; Yamashita, S.; Nakajima, N.; Arai, T.; Maruyama, T.; Yoshida, Y.; Ishigami, M.; Sakai, N.; Kameda-Takemura, K.; Matsuzawa, Y. Genetic cholesteryl ester transfer protein deficiency is extremely frequent in the Omagari area of Japan. Marked hyperalphalipoproteinemia caused by CETP gene mutation is not associated with longevity. *Arterioscler. Thromb. Vasc. Biol.* **1997**, *17*, 1053–1059. [CrossRef]
25. Yamashita, S.; Matsuzawa, Y. Re-evaluation of cholesteryl ester transfer protein function in atherosclerosis based upon genetics and pharmacological manipulation. *Curr. Opin. Lipidol.* **2016**, *27*, 459–472. [CrossRef]
26. Cimen, M.Y.B. Free radical metabolism in human erythrocytes. *Clin. Chim. Acta* **2008**, *390*, 1–11. [CrossRef] [PubMed]
27. Wallace, W.J.; Houtchens, R.A.; Maxwell, J.C.; Caughey, W.S. Mechanism of autooxidation for hemoglobins and myoglobins. Promotion of superoxide production by protons and anions. *J. Biol. Chem.* **1982**, *257*, 4966–4977. [CrossRef]
28. Andrés, C.M.C.; Pérez de la Lastra, J.M.; Andrés Juan, C.; Plou, F.J.; Pérez-Lebeña, E. Superoxide Anion Chemistry-Its Role at the Core of the Innate Immunity. *Int. J. Mol. Sci.* **2023**, *24*, 1841. [CrossRef] [PubMed]
29. Chatzinikolaou, P.N.; Margaritelis, N.V.; Paschalis, V.; Theodorou, A.A.; Vrabas, I.S.; Kyparos, A.; D'Alessandro, A.; Nikolaidis, M.G. Erythrocyte metabolism. *Acta Physiol.* **2024**, *240*, e14081. [CrossRef] [PubMed]
30. Klimov, A.N.; Kozhevnikova, K.A.; Kuzmin, A.A.; Kuznetsov, A.S.; Belova, E.V. On the ability of high density lipoproteins to remove phospholipid peroxidation products from erythrocyte membranes. *Biochemistry* **2001**, *66*, 300–304. [CrossRef]
31. Arrol, S.; Mackness, M.; Durrington, P. High-density-lipoprotein-associated enzymes and the prevention of lower density lipoprotein oxidation. *Eur. J. Lab. Med.* **1996**, *4*, 33–38.
32. el-Saadani, M.; Esterbauer, H.; el-Sayed, M.; Goher, M.; Nassar, A.Y.; Jürgens, G. A spectrophotometric assay for lipid peroxides in serum lipoproteins using a commercially available reagent. *J. Lipid Res.* **1989**, *30*, 627–630.
33. Mackness, M.I.; Abbott, C.; Arrol, S.; Durrington, P.N. The role of high-density lipoprotein and lipid-soluble antioxidant vitamins in inhibiting low-density lipoprotein oxidation. *Biochem. J.* **1993**, *294 Pt 3*, 829–834. [CrossRef] [PubMed]
34. Mackness, M.I.; Arrol, S.; Durrington, P.N. Paraoxonase prevents accumulation of lipoperoxides in low-density lipoprotein. *FEBS Lett.* **1991**, *286*, 152–154. [CrossRef] [PubMed]
35. Mackness, M.I.; Arrol, S.; Abbott, C.; Durrington, P.N. Protection of low-density lipoprotein against oxidative modification by high-density lipoprotein associated paraoxonase. *Atherosclerosis* **1993**, *104*, 129–135. [CrossRef] [PubMed]
36. Watson, A.; Berliner, J.A.; Hama, S.Y.; La Du, B.N.; Faull, K.F.; Fogelman, A.M.; Navab, M. Protective effect of high density lipoprotein associated paraoxonase. Inhibition of the biological activity of minimally oxidized low density lipoprotein. *J. Clin. Investig.* **1995**, *96*, 2882–2891. [CrossRef]
37. Hine, D.; Mackness, B.; Mackness, M. Cholesteryl-ester transfer protein enhances the ability of high-density lipoprotein to inhibit low-density lipoprotein oxidation. *IUBMB Life* **2011**, *63*, 772–774. [CrossRef]
38. Pantazi, D.; Tellis, C.; Tselepis, A.D. Oxidized phospholipids and lipoprotein-associated phospholipase A2 (Lp-PLA2) in atherosclerotic cardiovascular disease: An update. *Biofactors* **2022**, *48*, 1257–1270. [CrossRef]
39. Rodrigo, L.; Mackness, B.; Durrington, P.N.; Hernandez, A.; Mackness, M.I. Hydrolysis of platelet-activating factor by human serum paraoxonase. *Biochem. J.* **2001**, *354 Pt 1*, 1–7. [CrossRef]

40. Neary, R.; Bhatnagar, D.; Durrington, P.; Ishola, M.; Arrol, S.; Mackness, M. An investigation of the role of lecithin:cholesterol acyltransferase and triglyceride-rich lipoproteins in the metabolism of pre-beta high density lipoproteins. *Atherosclerosis* **1991**, *89*, 35–48. [CrossRef]
41. Rye, K.A.; Barter, P.J. Formation and metabolism of prebeta-migrating, lipid-poor apolipoprotein A-I. *Arterioscler. Thromb. Vasc. Biol.* **2004**, *24*, 421–428. [CrossRef]
42. Steinbrecher, U.P.; Parthasarathy, S.; Leake, D.S.; Witztum, J.L.; Steinberg, D. Modification of low density lipoprotein by endothelial cells involves lipid peroxidation and degradation of low density lipoprotein phospholipids. *Proc. Natl. Acad. Sci. USA* **1984**, *81*, 3883–3887. [CrossRef]
43. Morel, D.W.; DiCorleto, P.E.; Chisolm, G.M. Endothelial and smooth muscle cells alter low density lipoprotein in vitro by free radical oxidation. *Arteriosclerosis* **1984**, *4*, 357–364. [CrossRef] [PubMed]
44. Herb, M.; Schramm, M. Functions of ROS in Macrophages and Antimicrobial Immunity. *Antioxidants* **2021**, *10*, 313. [CrossRef] [PubMed]
45. Pepin, J.M.; O'Neil, J.A.; Hoff, H.F. Quantification of apo[a] and apoB in human atherosclerotic lesions. *J. Lipid Res.* **1991**, *32*, 317–327.
46. Packard, C.J. Triacylglycerol-rich lipoproteins and the generation of small, dense low-density lipoprotein. *Biochem. Soc. Trans.* **2003**, *31 Pt 5*, 1066–1069. [CrossRef]
47. Vekic, J.; Zeljkovic, A.; Cicero, A.F.; Janez, A.; Stoian, A.P.; Sonmez, A.; Rizzo, M. Atherosclerosis Development and Progression: The Role of Atherogenic Small, Dense LDL. *Medicina* **2022**, *58*, 299. [CrossRef]
48. Younis, N.; Charlton-Menys, V.; Sharma, R.; Soran, H.; Durrington, P.N. Glycation of LDL in non-diabetic people: Small dense LDL is preferentially glycated both in vivo and in vitro. *Atherosclerosis* **2009**, *202*, 162–168. [CrossRef]
49. Younis, N.N.; Soran, H.; Sharma, R.; Charlton-Menys, V.; Greenstein, A.; Elseweidy, M.M.; Durrington, P.N. Small-dense LDL and LDL glycation in metabolic syndrome and in statin-treated and non-statin-treated type 2 diabetes. *Diabetes Vasc. Dis. Res.* **2010**, *7*, 289–295. [CrossRef] [PubMed]
50. Younis, N.N.; Soran, H.; Pemberton, P.; Charlton-Menys, V.; Elseweidy, M.M.; Durrington, P.N. Small dense LDL is more susceptible to glycation than more buoyant LDL in Type 2 diabetes. *Clin. Sci.* **2013**, *124*, 343–349. [CrossRef]
51. Charlton-Menys, V.; Durrington, P. Apolipoproteins AI and B as therapeutic targets. *J. Intern. Med.* **2006**, *259*, 462–472. [CrossRef]
52. Soran, H.; Ho, J.H.; Adam, S.; Durrington, P.N. Non-HDL cholesterol should not generally replace LDL cholesterol in the management of hyperlipidaemia. *Curr. Opin. Lipidol.* **2019**, *30*, 263–272. [CrossRef]
53. Tames, F.J.; Mackness, M.I.; Arrol, S.; Laing, I.; Durrington, P.N. Non-enzymatic glycation of apolipoprotein B in the sera of diabetic and non-diabetic subjects. *Atherosclerosis* **1992**, *93*, 237–244. [CrossRef] [PubMed]
54. Younis, N.; Sharma, R.; Soran, H.; Charlton-Menys, V.; Elseweidy, M.; Durrington, P.N. Glycation as an atherogenic modification of LDL. *Curr. Opin. Lipidol.* **2008**, *19*, 378–384. [CrossRef]
55. Younis, N.N.; Soran, H.; Charlton-Menys, V.; Sharma, R.; Hama, S.; Pemberton, P.; Elseweidy, M.M.; Durrington, P.N. High-density lipoprotein impedes glycation of low-density lipoprotein. *Diab Vasc. Dis. Res.* **2013**, *10*, 152–160. [CrossRef]
56. Yim, M.B.; Yim, H.S.; Lee, C.; Kang, S.O.; Chock, P.B. Protein glycation: Creation of catalytic sites for free radical generation. *Ann. N. Y. Acad. Sci.* **2001**, *928*, 48–53. [PubMed]
57. Guimarães, E.L.M.; Empsen, C.; Geerts, A.; van Grunsven, L.A. Advanced glycation end products induce production of reactive oxygen species via the activation of NADPH oxidase in murine hepatic stellate cells. *J. Hepatol.* **2010**, *52*, 389–397. [CrossRef] [PubMed]
58. Lankin, V.Z.; Konovalova, G.G.; Tikhaze, A.K.; Nedosugova, L.V. The influence of glucose on the free radical peroxidation of low density lipoproteins in vitro and in vivo. *Biomed. Khim.* **2012**, *58*, 339–352. [CrossRef]
59. Moldogazieva, N.T.; Mokhosoev, I.M.; Mel'nikova, T.I.; Porozov, Y.B.; Terentiev, A.A. Oxidative Stress and Advanced Lipoxidation and Glycation End Products (ALEs and AGEs) in Aging and Age-Related Diseases. *Oxid. Med. Cell. Longev.* **2019**, *2019*, 3085756. [CrossRef]
60. Lindsay, R.M.; Smith, W.; Lee, W.K.; Dominiczak, M.H.; Baird, J.D. The effect of delta-gluconolactone, an oxidised analogue of glucose, on the nonenzymatic glycation of human and rat haemoglobin. *Clin. Chim. Acta* **1997**, *263*, 239–247. [CrossRef]
61. Gao, X.; Zhao, L.; Liu, S.; Li, Y.; Xia, S.; Chen, D.; Wang, M.; Wu, S.; Dai, Q.; Vu, H.; et al. γ-6-Phosphogluconolactone, a Byproduct of the Oxidative Pentose Phosphate Pathway, Contributes to AMPK Activation through Inhibition of PP2A. *Mol. Cell* **2019**, *76*, 857–871.e9. [CrossRef]
62. Thornalley, P.J.; Langborg, A.; Minhas, H.S. Formation of glyoxal, methylglyoxal and 3-deoxyglucosone in the glycation of proteins by glucose. *Biochem. J.* **1999**, *344 Pt 1*, 109–116.
63. Rabbani, N.; Godfrey, L.; Xue, M.; Shaheen, F.; Geoffrion, M.; Milne, R.; Thornalley, P.J. Glycation of LDL by methylglyoxal increases arterial atherogenicity: A possible contributor to increased risk of cardiovascular disease in diabetes. *Diabetes* **2011**, *60*, 1973–1980. [CrossRef]

64. Rabbani, N.; Thornalley, P.J. Dicarbonyl stress in cell and tissue dysfunction contributing to ageing and disease. *Biochem. Biophys. Res. Commun.* **2015**, *458*, 221–226. [CrossRef] [PubMed]
65. Allaman, I.; Bélanger, M.; Magistretti, P.J. Methylglyoxal, the dark side of glycolysis. *Front. Neurosci.* **2015**, *9*, 23. [CrossRef]
66. Rabbani, N.; Xue, M.; Thornalley, P.J. Dicarbonyls and glyoxalase in disease mechanisms and clinical therapeutics. *Glycoconj. J.* **2016**, *33*, 513–525. [CrossRef]
67. Lankin, V.Z.; Tikhaze, A.K.; Melkumyants, A.M. Dicarbonyl-Dependent Modification of LDL as a Key Factor of Endothelial Dysfunction and Atherosclerotic Vascular Wall Damage. *Antioxidants* **2022**, *11*, 1565. [CrossRef] [PubMed]
68. Uceda, A.B.; Mariño, L.; Casasnovas, R.; Adrover, M. An overview on glycation: Molecular mechanisms, impact on proteins, pathogenesis, and inhibition. *Biophys. Rev.* **2024**, *16*, 189–218. [CrossRef]
69. Hui, D.Y.; Noel, J.G.; Harmony, J.A. Binding of plasma low density lipoproteins to erythrocytes. *Biochim. Biophys. Acta* **1981**, *664*, 513–526. [CrossRef]
70. Durrington, P.N.; MacIver, J.E.; Holdsworth, G.; Galton, D.J. Severe hypertriglyceridemia associated with pancytopenia and lipoprotein lipase deficiency. *Ann. Intern. Med.* **1981**, *94*, 211–212. [CrossRef]
71. Sarin, H. Physiologic upper limits of pore size of different blood capillary types and another perspective on the dual pore theory of microvascular permeability. *J. Angiogenes Res.* **2010**, *2*, 14. [CrossRef]
72. Michel, C.C.; Nanjee, M.N.; Olszewski, W.L.; Miller, N.E. LDL and HDL transfer rates across peripheral microvascular endothelium agree with those predicted for passive ultrafiltration in humans. *J. Lipid Res.* **2015**, *56*, 122–128. [CrossRef]
73. Mackness, M.I.; Mackness, B.; Arrol, S.; Wood, G.; Bhatnagar, D.; Durrington, P.N. Presence of paraoxonase in human interstitial fluid. *FEBS Lett.* **1997**, *416*, 377–380. [CrossRef]
74. Goldberg, I.J.; Cabodevilla, A.G.; Younis, W. In the Beginning, Lipoproteins Cross the Endothelial Barrier. *J. Atheroscler. Thromb.* **2024**, *31*, 854–860. [CrossRef] [PubMed]
75. Pal, S.; Semorine, K.; Watts, G.F.; Mamo, J. Identification of lipoproteins of intestinal origin in human atherosclerotic plaque. *Clin. Chem. Lab. Med.* **2003**, *41*, 792–795. [CrossRef] [PubMed]
76. Nakano, T.; Nakajima, K.; Niimi, M.; Fujita, M.Q.; Nakajima, Y.; Takeichi, S.; Kinoshita, M.; Matsushima, T.; Teramoto, T.; Tanaka, A. Detection of apolipoproteins B-48 and B-100 carrying particles in lipoprotein fractions extracted from human aortic atherosclerotic plaques in sudden cardiac death cases. *Clin. Chim. Acta* **2008**, *390*, 38–43. [CrossRef]
77. Rapp, J.H.; Harris, H.W.; Hamilton, R.L.; Krupski, W.C.; Reilly, L.M.; Ehrenfeld, W.K.; Stoney, R.J.; Goldstone, J.; Kane, J.P. Particle size distribution of lipoproteins from human atherosclerotic plaque: A preliminary report. *J. Vasc. Surg.* **1989**, *9*, 81–88. [CrossRef] [PubMed]
78. Wissler, R.W.; Vesselinovitch, D.; Getz, G.S. Abnormalities of the arterial wall and its metabolism in atherogenesis. *Prog. Cardiovasc. Dis.* **1976**, *18*, 341–369. [CrossRef]
79. Schwartz, C.J.; Valente, A.J.; Sprague, E.A.; Kelley, J.L.; Nerem, R.M. The pathogenesis of atherosclerosis: An overview. *Clin. Cardiol.* **1991**, *14* (Suppl. S1), 1–16. [CrossRef]
80. Weinberg, P.D. Haemodynamic Wall Shear Stress, Endothelial Permeability and Atherosclerosis-A Triad of Controversy. *Front. Bioeng. Biotechnol.* **2022**, *10*, 836680. [CrossRef]
81. Gerhardt, T.; Ley, K. Monocyte trafficking across the vessel wall. *Cardiovasc. Res.* **2015**, *107*, 321–330. [CrossRef]
82. Medrano-Bosch, M.; Simón-Codina, B.; Jiménez, W.; Edelman, E.R.; Melgar-Lesmes, P. Monocyte-endothelial cell interactions in vascular and tissue remodeling. *Front. Immunol.* **2023**, *14*, 1196033. [CrossRef]
83. Libby, P. Inflammation during the life cycle of the atherosclerotic plaque. *Cardiovasc. Res.* **2021**, *117*, 2525–2536. [CrossRef]
84. Poznyak, A.V.; Grechko, A.V.; Orekhova, V.A.; Khotina, V.; Ivanova, E.A.; Orekhov, A.N. NADPH Oxidases and Their Role in Atherosclerosis. *Biomedicines* **2020**, *8*, 206. [CrossRef]
85. Harrison, D.G.; Widder, J.; Grumbach, I.; Chen, W.; Weber, M.; Searles, C. Endothelial mechanotransduction, nitric oxide and vascular inflammation. *J. Intern. Med.* **2006**, *259*, 351–363. [CrossRef] [PubMed]
86. Gisterå, A.; Ketelhuth, D.F.J.; Malin, S.G.; Hansson, G.K. Animal Models of Atherosclerosis-Supportive Notes and Tricks of the Trade. *Circ. Res.* **2022**, *130*, 1869–1887. [CrossRef] [PubMed]
87. Klimov, A.N.; Nagornev, V.A. Current concepts of the pathogenesis of atherosclerosis in light of the development of N.N. Anichkov's theory (on the centenary of his birth). *Arkhiv Patol.* **1985**, *47*, 12–23.
88. Dai, G.; Kaazempur-Mofrad, M.R.; Natarajan, S.; Zhang, Y.; Vaughn, S.; Blackman, B.R.; Kamm, R.D.; García-Cardeña, G.; Gimbrone, M.A., Jr. Distinct endothelial phenotypes evoked by arterial waveforms derived from atherosclerosis-susceptible and -resistant regions of human vasculature. *Proc. Natl. Acad. Sci. USA* **2004**, *101*, 14871–14876. [CrossRef] [PubMed]
89. Cancel, L.M.; Fitting, A.; Tarbell, J.M. In vitro study of LDL transport under pressurized (convective) conditions. *Am. J. Physiol. Heart Circ. Physiol.* **2007**, *293*, H126–H132. [CrossRef]
90. Dabagh, M.; Jalali, P.; Tarbell, J.M. The transport of LDL across the deformable arterial wall: The effect of endothelial cell turnover and intimal deformation under hypertension. *Am. J. Physiol. Heart Circ. Physiol.* **2009**, *297*, H983–H996. [CrossRef] [PubMed]

91. Strong, J.P.; Zieske, A.W.; Malcom, G.T. Lipoproteins and atherosclerosis in children: An early marriage? *Nutr. Metab. Cardiovasc. Dis.* **2001**, *11* (Suppl. S5), 16–22.
92. Chen, Z.; Peto, R.; Collins, R.; MacMahon, S.; Lu, J.; Li, W. Serum cholesterol concentration and coronary heart disease in population with low cholesterol concentrations. *BMJ* **1991**, *303*, 276–282. [CrossRef]
93. Lorey, M.B.; Öörni, K.; Kovanen, P.T. Modified Lipoproteins Induce Arterial Wall Inflammation During Atherogenesis. *Front. Cardiovasc. Med.* **2022**, *9*, 841545. [CrossRef] [PubMed]
94. Zhang, X.; Sessa, W.C.; Fernández-Hernando, C. Endothelial Transcytosis of Lipoproteins in Atherosclerosis. *Front. Cardiovasc. Med.* **2018**, *5*, 130. [CrossRef]
95. Huang, L.; Chambliss, K.L.; Gao, X.; Yuhanna, I.S.; Behling-Kelly, E.; Bergaya, S.; Ahmed, M.; Michaely, P.; Luby-Phelps, K.; Darehshouri, A.; et al. SR-B1 drives endothelial cell LDL transcytosis via DOCK4 to promote atherosclerosis. *Nature* **2019**, *569*, 565–569. [CrossRef] [PubMed]
96. Zhang, X.; Fernández-Hernando, C. Transport of LDLs into the arterial wall: Impact in atherosclerosis. *Curr. Opin. Lipidol.* **2020**, *31*, 279–285. [CrossRef]
97. Ghaffari, S.; Jang, E.; Naderinabi, F.; Sanwal, R.; Khosraviani, N.; Wang, C.; Steinberg, B.E.; Goldenberg, N.M.; Ikeda, J.; Lee, W.L. Endothelial HMGB1 Is a Critical Regulator of LDL Transcytosis via an SREBP2-SR-BI Axis. *Arterioscler. Thromb. Vasc. Biol.* **2021**, *41*, 200–216. [CrossRef] [PubMed]
98. Jang, E.; Robert, J.; Rohrer, L.; von Eckardstein, A.; Lee, W.L. Transendothelial transport of lipoproteins. *Atherosclerosis* **2020**, *315*, 111–125. [CrossRef]
99. Ho, T.W.W.; Henry, A.; Lee, W.L. LDL Transcytosis by the Arterial Endothelium-Atherosclerosis by a Thousand Cuts? *Curr. Atheroscler. Rep.* **2023**, *25*, 457–465. [CrossRef]
100. Ma, B.; Jia, J.; Wang, X.; Zhang, R.; Niu, S.; Ni, L.; Di, X.; Liu, C. Differential roles of Scavenger receptor class B type I: A protective molecule and a facilitator of atherosclerosis (Review). *Mol. Med. Rep.* **2020**, *22*, 2599–2604. [CrossRef]
101. Shen, W.J.; Azhar, S.; Kraemer, F.B. SR-B1: A Unique Multifunctional Receptor for Cholesterol Influx and Efflux. *Annu. Rev. Physiol.* **2018**, *80*, 95–116. [CrossRef]
102. Luchetti, F.; Crinelli, R.; Nasoni, M.G.; Benedetti, S.; Palma, F.; Fraternale, A.; Iuliano, L. LDL receptors, caveolae and cholesterol in endothelial dysfunction: oxLDLs accomplices or victims? *Br. J. Pharmacol.* **2021**, *178*, 3104–3114. [CrossRef]
103. Tian, K.; Ogura, S.; Little, P.J.; Xu, S.W.; Sawamura, T. Targeting LOX-1 in atherosclerosis and vasculopathy: Current knowledge and future perspectives. *Ann. N. Y. Acad. Sci.* **2019**, *1443*, 34–53. [CrossRef]
104. Akhmedov, A.; Sawamura, T.; Chen, C.H.; Kraler, S.; Vdovenko, D.; Lüscher, T.F. Lectin-like oxidized low-density lipoprotein receptor-1 (LOX-1): A crucial driver of atherosclerotic cardiovascular disease. *Eur. Heart J.* **2021**, *42*, 1797–1807. [CrossRef]
105. Barreto, J.; Karathanasis, S.K.; Remaley, A.; Sposito, A.C. Role of LOX-1 (Lectin-Like Oxidized Low-Density Lipoprotein Receptor 1) as a Cardiovascular Risk Predictor: Mechanistic Insight and Potential Clinical Use. *Arterioscler. Thromb. Vasc. Biol.* **2021**, *41*, 153–166. [CrossRef] [PubMed]
106. Cheng, W.; Shu, M.; Kuang, L.; Bai, X.; Jia, X.; Zhao, Y.; Lu, Y.; Zhu, L.; Wang, L.; Zhu, Y.; et al. Scavenger receptor a mediates glycated LDL transcytosis across endothelial cells to promote atherosclerosis. *Int. J. Biol. Macromol.* **2023**, *235*, 123836. [CrossRef]
107. Shu, M.; Cheng, W.; Jia, X.; Bai, X.; Zhao, Y.; Lu, Y.; Zhu, L.; Zhu, Y.; Wang, L.; Shu, Y.; et al. AGEs promote atherosclerosis by increasing LDL transcytosis across endothelial cells via RAGE/NF-κB/Caveolin-1 pathway. *Mol. Med.* **2023**, *29*, 113. [CrossRef]
108. Goldberg, D.; Khatib, S. Atherogenesis, Transcytosis, and the Transmural Cholesterol Flux: A Critical Review. *Oxid. Med. Cell. Longev.* **2022**, *2022*, 2253478. [CrossRef] [PubMed]
109. Fung, K.Y.; Ho, T.W.W.; Xu, Z.; Neculai, D.; Beauchemin, C.A.; Lee, W.L.; Fairn, G.D. Apolipoprotein A1 and high-density lipoprotein limit low-density lipoprotein transcytosis by binding SR-B1. *J. Lipid Res.* **2024**, *65*, 100530. [CrossRef]
110. Miller, N.E.; Weinstein, D.B.; Carew, T.E.; Koschinsky, T.; Steinberg, D. Interaction between high density and low density lipoproteins uptake and degradation by cultured human fibroblasts. *J. Clin. Investig.* **1977**, *60*, 78–88. [CrossRef]
111. Chistiakov, D.A.; Melnichenko, A.A.; Myasoedova, V.A.; Grechko, A.V.; Orekhov, A.N. Mechanisms of foam cell formation in atherosclerosis. *J. Mol. Med.* **2017**, *95*, 1153–1165. [CrossRef]
112. Gui, Y.; Zheng, H.; Cao, R.Y. Foam Cells in Atherosclerosis: Novel Insights Into Its Origins, Consequences, and Molecular Mechanisms. *Front. Cardiovasc. Med.* **2022**, *9*, 845942. [CrossRef]
113. Cuthbert, G.A.; Shaik, F.; Harrison, M.A.; Ponnambalam, S.; Homer-Vanniasinkam, S. Scavenger Receptors as Biomarkers and Therapeutic Targets in Cardiovascular Disease. *Cells* **2020**, *9*, 2453. [CrossRef] [PubMed]
114. Getz, G.S.; Reardon, C.A. Apoprotein E and Reverse Cholesterol Transport. *Int. J. Mol. Sci.* **2018**, *19*, 3479. [CrossRef] [PubMed]
115. Rosenblat, M.; Vaya, J.; Shih, D.; Aviram, M. Paraoxonase 1 (PON1) enhances HDL-mediated macrophage cholesterol efflux via the ABCA1 transporter in association with increased HDL binding to the cells: A possible role for lysophosphatidylcholine. *Atherosclerosis* **2005**, *179*, 69–77. [CrossRef] [PubMed]
116. Deakin, S.P.; Bioletto, S.; Bochaton-Piallat, M.L.; James, R.W. HDL-associated paraoxonase-1 can redistribute to cell membranes and influence sensitivity to oxidative stress. *Free Radic. Biol. Med.* **2011**, *50*, 102–109. [CrossRef]

117. Evans, C.E.; Mylchreest, S.; Charlton-Menys, V.; Durrington, P. The role of hydrostatic pressure in foam cell formation upon exposure of macrophages to LDL and oxidized LDL. *Atherosclerosis* **2008**, *197*, 596–601. [CrossRef]
118. Durrington, P.; Soran, H. Paraoxonase 1: Evolution of the enzyme and of its role in protecting against atherosclerosis. *Curr. Opin. Lipidol.* **2024**, *35*, 171–178. [CrossRef]
119. Aldridge, W.N Serum esterases. II. An enzyme hydrolysing diethyl p-nitrophenyl phosphate (E600) and its identity with the A-esterase of mammalian sera. *Biochem. J.* **1953**, *53*, 117–124. [CrossRef]
120. Augustinsson, K.B. Arylesterases. *J. Histochem. Cytochem.* **1964**, *12*, 744–747. [CrossRef]
121. Brogen, C.-H.; Bøg-Hansen, T.C. Enzyme Characterization in Quantitative Immunoelectrophoresis. *Scand. J. Immunol.* **1975**, *4*, 37–51. [CrossRef]
122. Mackness, M.I.; Hallam, S.D.; Peard, T.; Warner, S.; Walker, C.H. The separation of sheep and human serum "A"-esterase activity into the lipoprotein fraction by ultracentrifugation. *Comp. Biochem. Physiol. B* **1985**, *82*, 675–677. [CrossRef]
123. Furlong, C.E.; Costa, L.G.; Hassett, C.; Richter, R.J.; Sundstrom, J.A.; Adler, D.A.; Disteche, C.M.; Omiecinski, C.J.; Chapline, C.; Crabb, J.W.; et al. Human and rabbit paraoxonases: Purification, cloning, sequencing, mapping and role of polymorphism in organophosphate detoxification. *Chem. Biol. Interact.* **1993**, *87*, 35–48. [CrossRef] [PubMed]
124. Draganov, D.I.; La Du, B.N. Pharmacogenetics of paraoxonases: A brief review. *Naunyn Schmiedebergs Arch. Pharmacol.* **2004**, *369*, 78–88. [CrossRef]
125. Mackness, B.; Hunt, R.; Durrington, P.N.; Mackness, M.I. Increased immunolocalization of paraoxonase, clusterin, and apolipoprotein A-I in the human artery wall with the progression of atherosclerosis. *Arterioscler. Thromb. Vasc. Biol.* **1997**, *17*, 1233–1238. [CrossRef]
126. McElveen, J.; Mackness, M.I.; Colley, C.M.; Peard, T.; Warner, S.; Walker, C.H. Distribution of paraoxon hydrolytic activity in the serum of patients after myocardial infarction. *Clin. Chem.* **1986**, *32*, 671–673. [PubMed]
127. Ayub, A.; Mackness, M.I.; Arrol, S.; Mackness, B.; Patel, J.; Durrington, P.N. Serum paraoxonase after myocardial infarction. *Arterioscler. Thromb. Vasc. Biol.* **1999**, *19*, 330–335. [CrossRef]
128. Mackness, B.; Davies, G.K.; Turkie, W.; Lee, E.; Roberts, D.H.; Hill, E.; Roberts, C.; Durrington, P.N.; Mackness, M.I. Paraoxonase status in coronary heart disease: Are activity and concentration more important than genotype? *Arterioscler. Thromb. Vasc. Biol.* **2001**, *21*, 1451–1457. [CrossRef] [PubMed]
129. Mackness, B.; Durrington, P.; McElduff, P.; Yarnell, J.; Azam, N.; Watt, M.; Mackness, M. Low paraoxonase activity predicts coronary events in the Caerphilly Prospective Study. *Circulation* **2003**, *107*, 2775–2779. [CrossRef]
130. Mackness, M.I.; Harty, D.; Bhatnagar, D.; Winocour, P.H.; Arrol, S.; Ishola, M.; Durrington, P.N. Serum paraoxonase activity in familial hypercholesterolaemia and insulin-dependent diabetes mellitus. *Atherosclerosis* **1991**, *86*, 193–199. [CrossRef]
131. Abbott, C.A.; Mackness, M.I.; Kumar, S.; Boulton, A.J.; Durrington, P.N. Serum paraoxonase activity, concentration, and phenotype distribution in diabetes mellitus and its relationship to serum lipids and lipoproteins. *Arterioscler. Thromb. Vasc. Biol.* **1995**, *15*, 1812–1818. [CrossRef]
132. Mackness, B.; Durrington, P.N.; Boulton, A.J.M.; Hine, D.; Mackness, M.I. Serum paraoxonase activity in patients with type 1 diabetes compared to healthy controls. *Eur. J. Clin. Investig.* **2002**, *32*, 259–264. [CrossRef]
133. Liu, Y. Clinical Study on Apolipoprotein E Distribution, Metabolism and Glycation. Ph.D. Thesis, University of Manchester, Manchester, UK, 2015.
134. Garin, M.C.B.; Kalix, B.; Morabia, A.; James, R.W. Small, dense lipoprotein particles and reduced paraoxonase-1 in patients with the metabolic syndrome. *J. Clin. Endocrinol. Metab.* **2005**, *90*, 2264–2269. [CrossRef] [PubMed]
135. Sentí, M.; Tomás, M.; Fitó, M.; Weinbrenner, T.; Covas, M.I.; Sala, J.; Masiá, R.; Marrugat, J. Antioxidant paraoxonase 1 activity in the metabolic syndrome. *J. Clin. Endocrinol. Metab.* **2003**, *88*, 5422–5426. [CrossRef] [PubMed]
136. Mackness, B.; Quarck, R.; Verreth, W.; Mackness, M.; Holvoet, P. Human paraoxonase-1 overexpression inhibits atherosclerosis in a mouse model of metabolic syndrome. *Arterioscler. Thromb. Vasc. Biol.* **2006**, *26*, 1545–1550. [CrossRef] [PubMed]
137. Adhe-Rojekar, A.; Mogarekar, M.R.; Rojekar, M.V. Paraoxonase activity in metabolic syndrome in children and adolescents. *Casp. J. Intern. Med.* **2018**, *9*, 116–120. [CrossRef]
138. Ferré, N.; Feliu, A.; García-Heredia, A.; Marsillach, J.; París, N.; Zaragoza-Jordana, M.; Mackness, B.; Mackness, M.; Escribano, J.; Closa-Monasterolo, R.; et al. Impaired paraoxonase-1 status in obese children. Relationships with insulin resistance and metabolic syndrome. *Clin. Biochem.* **2013**, *46*, 1830–1836. [CrossRef]
139. Kappelle, P.J.W.H.; Bijzet, J.; Hazenberg, B.P.; Dullaart, R.P.F. Lower serum paraoxonase-1 activity is related to higher serum amyloid a levels in metabolic syndrome. *Arch. Med. Res.* **2011**, *42*, 219–225. [CrossRef]
140. Adam, S.; Ho, J.H.; Liu, Y.; Siahmansur, T.; Siddals, K.; Iqbal, Z.; Azmi, S.; Senapati, S.; New, J.; Jeziorska, M.; et al. Bariatric Surgery-induced High-density Lipoprotein Functionality Enhancement Is Associated With Reduced Inflammation. *J. Clin. Endocrinol. Metab.* **2022**, *107*, 2182–2194. [CrossRef]

141. Jiang, X.; Ding, C.; Wang, C.; Yu, J.; Hua, Z.; Chen, X.; Ma, J.; Chen, W. Association of Paraoxonase 1 Gene Polymorphisms and Polycystic Ovarian Syndrome Susceptibility: A Systematic Review and Meta-Analysis. *Gynecol. Obstet. Investig.* **2020**, *85*, 167–177. [CrossRef]
142. Samouilidou, E.C.; Liaouri, A.; Kostopoulos, V.; Nikas, D.; Grapsa, E. The importance of paraoxonase 1 activity in chronic kidney disease. *Ren. Fail.* **2024**, *46*, 2376930. [CrossRef]
143. Mackness, B.; Mackness, M.I.; Arrol, S.; Turkie, W.; Durrington, P.N. Effect of the human serum paraoxonase 55 and 192 genetic polymorphisms on the protection by high density lipoprotein against low density lipoprotein oxidative modification. *FEBS Lett.* **1998**, *423*, 57–60. [CrossRef]
144. Zeng, Q.; Zeng, J. A meta-analysis on relationship between paraoxonase 1 polymorphisms and atherosclerotic cardiovascular diseases. *Life Sci.* **2019**, *232*, 116646. [CrossRef]
145. Ashiq, S.; Ashiq, K. The Role of Paraoxonase 1 (PON1) Gene Polymorphisms in Coronary Artery Disease: A Systematic Review and Meta-Analysis. *Biochem. Genet.* **2021**, *59*, 919–939. [CrossRef] [PubMed]
146. Zuin, M.; Trentini, A.; Marsillach, J.; D'Amuri, A.; Bosi, C.; Roncon, L.; Passaro, A.; Zuliani, G.; Mackness, M.; Cervellati, C. Paraoxonase-1 (PON-1) Arylesterase Activity Levels in Patients with Coronary Artery Disease: A Meta-Analysis. *Dis. Markers* **2022**, *2022*, 4264314. [CrossRef]
147. Mahrooz, A. Pleiotropic functions and clinical importance of circulating HDL-PON1 complex. *Adv. Clin. Chem.* **2024**, *121*, 132–171. [CrossRef] [PubMed]
148. James, R.W.; Garin, M.C.B.; Calabresi, L.; Miccoli, R.; von Eckardstein, A.; Tilly-Kiesi, M.; Taskinen, M.R.; Assmann, G.; Franceschini, G. Modulated serum activities and concentrations of paraoxonase in high density lipoprotein deficiency states. *Atherosclerosis* **1998**, *139*, 77–82. [CrossRef]
149. Bar-Rogovsky, H.; Hugenmatter, A.; Tawfik, D.S. The evolutionary origins of detoxifying enzymes: The mammalian serum paraoxonases (PONs) relate to bacterial homoserine lactonases. *J. Biol. Chem.* **2013**, *288*, 23914–23927. [CrossRef] [PubMed]
150. Kunutsor, S.K.; Bakker, S.J.L.; James, R.W.; Dullaart, R.P.F. Serum paraoxonase-1 activity and risk of incident cardiovascular disease: The PREVEND study and meta-analysis of prospective population studies. *Atherosclerosis* **2016**, *245*, 143–154. [CrossRef]
151. Bhattacharyya, T.; Nicholls, S.J.; Topol, E.J.; Zhang, R.; Yang, X.; Schmitt, D.; Fu, X.; Shao, M.; Brennan, D.M.; Ellis, S.G.; et al. Relationship of paraoxonase 1 (PON1) gene polymorphisms and functional activity with systemic oxidative stress and cardiovascular risk. *JAMA* **2008**, *299*, 1265–1276. [CrossRef]
152. Corsetti, J.P.; Sparks, C.E.; James, R.W.; Bakker, S.J.L.; Dullaart, R.P.F. Low Serum Paraoxonase-1 Activity Associates with Incident Cardiovascular Disease Risk in Subjects with Concurrently High Levels of High-Density Lipoprotein Cholesterol and C-Reactive Protein. *J. Clin. Med.* **2019**, *8*, 1357. [CrossRef]
153. Soran, H.; Younis, N.N.; Charlton-Menys, V.; Durrington, P. Variation in paraoxonase-1 activity and atherosclerosis. *Curr. Opin. Lipidol.* **2009**, *20*, 265–274. [CrossRef]
154. Mahrooz, A.; Mackness, M.; Bagheri, A.; Ghaffari-Cherati, M.; Masoumi, P. The epigenetic regulation of paraoxonase 1 (PON1) as an important enzyme in HDL function: The missing link between environmental and genetic regulation. *Clin. Biochem.* **2019**, *73*, 1–10. [CrossRef]
155. Mackness, B.; Durrington, P.N.; Mackness, M.I. Lack of protection against oxidative modification of LDL by avian HDL. *Biochem. Biophys. Res. Commun.* **1998**, *247*, 443–446. [CrossRef]
156. Shih, D.M.; Gu, L.; Xia, Y.R.; Navab, M.; Li, W.F.; Hama, S.; Castellani, L.W.; Furlong, C.E.; Costa, L.G.; Fogelman, A.M.; et al. Mice lacking serum paraoxonase are susceptible to organophosphate toxicity and atherosclerosis. *Nature* **1998**, *394*, 284–287. [CrossRef] [PubMed]
157. Shih, D.M.; Xia, Y.R.; Wang, X.P.; Miller, E.; Castellani, L.W.; Subbanagounder, G.; Cheroutre, H.; Faull, K.F.; Berliner, J.A.; Witztum, J.L.; et al. Combined serum paraoxonase knockout/apolipoprotein E knockout mice exhibit increased lipoprotein oxidation and atherosclerosis. *J. Biol. Chem.* **2000**, *275*, 17527–17535. [CrossRef]
158. Tward, A.; Xia, Y.R.; Wang, X.P.; Shi, Y.S.; Park, C.; Castellani, L.W.; Lusis, A.J.; Shih, D.M. Decreased atherosclerotic lesion formation in human serum paraoxonase transgenic mice. *Circulation* **2002**, *106*, 484–490. [CrossRef] [PubMed]
159. Guns, P.J.; Van Assche, T.; Verreth, W.; Fransen, P.; Mackness, B.; Mackness, M.; Holvoet, P.; Bult, H. Paraoxonase 1 gene transfer lowers vascular oxidative stress and improves vasomotor function in apolipoprotein E-deficient mice with pre-existing atherosclerosis. *Br. J. Pharmacol.* **2008**, *153*, 508–516. [CrossRef] [PubMed]
160. She, Z.G.; Zheng, W.; Wei, Y.S.; Chen, H.Z.; Wang, A.B.; Li, H.L.; Liu, G.; Zhang, R.; Liu, J.J. Human paraoxonase gene cluster transgenic overexpression represses atherogenesis and promotes atherosclerotic plaque stability in ApoE-null mice. *Circ. Res.* **2009**, *104*, 1160–1168. [CrossRef]
161. Zhang, C.; Peng, W.; Wang, M.; Zhu, J.; Zang, Y.; Shi, W.; Zhang, J.; Qin, J. Studies on protective effects of human paraoxonases 1 and 3 on atherosclerosis in apolipoprotein E knockout mice. *Gene Ther.* **2010**, *17*, 626–633. [CrossRef]
162. Rohatgi, A.; Westerterp, M.; von Eckardstein, A.; Remaley, A.; Rye, K.A. HDL in the 21st Century: A Multifunctional Roadmap for Future HDL Research. *Circulation* **2021**, *143*, 2293–2309. [CrossRef]

163. Rosenson, R.S.; Brewer Jr, H.B.; Ansell, B.J.; Barter, P.; Chapman, M.J.; Heinecke, J.W.; Kontush, A.; Tall, A.R.; Webb, N.R. Dysfunctional HDL and atherosclerotic cardiovascular disease. *Nat. Rev. Cardiol.* **2016**, *13*, 48–60. [CrossRef]
164. Kriska, T.; Marathe, G.K.; Schmidt, J.C.; McIntyre, T.M.; Girotti, A.W. Phospholipase action of platelet-activating factor acetylhydrolase, but not paraoxonase-1, on long fatty acyl chain phospholipid hydroperoxides. *J. Biol. Chem.* **2007**, *282*, 100–108. [CrossRef] [PubMed]
165. Teiber, J.F.; Draganov, D.I.; La Du, B.N. Purified human serum PON1 does not protect LDL against oxidation in the in vitro assays initiated with copper or AAPH. *J. Lipid Res.* **2004**, *45*, 2260–2268. [CrossRef] [PubMed]
166. Khattib, A.; Musa, S.; Halabi, M.; Hayek, T.; Khatib, S. Lyso-DGTS Lipid Derivatives Enhance PON1 Activities and Prevent Oxidation of LDL: A Structure-Activity Relationship Study. *Antioxidants* **2022**, *11*, 2058. [CrossRef]
167. Mishra, V.K.; Palgunachari, M.N.; McPherson, D.T.; Anantharamaiah, G.M. Lipid complex of apolipoprotein A-I mimetic peptide 4F is a novel platform for paraoxonase-1 binding and enhancing its activity and stability. *Biochem. Biophys. Res. Commun.* **2013**, *430*, 975–980. [CrossRef] [PubMed]
168. Seddon, A.M.; Curnow, P.; Booth, P.J. Membrane proteins, lipids and detergents: Not just a soap opera. *Biochim. Biophys. Acta* **2004**, *1666*, 105–117. [CrossRef]
169. James, R.W.; Deakin, S.P. The importance of high-density lipoproteins for paraoxonase-1 secretion, stability, and activity. *Free Radic. Biol. Med.* **2004**, *37*, 1986–1994. [CrossRef]
170. Rochu, D.; Renault, F.; Cléry-Barraud, C.; Chabrière, E.; Masson, P. Stability of highly purified human paraoxonase (PON1): Association with human phosphate binding protein (HPBP) is essential for preserving its active conformation(s). *Biochim. Biophys. Acta* **2007**, *1774*, 874–883. [CrossRef]
171. Tavori, H.; Aviram, M.; Khatib, S.; Musa, R.; Nitecki, S.; Hoffman, A.; Vaya, J. Human carotid atherosclerotic plaque increases oxidative state of macrophages and low-density lipoproteins, whereas paraoxonase 1 (PON1) decreases such atherogenic effects. *Free Radic. Biol. Med.* **2009**, *46*, 607–615. [CrossRef]
172. Aharoni, A.; Gaidukov, L.; Yagur, S.; Toker, L.; Silman, I.; Tawfik, D.S. Directed evolution of mammalian paraoxonases PON1 and PON3 for bacterial expression and catalytic specialization. *Proc. Natl. Acad. Sci. USA* **2004**, *101*, 482–487. [CrossRef]
173. Graham, A.; Hassall, D.G.; Rafique, S.; Owen, J.S. Evidence for a paraoxonase-independent inhibition of low-density lipoprotein oxidation by high-density lipoprotein. *Atherosclerosis* **1997**, *135*, 193–204. [CrossRef]
174. Aviram, M.; Billecke, S.; Sorenson, R.; Bisgaier, C.; Newton, R.; Rosenblat, M.; Erogul, J.; Hsu, C.; Dunlop, C.; La Du, B. Paraoxonase active site required for protection against LDL oxidation involves its free sulfhydryl group and is different from that required for its arylesterase/paraoxonase activities: Selective action of human paraoxonase allozymes Q and R. *Arterioscler. Thromb. Vasc. Biol.* **1998**, *18*, 1617–1624. [CrossRef] [PubMed]
175. Wheeler, J.G.; Keavney, B.D.; Watkins, H.; Collins, R.; Danesh, J. Four paraoxonase gene polymorphisms in 11212 cases of coronary heart disease and 12786 controls: Meta-analysis of 43 studies. *Lancet* **2004**, *363*, 689–695. [CrossRef] [PubMed]
176. Ross, R.S. A parlous state of storm and stress. The life and times of James B. Herrick. *Circulation* **1983**, *67*, 955–959. [CrossRef]
177. Perła-Kaján, J.; Borowczyk, K.; Głowacki, R.; Nygård, O.; Jakubowski, H. Paraoxonase 1 Q192R genotype and activity affect homocysteine thiolactone levels in humans. *FASEB J.* **2018**, *32*, 6019–6024. [CrossRef] [PubMed]

antioxidants

MDPI

Review

The Molecular Bases of Anti-Oxidative and Anti-Inflammatory Properties of Paraoxonase 1

Hieronim Jakubowski [1,2]

[1] Department of Biochemistry and Biotechnology, University of Life Sciences, 60-637 Poznań, Poland; jakubows@rutgers.edu; Tel.: +1-973-972-8733; Fax: 973-972-8981
[2] Department of Microbiology, Biochemistry and Molecular Genetics, International Center for Public Health, New Jersey Medical School, Rutgers University, Newark, NJ 07103, USA

Abstract: The anti-oxidative and anti-inflammatory properties of high-density lipoprotein (HDL) are thought to be mediated by paraoxonase 1 (PON1), a calcium-dependent hydrolytic enzyme carried on a subfraction of HDL that also carries other anti-oxidative and anti-inflammatory proteins. In humans and mice, low PON1 activity is associated with elevated oxidized lipids and homocysteine (Hcy)-thiolactone, as well as proteins that are modified by these metabolites, which can cause oxidative stress and inflammation. PON1-dependent metabolic changes can lead to atherothrombotic cardiovascular disease, Alzheimer's disease, and cancer. The molecular bases underlying these associations are not fully understood. Biochemical, proteomic, and metabolic studies have significantly expanded our understanding of the mechanisms by which low PON1 leads to disease and high PON1 is protective. The studies discussed in this review highlight the changes in gene expression affecting proteostasis as a cause of the pro-oxidative and pro-inflammatory phenotypes associated with attenuated PON1 activity. Accumulating evidence supports the conclusion that PON1 regulates the expression of anti-oxidative and anti-inflammatory proteins, and that the disruption of these processes leads to disease.

Keywords: PON1 physiological substrates; homocysteine thiolactone; 5-(3′,4′-dihydroxyphenyl)-γ-valerolactone; PON1 proteomics; anti-oxidant proteins; anti-inflammatory proteins; cardiovascular disease; Alzheimer's disease; cancer

1. Introduction

Atherosclerosis is the main cause of morbidity and mortality in the Western world. It is a multifactorial chronic inflammatory disease that involves a complex interaction of circulating cells and blood factors with the blood vessels. The disease starts with endothelial dysfunction, which leads to accumulation of oxidized lipids in the artery wall [1,2]. Lipid oxidation plays a central role in atherogenesis [3] by inducing a pro-inflammatory phenotype in the arterial wall that underlies the development and progression of atherosclerosis [4].

High-density lipoprotein (HDL) is an established protective factor against atherosclerosis due to its ability to mediate reverse cholesterol transport as well as anti-oxidative, anti-inflammatory, and endothelial protective functions [4–6]. HDL can inhibit endothelial cell adhesion molecules, such as the vascular cell adhesion molecule 1 (VCAM-1), the intercellular adhesion molecule-1 (ICAM-1), and E-selectin, that enable monocytes to bind at the sites of developing atherosclerosis [7]. HDL can remove peroxidized lipids from LDL and, subsequently, reduce them in a reaction with methionine residues of apolipoprotein A1 (APOA1) [8]. Lipid-free APOA1 can also remove lipid peroxide molecules from low density lipoprotein (LDL) [9]. Reconstituted HDL containing only APOA1 and phospholipids inhibits LDL oxidation like the native HDL3b and HDL3c particles do [8]. Other HDL-associated lipoproteins and enzymes, including paraoxonase 1 (PON1), have also been implicated in HDL's anti-oxidative, anti-inflammatory, and endothelial protective functions [10,11].

PON1, a hydrolytic enzyme that requires calcium for activity, is expressed in the liver, kidney, colon [12], and brain [13–15], and circulates attached to HDL in the blood. It is a minor HDL protein with potential clinical significance. Proteomic studies revealed that HDL particles carrying PON1 are enriched in several other important proteins such as A2M, ALB, CLU, IGHG1, IGLC2, PROS1, and TF [16].

Studies over the last decade have significantly expanded our knowledge regarding the natural substrates of PON1 and their role in human disease. Other studies have shown that the protective function of PON1 in human health is due to the ability of PON1 to affect the expression of genes involved in anti-oxidative and anti-inflammatory processes. These studies are discussed in the present review, highlighting the involvement of reduced PON1 expression/activity in the pro-oxidative, pro-atherogenic, pro-amyloidogenic, and pro-cancerogenic phenotypes.

2. Hydrolytic Activities of the PON1 Enzyme

The *PON1* gene is located on the long arm of chromosome 3 in the *PON* cluster together with *PON2* and *PON3* genes. Its polymorphic variants include *PON1-Q192R* [17], which involves the glutamine (Q) to arginine (R) change at position 192 of the amino acid sequence of the PON1 protein and affects its hydrolytic activity. Historically, the hydrolytic activity of PON1 has been assayed with non-natural substrates such as the organophosphate paraoxon (for which the PON1 enzyme has been named) and phenyl acetate [18] (Figure 1).

Studies of homocysteine (Hcy) metabolism have led to the discovery that PON1 is responsible for the enzymatic hydrolysis of Hcy-thiolactone to Hcy (Figure 1) in human serum, thus identifying the first natural substrate of PON1 [19]. Hcy-thiolactone, a cyclic chemically reactive thioester, is a product of Hcy editing by methionyl-tRNA synthetase during protein biosynthesis [20–22].

PON1 is the only Hcy-thiolactone hydrolyzing enzyme in the human blood [19,23]. The Hcy-thiolactonase activity of the PON1 enzyme shows an interindividual variability of over 10-fold [24,25], similar to the interindividual variability in the paraoxonase activity [17]. This variability is mostly due to polymorphisms in the human *PON1* gene [17]. For example, the *PON1-192RR* variant exhibits high activity while *PON1-192QQ* variant has low activity towards Hcy-thiolactone [23] and paraoxon [17]. In contrast, the *PON1-Q192R* polymorphism has an opposite effect on the arylesterase activity: The *PON1-192RR* variant exhibits low arylesterase activity while the PON1-192QQ variant has high arylesterase activity [16,26–29]. Individuals who have the low-activity *PON1-192QQ* polymorphic variant produce significantly more Hcy-thiolactone than those who have the high-activity *PON1-192RR* polymorphic variant [26].

Low PON1 expression/activity is accompanied by increased oxidative stress and predicts adverse outcomes in cardiovascular disease (CVD) [28,30], diabetes [31,32], neurological disease [33], and cancer [34]. This has been suggested to be due to the mediation by PON1 of anti-oxidative and anti-inflammatory effects of HDL [35,36]. Many other HDL components have also been shown to mediate the anti-oxidative activity of HDL [10,11,37], including APOA1, which accounts for 70% of the HDL protein mass [37] and anti-apoptotic activity [38] and most of the HDL anti-oxidative activity [8]. Accumulating evidence suggests that influence of PON1 on oxidative stress and inflammation is indirect rather than direct [39].

Hcy-thiolactone is harmful because it reacts with the ε-amino group of protein lysine residues, forming *N*-homocysteinylated-proteins, which impairs protein's structure and function [22]. Hydrolytic detoxification of Hcy-thiolactone by PON1 is beneficial because it prevents protein damage by *N*-homocysteinylation [19,24,40]. For example, serum from donors with the *PON1-LL55/RR192* genotype hydrolyzed Hcy-thiolactone (Figure 2A) to Hcy (Figure 2B) faster and afforded better protection from protein *N*-

homocysteinylation than serum from donors with the *PON1-MM55/QQ192* genotype (Figure 2C). Notably, PON1 in rabbit serum hydrolyzed Hcy-thiolactone (Figure 2A) even faster and afforded much better protection from protein *N*-homocysteinylation than any human serum (Figure 2C).

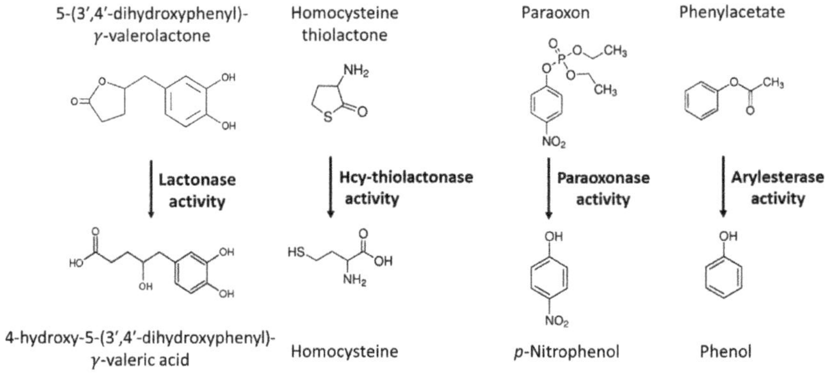

Figure 1. Hydrolytic activities of the PON1 enzyme. Hcy-thiolactone [19,23–25] and 5-(3′,4′-dihydroxyphenyl)-γ-valerolactone [41] are biological substrates of PON1; paraoxon and phenylacetate are nonbiological substrates of PON1 [17,18].

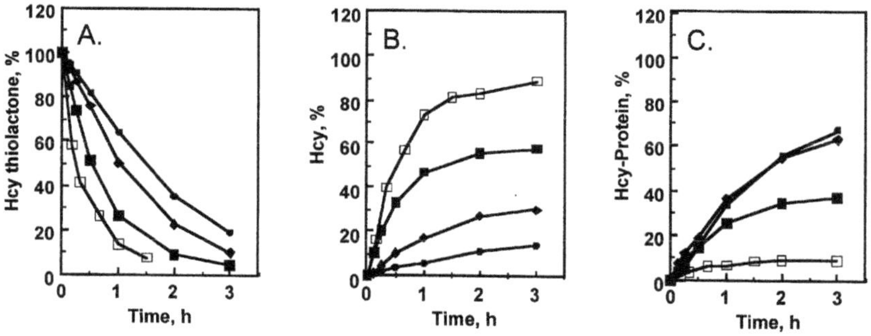

Figure 2. Turnover of Hcy-thiolactone and accumulation of *N*-Hcy-protein in serum at 37 °C. Changes in Hcy thiolactone (3.5 μM at time zero) (**A**), Hcy (**B**), and *N*-Hcy-protein (**C**) levels in human serum from individuals with *PON1-LL55/RR192* genotype (■, $t_{1/2}$ = 0.5 h), *PON1-MM55/QQ192* genotype (♦, $t_{1/2}$ = 1 h), human serum with the PON1 enzyme inactivated by 5 mM EDTA/2 mM D-penicillamine (•, 1.5 h), and rabbit serum (□, 0.25 h). Reproduced with permission from ref. [24]. Copyright 2001 by John Wiley and Sons.

In a large randomized clinical trial, urinary Hcy-thiolactone was associated with myocardial infarction in coronary artery disease patients [42]. In a mouse and cellular models of Alzheimer's disease (AD), Hcy-thiolactone promoted the accumulation of amyloid beta (Aβ) by inhibiting autophagy [15]. Hcy-thiolactone can promote the progression to AD by upregulating amyloid precursor protein (APP), which results in increased generation of Aβ [15].

The involvement of Hcy-thiolactone in disease can also be explained by its ability to impair protein structure/function via the *N*-homocystinylation of protein lysine residues [22]. For example, the *N*-homocysteinylation of fibrinogen by Hcy-thiolactone, which impairs the lysis of fibrin clots in vitro [43], explains the association of Hcy-thiolactone with the impaired lysis of fibrin clots in vivo in humans (manifested by a longer time of fibrinolysis), as we have recently shown in a large randomized controlled trial [44].

Enzymological studies in vitro led to a contention that the lactonase activity is a native physiological activity of PON1, but no physiological evidence was provided [45,46]. Other studies repeated this contention by stating that the lactonase activity is "the established native physiological activity of PONs" [47] even though no physiological evidence supporting such statement has been reported either. A study that attempted to identify endogenous lipophilic lactones as possible in vivo substrates for PON1 in human serum, found none [48]. The possible involvement of PON1 in metabolism of endogenous lipophilic lactones in vivo as proposed in refs. [45,46] remains to be proven.

Nevertheless, recent findings showed that some phenyl-γ-valerolactones (PVLs), phase 2 metabolites derived from dietary flavan-3-ols, are substrates for PON1 and PON3 in vivo [41]. Flavan-3-ols constitute the main class of polyphenolic bioactive compounds present in the food and beverages such as tea, pome fruits, cocoa products, and berries. Large-scale randomized clinical trials show that flavan-3-ol intake was associated with beneficial cardiovascular effects [49] but had no effect on cognition [50]. After intake, flavan-3-ols are catabolized by gut microbiota to PVLs and phenyl-γ-valeric acids (PVAs), which enter the circulation and are distributed throughout the human body [51]. After the intraperitoneal administration of 5-(3′,4′-dihydroxyphenyl)-γ-valerolactone (γVL), the sulfated form of γVL was detected in the brain, while γVL aglycon was not detected [52]. In TNF-α stimulated human brain primary microvascular endothelial cells, 5-(4′-hydroxyphenyl)-γ-valerolactone-3′-sulfate and 5-(4′-hydroxyphenyl)-γ-valerolactone-3′-*O*-glucuronide were biologically active at low nanomolar concentrations and influenced the expression of genes involved in biological pathways such as cell adhesion, cytoskeleton organization, focal adhesion, signaling pathways, pathways regulating endothelial permeability, and interaction with immune cells [53]. However, it is not known whether corresponding PVAs (i.e., products of PVLs hydrolysis by PON1) can also influence gene expression.

In human serum, γVL was rapidly hydrolyzed to the corresponding γ-substituted valeric acid (γVA) by PON1 and PON3 ($t_{1/2}$ = 9.8 min) (Figure 3B) [41]. The hydrolysis was prevented by treatments with EGTA (calcium chelator and an inhibitor of PON1) or with heat (Figure 3A). Km was 269 μM (Figure 3C), way above sub-micromolar γVL concentrations in humans [50]. Some, but not all, phase 2 metabolites (sulfated or glucuronidated γVL) were also hydrolyzed by PON1/PON3 in serum. In general, conjugated γVLs were worse substrates of PON than unconjugated γVL. Additional conjugations of γVL significantly reduced or prevented the hydrolysis of γVL metabolites by PON. Another polyphenol-derived lactone, enterolactone, was not a substrate [41].

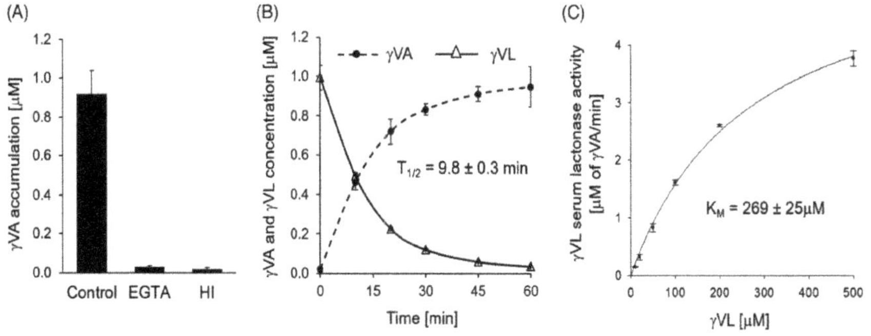

Figure 3. Turnover of 5-(3′,4′-dihydroxyphenyl)-γ-valerolactone (γVL) and accumulation of 5-(3′,4′-dihydroxyphenyl)-γ-valeric acid (γVA) in human serum at 37 °C. (**A**) Accumulation of γVA in control serum supplemented with 1 μM γVL after 1 h, serum + 5 mM EGTA, and heat-inactivated serum (57 °C, 30 min; HI). Data represent mean ± standard deviation (*n* = 6). (**B**) Kinetics of γVL disappearance and γVA generation in serum. (**C**) Serum γVL-hydrolyzing activity as a function of γVL concentration. Data represent mean ± standard deviation (*n* = 4 per time point or concentration). Reproduced from ref. [41].

In contrast to the established influence of the PON1 genotype on the hydrolysis of Hcy-thiolactone [23,39], the EPIC-Norfolk sub-cohort study found that the sum of urinary conjugated γVLs was not influenced by the *PON1* genotype (*Q192R*, rs662 in the coding region; −162A/G rs705381 in the promoter region) in males but there was a small effect in females [47]. These findings suggest that the *PON1* genotype has a minor sex-dependent effect on the hydrolysis of conjugated γVLs; this, however, remains to be examined in future studies.

3. Association of PON1 with Human Disease

PON1 has been studied in the fields of toxicology, CVD, renal disease, liver disease, Alzheimer's disease, and cancer. Initial studies have shown that $Pon1^{-/-}$ mice are highly susceptible to the toxicity of organophosphate insecticides [54] and to atherosclerosis induced by the metabolic stress of a high-fat diet [55], or by *ApoE* depletion [56]. The molecular basis of PON1's protective role in organophosphate poisoning is well understood [54]. In contrast, the nature of PON1 targets in atherosclerosis and other human diseases is not fully understood. Elevated oxidative stress and inflammation, associated with CVD [5], are also observed in Pon1-deficient mice [55,56] and humans with attenuated PON1 activity [28].

Reduced PON1 activity accompanied by increased oxidative stress and inflammation is a common finding in patients with CVD [28,30,57,58], diseases of the kidney [31,32] and liver [59], Alzheimer's disease [33,60,61], and cancer [34,62] (Table 1). This has been suggested to be due to the mediation by PON1 of anti-oxidative and anti-inflammatory effects of HDL [35,36]. Many other HDL components have also been shown to mediate the anti-oxidative and anti-inflammatory activity of HDL [10,11,37], including APOA1, which accounts for 70% of HDL protein mass [37] and anti-apoptotic activity [38], and for most of the HDL anti-oxidative activity [8]. Although how attenuated PON1 expression or activity can induce oxidative stress and inflammation is not clear, accumulating evidence, discussed below, suggests that the influence of PON1 on oxidative stress and inflammation is indirect rather than direct [39].

Table 1. Association of PON1 with oxidative stress, inflammation, and human disease *.

Disease	PON1 Activity	*PON1* Genotype	Oxidative Stress	Inflammation	References
Cardiovascular disease	↓	*PON1-192QQ*	↑	↑	[28,30,57,58]
Kidney disease	↓	ND	ND	↑	[31,32]
Fatty liver disease	↓	ND	↑	↑	[59]
Alzheimer's disease	↓	*PON1-107TT*	↑	ND	[33,60,61,63]
Hepatocellular carcinoma	↓	ND	↑	↑	[34,62]

* ND, not determined. Up and down arrows indicate the direction of change.

3.1. PON1, Oxidative Stress, Inflammation, and CVD

In $Pon1^{-/-}$ mice fed with a high-fat diet, the enhancement of atherosclerosis is accompanied by the upregulation of oxidative stress, which is manifested by elevated levels of lipid peroxides in purified HDL [55]. In $Pon1^{-/-}ApoE^{-/-}$ mice, elevated oxidized phospholipid epitopes in plasma, bioactive oxidized phospholipids in purified endogenous intermediate density lipoprotein/LDL, and the upregulated expression of oxidative stress-responsive genes such as heme oxygenase-1 (HO1), peroxisome proliferator-activated receptor gamma (PPARγ), and oxLDL receptor (oxLDL-R) in the liver were observed [56]. Although no lipid hydroperoxides were found in fresh purified LDL from any Pon1 genotype, the LDL from $Pon1^{-/-}$ mice nevertheless stimulated lipid hydroperoxide generation and monocyte transmigration better than did the LDL from $Pon1^{+/+}$ mice in a coculture model. These results suggested that the LDL from *Pon1*$^{-/-}$ mice was changed somehow to become prone to oxidation. Lipid hydroperoxide formation in LDL was inhibited by the pretreatment with purified human PON1 [55].

The overexpression in mice of human PON1 using bacterial artificial chromosome genomic clones increased plasma PON1 levels 2- to 4-fold and significantly reduced aortic lesions in dietary as well as *ApoE*$^{-/-}$ models [64]. The overexpression of human PON1 in a *LDL*$^{-/-}$ mouse model of metabolic syndrome via adenovirus-mediated PON1 gene transfer increased the paraoxonase activity of PON1 4.4-fold and significantly reduced the plaque-associated oxLDL, titer of auto-antibodies against LDL modified by malondialdehyde (MDA) (a proxy for oxLDL), and plaque volume by 80% [65]. Unfortunately, how Pon1 overexpression influences the expression of genes involved in inflammation and oxidative stress has not been studied in these two mouse models.

The overexpression of the human PON gene cluster (PC Tg) in *ApoE*$^{-/-}$ mice using bacterial artificial chromosome increased the enzymatic activity towards the paraoxon substrate in isolated HDL by 60%, stabilized atherosclerotic lesions, and significantly attenuated (by 20–30%) plaque area [66]. PC Tg HDL significantly inhibited oxLDL production (by 40–67%) compared to wild-type HDL. The inflammation markers ICAM-1 and MCP-1 were significantly downregulated (by 31–51%) in PC Tg/*ApoE*$^{-/-}$ mice compared to *ApoE*$^{-/-}$ mice. The inflammatory response of isolated PC Tg macrophages (due to human PON2 overexpression) was significantly attenuated compared to macrophages isolated from *ApoE*$^{-/-}$ mice, as shown by the quantification of TNF-α and IL-6. Human PON2 inhibited also macrophage MMP-9 expression and foam cell formation from PC Tg macrophages compared to macrophages from *ApoE*$^{-/-}$ mice [66]. These findings show that PON gene cluster overexpression protects from atherosclerosis by ameliorating oxidative stress and downregulating the expression of genes involved in inflammation.

The first large-scale prospective study that evaluated the relationship between oxidative stress and the PON1 genotype, and their activity and prognostic value as predictors of future CVD, involved 1339 patients (65 years old, 72% male) and 283 controls without CVD (57 years old, 48% male) who underwent coronary angiography [28]. The study found, at baseline, that the low paraoxonase or arylesterase activity of PON1 as well as the *PON1-192QQ* polymorphic variant were associated with elevated various oxidized fatty acids (5-, 8-, 9-, 11-, 12-, 15-hydroxyeicosatetraenoic acids (HETEs), 9-, 13-hydroxyoctadecadienoic acids (HODEs), 8-isoprostane prostaglandin $F_{2\alpha}$ (8-isoPGF$_{2\alpha}$)) in patients ($n = 150$) (Table 1). Participants carrying *PON1-192QQ* alleles had a significantly increased risk of adverse CVD outcomes such as death, myocardial infarction (MI), and stroke, compared with *PON1-192RR* and *PON1-192QR* carriers over a 3-year-followup (18.0% vs. 13.6%, adjusted hazard ratio 1.48, $p = 0.01$) and all-cause mortality (11.1% vs. 6.75%, adjusted hazard ratio 2.05, $p = 0.001$). Although the *PON1-192QQ* genotype was not associated with nonfatal stroke or MI, the low activity of PON1predicated an increased frequency of stroke and MI, all-cause mortality, and the sum of adverse CVD outcomes. Specifically, participants with the lowest paraoxonase or arylesterase activity of PON1 (1st quartile) showed an increased frequency of adverse CVD outcomes (paraoxonase: 25.1%; arylesterase 23.5%) compared to participants with the highest activities of PON1 (4th quartile) (7.3% or 7.7%, respectively). The adjusted hazard ratios for nonfatal MI and stroke, all-cause mortality, and the sum of in the lowest vs. highest PON1 activity quartiles were 4.4, 2.4, and 3.4, respectively, for paraoxonase and 4.5, 2.2, and 2.9 for arylesterase, respectively, they were independent in multivariate analysis in models (separate for paraoxonase and arylesterase) adjusted for all traditional cardiac risk factors and medications). These findings demonstrate that the PON1 genotype/activity affects oxidative stress and predicts future CVD risk.

However, it should be noted that the *PON1-Q192R* polymorphism, associated with indices of oxidative stress in vivo [28], has opposite effects on the paraoxonase and arylesterase activities of PON1: The *192Q* allele associates with low paraoxonase and high arylesterase activity, while the *192R* allele associates with high paraoxonase and low arylesterase activities [23,26,29,67]. In this context, it is not clear why the low paraoxonase and arylesterase activities of PON1 were associated with nonfatal stroke and MI, but the *PON1-192QQ* genotype was not [28].

A population-based cross-sectional study of 1,895 participants (32-year-old, 46% male) examined a relationship between rs669 SNP (*PON1-Q192R*), PON1 activity, and conjugated dienes in lipoprotein lipids [68] as a measure of oxLDL lipids [69] that is known to correlate with lipid hydroperoxides and MDA [70]. In multiple regression models, the paraoxonase activity of PON1was inversely correlated with oxLDL lipids ($p = 0.0001$) but not with oxHDL lipids, and tended to be associated with oxLDL protein ($p = 0.08$). A stronger association between PON1 activity and oxLDL lipids was seen in the *PON1-192RR* carriers than in the *PON1-192QQ* carriers. Although *PON1 rs662* SNP was strongly associated with paraoxonase activity of PON1, it was not associated with oxHDL lipids or protein.

A case-control study found that CAD patients confirmed by angiography ($n = 105$) had significantly increased plasma 8-isoprostane F2 (8-iso-PGF2α, produced by the non-enzymatic peroxidation of arachidonic acid in membrane phospholipids) and reduced paraoxonase and arylesterase activities of PON1 compared to healthy controls ($n = 45$) [58]. Paraoxonase and arylesterase activities of PON1 were significantly negatively associated with the severity of CAD (Gensini score) in univariate analyses, while 8-iso-PGF2α was associated positively. Such associations were also seen in multiple regression models adjusted for traditional risk factors. These findings suggest that PON1 may protect phospholipids from oxidation [58]. However, the mechanism underlying these findings remains to be elucidated.

One study examined how *PON1* SNPs and PON1 arylesterase activity are related to the oxidation susceptibility of LDL isolated from male CAD patients and healthy control participants [71]. The susceptibility of LDL to oxidation was measured using an assay, in which LDL is oxidized by copper and the resulting conjugated dienes are monitored by absorbance at 234 nm. During LDL preparation from each participant, HDL/PON1 was removed. The study involved CAD patients ($n = 205$, 70-year-old, >80% stenosis) and control participants ($n = 232$, 66 years old, <15% stenosis). It was found that the susceptibility of LDL to oxidation was not correlated with arylesterase activity of PON1, although it was correlated with CAD. In contrast, PON1 promoter SNP, *PON1 -108C/T*, which affects PON1 expression, and other *PON1* SNPs, were associated with the susceptibility of LDL to copper induced. The absence of congruency in the relationships between the susceptibility of LDL to oxidation and CAD, PON1 arylesterase activity, and *PON1 -108C/T* SNP raises doubts regarding validity of the experimental approach used in this study.

3.2. PON1, Lipid Oxidation, Hcy-Thiolactone, and Alzheimer's Disease

OxLDL lipids increase β-amyloid production by SH-SY5Y cells [72]. Importantly, amyloid beta binds to oxLDL and accelerates the formation of macrophage foam cells [73], suggesting that oxLDL can directly participate in the development of AD.

PON1 plays an important role in the detoxification of neurotoxins including organophosphate pesticides, potent inhibitors of acetylcholinesterase; people with low PON1 activity show increased sensitivity to neurotoxins while those with high PON1 activity are less susceptible [55]. Notably, exposure to organophosphates increases the risk of developing AD [74,75]. Treatments with doses of chlorpyrifos oxone that do not affect wild-type *Pon1*$^{+/+}$ mice are known to induce seizures and death in *Pon1* knockout mice [55]. Importantly, Pon1 is also known to detoxify Hcy-thiolactone in mice. For example, treatments with Hcy-thiolactone induce seizures significantly faster (Figure 4A) and with increased incidence (Figure 4B) in *Pon1*$^{-/-}$ mice compared to wild type *Pon1*$^{+/+}$ mice. Death incidence was also higher in *Pon1*$^{-/-}$ mice (Figure 4C) [40].

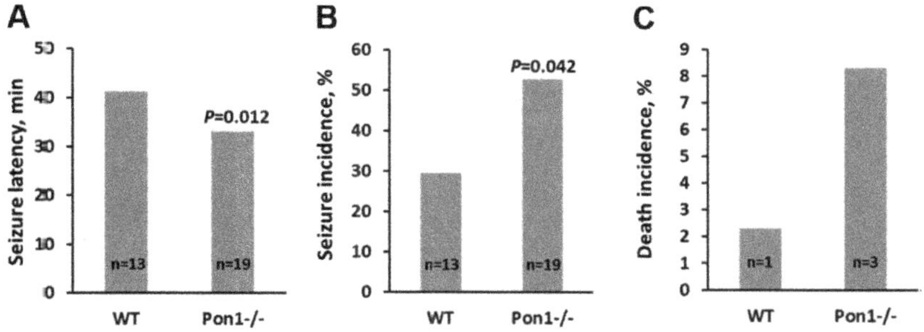

Figure 4. Latency (**A**), incidence of seizures (**B**), and death (**C**) in *L*-Hcy-thiolactone-injected (intraperitoneally, 3.7 µmol/g body weight) $Pon1^{-/-}$ mice (n = 19) and their $Pon1^{+/+}$ siblings (WT, n = 13) monitored for 90 min after injection. The figure was drawn based on data from Borowczyk et al. [40].

3.2.1. Mice

Proteomic analyzes of $Pon1^{-/-}$ and $Pon1^{+/+}$ mice have shown that Pon1 plays an important role in maintaining cellular proteostasis [60], in addition to controlling Hcy-thiolactone and *N*-Hcy-protein levels [40]. *Pon1* gene deletion affects the expression of cellular proteins in an organ-specific way, with the patterns of expression modulated by hyperhomocysteinemia (HHcy). In the brains of $Pon1^{-/-}$ mice, proteins involved in anti-oxidant defenses (Sod1, DJ-1), brain-specific function (Nrgn), and the assembly of cytoskeleton (Tbcb) were significantly downregulated, while the CapZa2 protein involved in the assembly of cytoskeleton was significantly upregulated compared to wild-type $Pon1^{+/+}$ mouse brain [60].

In the brains of HHcy $Pon1^{-/-}$ mice that were fed with high methionine diet, Prdx2 and DJ-1proteins participating in anti-oxidant defense; Ncald, Nrgn, and Stmn1 proteins involved in brain-specific function; energy metabolism protein Ak1; cell cycle GDI1 and Ran proteins; cytoskeleton assembly Tbcb protein; and Hdhd2 protein of unknown function were all upregulated (Table 2). Notably, *Pon1* gene deletion affected the expression of DJ-1 (Park7), Sod1, and Prdx2 proteins involved in the oxidative stress response that are also known to be associated with AD [60].

Table 2. Brain proteins affected by *Pon1* depletion and/or HHcy in mice are also affected in AD and other neuropathies.

Protein Name	Change in $Pon1^{-/-}$ vs. $Pon1^{+/+}$ Brain *		Change in Human AD Brain (Another Neuropathy or Animal Model) **
	Std. Diet	1%-Met Diet	
	Brain-specific		
Ncald	–	↑	↓, (↓ $Gls^{-/-}$ mouse)
Nrgn	↓	↑	↓
Stmn1	–	↑	↓, (↑ MS, TLE, SMA, schizophrenia), (↑ HD4 mouse model)
	Anti-oxidant defense		
Sod1	↓	–	(↑ ALS)
Prdx2	–	↑	↑
DJ-1 (Park7)	↓	↑	↑

Table 2. *Cont.*

Protein Name	Change in $Pon1^{-/-}$ vs. $Pon1^{+/+}$ Brain *		Change in Human AD Brain (Another Neuropathy or Animal Model) **
	Std. Diet	**1%-Met Diet**	
	Energy metabolism		
Ak1	–	↑	↑
	Cell cycle		
GDI1	–	↑	(↑ rat ischemic brain)
Ran	–	↑	↑
	Cytoskeleton assembly		
Tbcb	↓	↑	(↑ GAN)
CapZa2	↑	–	↑ CapZb2 #
	Other proteins		
Hdhd2	–	↑	

* The up '↑' and down '↓' arrows indicate up-regulated and down-regulated proteins, respectively. No significant change is indicated by dash '–'. ** AD, Alzheimer's disease; MS, multiple sclerosis; HD, Huntington disease; GAN, giant axon neuropathy; TLE, temporal lobe epilepsy; SMA, spinal muscular atrophy. # The b2 subunit of the CapZ heterodimer. Adapted from ref. [60].

Clusterin (CLU or APOJ), involved in the transport of amyloid beta (Aβ) from plasma to the brain in humans (reviewed in [76]), is carried on a minor HDL subspecies that contains two other proteins: APOA1 and PON1 [77]. Importantly, Clu (ApoJ) levels are significantly elevated in the plasma of $Pon1^{-/-}$ mice compared to wild-type $Pon1^{+/+}$ animals [23].

PON1 involvement in AD was examined using $Pon1^{-/-}$5xFAD mice and in Aβ-overexpressing mouse neuroblastoma N2a-APP_{swe} cells [15]. 5xFAD mice overexpress the K670N/M671L (Swedish), I716V (Florida), and V717I (London) mutations in human APP (695) and the M146L and L286V mutations in human PS1 and start to accumulate high levels of Aβ42 at about 2 months old [78]. The dysregulation of mTOR signaling and autophagy are linked to Aβ accumulation in AD patients [79,80], while histone H4K20me1 demethylation by the histone demethylase PHF8 maintains the homeostasis of mTOR signaling [81].

The study revealed that Pon1 plays an important role in protecting from the amyloidogenic processing of APP to Aβ in brains of mice and identified mechanism of this new function of Pon1 in the central nervous system (Figure 5). Specifically, Pon1 depletion in $Pon1^{-/-}$5xFAD mice significantly downregulated Phf8 and upregulated the methylated histone H4K20me1 mark. This led to the upregulation of mTOR expression and increased its active form, phospho-mTOR, which impaired autophagy by downregulating Bcln1, Atg5, and Atg7 proteins in $Pon1^{-/-}$5xFAD mouse brains compared to $Pon1^{+/+}$5xFAD brains. Silencing of the *Pon1* gene in N2a-APP_{swe} cells by RNA interference using the siRNA targeting *Pon1* gene led to Phf8 downregulation, which increased histone H4K20me1 binding at the *mTOR* promoter, thereby upregulating mTOR expression and signaling. Upregulated mTOR signaling impaired autophagy and significantly elevated APP expression and Aβ levels. Hcy-thiolactone or *N*-Hcy-protein (metabolites known to accumulated $Pon1^{-/-}$ mice), or Phf8 depletion by RNA interference, elevated Aβ levels in N2a-APP_{swe} cells [15]. Notably, *Phf8* gene silencing did not influence the expression of APP, indicating that Aβ levels increased independently of APP [82].

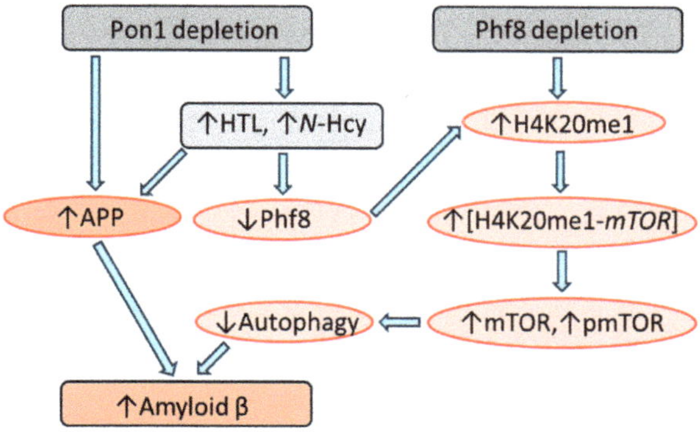

Figure 5. Proposed mechanism of Aβ generation in *Pon1*$^{-/-}$5xFAD mice. Pon1, paraoxonase 1; Hcy, homocysteine; HTL, Hcy-thiolactone; APP, amyloid β precursor protein; mTOR, mammalian target of rapamycin; pmTOR, phospho-mTOR; Phf8, plant homeodomain finger protein 8. [H4K20me1-*mTOR*] represents H4K20me1 bound at the *mTOR* promoter. The thick arrows indicate the influence of the change in one process/protein/metabolite on another. The thin up and down arrows indicate the direction of change. Reprinted from ref. [83].

Pon1 depletion induced changes in the Phf8->H4K20me1->mTOR->autophagy pathway (Figure 5) that were similar to the changes induced by HHcy [15], suggesting that the same Hcy metabolites were involved. This suggestion is supported by our previous findings showing that a common primary physiological outcome of Pon1 depletion and of HHcy was essentially the same: Pon1 depletion [40,84] and HHcy [85] each increased Hcy-thiolactone and *N*-Hcy-protein levels. Taken together, our findings show that Aβ generation in the *Pon1*$^{-/-}$ brain is mediated by the influence of Hcy-related metabolites on mTOR signaling/autophagy [15]. These findings provide a mechanistic explanation for the link between attenuated PON1 activity [36] or elevated Hcy [86] and AD.

3.2.2. Humans

A few studies have examined PON1 activity in relation to oxidative stress in AD patients. In one study, PON1 activities were found to be significantly decreased (Table 1) while PAF-AH activity and oxLDL levels were significantly increased in 49 AD patients (74 years old, 59% female, MMSE score = 21 ± 5) compared to 34 age/sex-matched control individuals [63]. The study found a significant inverse correlation of oxLDL with PON1 activities (but not with activity of PAF-AH) in AD patients and non-AD control individuals. Further, the activities of PON1 and levels of oxLDL were associated with the severity of AD (assessed by using the MMSE test, which quantifies global cognition). Patients with moderate (MMSE score of 11 to 24) and severe (MMSE score < 10) AD had significantly decreased activities of PON1 and increased oxLDL levels compared to patients with mild AD (MMSE score > 24). Even though PAF and oxidized phospholipids hydrolysis by PAF-AH generates free oxidized fatty acids, which have potent biological activity, PAF-AH activity was not correlated with the oxLDL nor with the severity of AD. Although these findings suggest that PON1 may participate in oxLDL metabolism in AD, the nature of this participation is not clear.

Another study evaluated oxLDL in 54 late-onset AD patients (aged 77 years, 81% female, MMSE score = 18) and 51 healthy elderly individuals (aged 77 years, 73% male, MMSE score = 29) and a relationship between oxLDL and *PON1-107C/T* polymorphism and the *APOE* genotype [87]. Patients with AD and control individuals with the *PON1-107TT* genotype had significantly elevated levels of plasma oxLDL compared to those with the *PON1-107CC/CT* genotype. The distribution of lipoprotein cholesterol in patients with AD was shifted toward a greater prevalence of smaller, denser LDL. In AD patients, the smaller, denser LDL levels were significantly associated with the levels of oxLDL. Lipoprotein distribution was not influenced by *APOE* genotype. These findings suggest that plasma oxLDL levels could modulate the association of *PON1-107TT* polymorphism with AD [87].

A study that examined relationships among PON1, lipid peroxidation, and dementia with AD patients ($n = 63$), vascular dementia patients ($n = 40$), and mixed dementia patients ($n = 33$) found that MDA/thiobarbituric acid-reactive substances were elevated to a greater extent in vascular dementia than in AD [61]. In patients with vascular involvement, the increase in MDA/TBARS reflected the extent of global cortical atrophy. The arylesterase activity of PON1 was significantly attenuated in patients with dementia, more so in patients with severe cognitive deficits. In patients with vascular dementia, the low arylesterase activity of PON1 was associated with increased brain ischemia and medial temporal lobe atrophy. These findings show that the reduced activity of PON1 and increased levels of the MDA/TBARS oxidative stress marker are associated with brain atrophy and vascular dementia rather than with cognitive decline. However, it is not clear how reduced PON1 activity can lead to oxidative stress and impaired cognition.

3.3. PON1 Depletion, Dysregulation of Signaling Pathways, and Cancer

Hepatocellular carcinoma (HCC) is one of the most common neoplasms, the third leading cause of cancer death, and a leading cause of death among patients with cirrhosis [88]. Liver cirrhosis is widely prevalent worldwide and can be a consequence of different causes, such as obesity, non-alcoholic fatty liver disease, high alcohol consumption, hepatitis B or C infection, autoimmune diseases, cholestatic diseases, and iron or copper overload [59].

Recent studies show that PON1 activity and expression are compromised in HCC patients. Specifically, serum PON1 activity, measured with 4-nitrophenylacetate as a substrate, was significantly reduced in HCC patients [62]. Transcriptomic analysis showed that the expression of PON1was significantly downregulated in HCC tissues compared to normal tissues [34]. However, there was also a significant variation in PON1 expression between HCC patients. Patients with low PON1 expression manifested significant differences in pathology severity and tumor size and grade. Female HCC patients with low PON1 expression had a higher degree of tumor malignancy.

Differences in PON1 expression influenced the clinical manifestations, biological processes, immune infiltration, and expression of immune checkpoints in HCC, suggesting that PON1 plays an important role in modulating tumor progression and immune cell infiltration, thus establishing PON1 as a new biomarker important for prognosis, targeted therapy, and immunotherapy in HCC patients [34].

Bioinformatic analysis of pathway enrichment in the high and low PON1 mRNA expression groups showed that the *PON1* gene inhibits key signaling pathways, such as the PI3K/Akt/mTOR signaling, the cell cycle G2 checkpoint, the TGF-β signaling, and the Wnt/β-catenin signaling, which play a crucial role in pathogenesis and progression of HCC [34]. Interestingly, we found that Pon1 depletion upregulated mTOR signaling and inhibited autophagy via Pcft/H4K20me1 in mouse brain and neuroblastoma cells [15], suggesting that effects of Pon1 depletion on gene expression are disease/tissue-specific.

4. PON1 Has No Intrinsic Anti-Oxidant Activity: Don't Waste Clean Thoughts on Dirty Enzymes

PON1 has been stated to hydrolyze oxidized lipids and, thus, to promote athero-protective effects, e.g., refs. [28,89], which incorrectly implies that PON1 has an intrinsic anti-oxidant function. That PON1 has the ability to hydrolyze oxidized lipids was originally proposed by a study that reported the ability of purified native human PON1 to inhibit copper-induced oxidation of LDL in an in vitro assay that quantified lipo-peroxides and TBARS [90].

The availability of an assay for a biological event in a cell-free system usually facilitates studies of its molecular mechanism. Indeed, this assay has been used in many in vitro studies using purified native (e.g., refs. [91–94]) and recombinant [95,96] PON1 preparations. Unfortunately, these and other studies in the PON1 field did not follow the maxim "don't waste clean thoughts on dirty enzymes" attributed by Arthur Kornberg in his 'ten commandments of enzymology' [97] to Efraim Racker, a pioneer in the enzymology of oxidative phosphorylation [98].

Some labs did not replicate the finding that purified PON1 protects LDL from oxidation [46,99] while those that did [100–102] went on to correct themselves by showing, in more rigorous and well-controlled studies, that their earlier findings were due to PAF-AH contamination in PON1 preparations and that PAF-AH-free PON1 does not protect lipoproteins from oxidation nor hydrolyze oxidized lipids [46,103,104]. Rigorously purified PON1, or plasma from an individual with a mutation in the *PAF-AH* gene, did not hydrolyze PAF nor the oxidized phospholipids from oxLDL [99].

One study purported to show that purified PON1 was capable of hydrolyzing PAF. In that study [105], purified PON1 preparations were tested by Western blotting (20 μg) and amino acid sequencing (50 μg, or about 1 nmol PON1) and found not to have any detectable PAF-AH contamination. However, such evidence does not exclude PAF-AH contamination, considering that as little as 5 to 10 ng of PAF-AH (undetectable by Western blotting and not sufficient for sequencing) is sufficient to account for all the phospholipase activity in purified PON1 preparations [99]. In fact, other labs have shown that purified PON1 has no phospholipase A2-like activity toward PAF or pro-atherogenic oxidized phospholipids and that PAF-AH is the sole phospholipase A2 of HDL [99,103]. Rigorously purified PON1, or plasma from an individual with a mutation in the *PAF-AH* gene, did not hydrolyze PAF nor the oxidized phospholipids from oxLDL [99].

Although Aviram et al. [95] and Liu et al. [96] reported that PON1, PON2, and PON3 protect LDL from oxidative modification, Draganov et al. found no protection [46]. Re5combinant human PON1 was expressed from a baculovirus vector in insect cells and purified. When PON1 hydrolytic activity and a putative anti-oxidant activity were monitored during PON1 purification, the two activities did not co-purify at any stage and in any of the preparations. The putative anti-oxidant activity was shown to be associated with a low mass contaminant and the detergent used in PON1 purification [46]. That putative anti-oxidant activity in PON1 preparations was associated with the detergent present in these preparations was confirmed by another lab that also showed that anti-oxidant activity was not associated with hydrolytic PON1 activities such as arylesterase and lactonase, nor with phospholipase activity [103]. Unfortunately, it appears that many other laboratories did not seem bothered to control their PON1 preparations for contaminants.

Studies that examined the contribution of individual protein components to the ability of HDL to inhibit LDL oxidation showed that APOA1 is the major anti-oxidant protein in HDL [10]. APOA1 is also the major factor responsible for the protection of human endothelial cells from oxLDL-induced apoptosis, accounting for 70% of HDL antiapoptotic activity [37]. APOA1 is one of the two phosphatidylcholine peroxide-reducing enzymes isolated from human plasma (the other is glutathione peroxidase) [106]. APOA1 is essential for HDL structure and for activation of the HDL-associated enzymes PON1 and LCAT [107]. Two methionine residues in APOA1 (Met112, Met148) are oxidized to sulfoxides during the reduction of lipid peroxides to redox-inactive hydroxides [108,109]. Reconstituted HDL containing only purified APOA1 and phospholipids (palmitoyloleoyl phosphatidylcholine at a molar ratio of 1.0/77.1) has the capacity to inhibit LDL oxidation like that of native normolipidemic small, dense HDL3b and 3c isolated from normal human plasma. The oxidation of APOA1 Met residues in HDL3 incubated with oxLDL is accompanied by the concomitant reduction of lipid peroxides to lipid hydroxides [8].

To assess a role of HDL-associated enzymes, such as PON1, PAF-AH, and LCAT, in oxLDL inactivation, HDL3 was pretreated with inhibitors such as DFP, which inhibits the 3 enzymes, Pefabloc, which inhibits only PAF-AH, or EDTA, which inhibits only PON1, and then incubated with oxLDL. As expected, pretreatment significantly reduced the activities of LCAT (by 50%), PAF-AH (by 90%), and PON1 (by 99%). In contrast, the capacity of HDL3 to inactivate lipid peroxides in oxLDL or to delay LDL oxidation was not affected. None of the inhibitors impaired the capacity of HDL3 to delay the accumulation of conjugated dienes in LDL [8]. Two earlier studies have also reported that the inactivation of PON1 activity by EDTA did not affect the anti-oxidant activity of HDL3 [110] or PON1 preparations [93] in the copper-induced LDL oxidation assay. These findings do not support the contention that paraoxonase activity inhibits the formation of 'minimally oxidized' LDL by hydrolyzing biologically active oxidized phospholipids [9,91].

5. Mechanistic Bases of PON1 Involvement in Human Disease

The findings that PON1 is associated with oxidative stress and inflammation in humans and in mouse models (discussed in Section 2) but cannot be directly linked to these processes (discussed in Section 3), suggest that the influence of PON1 on oxidative stress and inflammation is indirect.

Studies of proteomic and transcriptomic changes in mice and humans in relation to changes in PON1 expression and activity (listed in Table 3 and discussed below) support this suggestion and provide insights into the biological function of PON1. Specifically, these studies suggest that vascular inflammation and oxidative stress that are associated with PON1 depletion are caused by the dysregulation of genes involved in these processes. The majority of studies discussed in this section are related to CVD, with two related to kidney disease and one to brain disease. Studies related to AD and cancer are discussed in Section 2.

Table 3. PON1 influences oxidative stress- and inflammation-related gene expression.

Model	Treatment	Gene Expression Assessment		Outcome		References
		Methods	Tissue	In Vivo	In Vitro	
Pon1$^{-/-}$ vs. *Pon1*$^{+/+}$mice, high fat diet	Pon1 deletion in WT mice	Enzymatic activity assay, Northern blot, RT-qPCR, Western blot	Liver, plasma	Pon1 protein absent in *Pon1*$^{-/-}$ mice, ↑lipid peroxides in HDL, no lipid peroxides in LDL, ↑atherosclerosis; no atherosclerosis in *Pon1*$^{-/-}$ mice on a chow diet	↑Lipid peroxides in hLDL, ↑MCP1, ↑monocyte migration ameliorated by *Pon1*$^{+/+}$ HDL in a cell co-culture model of the arterial wall; Pon1$^{-/-}$ HDL does not prevent hLDL oxidation	Shih D.M. et al. [55]
Pon1$^{-/-}$*ApoE*$^{-/-}$ vs. *Pon1*$^{+/+}$*ApoE*$^{-/-}$ mice, std chow diet	Pon1 deletion in *ApoE*$^{-/-}$ mice	Enzymatic activity assay, Northern blot, RT-qPCR	Liver, plasma	↑Lipid peroxides in LDL, ↑oxidized phospholipid epitopes in plasma; ↑HO1, PPARγ, ↑oxLDL receptors (SRA, CD36, macrosialin), but not HDL receptor SR-BI, in the liver; no change in anti-oxLDL and anti-MDA-LDL autoantibody levels; ↑atherosclerosis	LDL from *Pon1*$^{-/-}$ mice elevated lipid hydroperoxide and monocyte transmigration	Shih D.M. et al. [56]
Human *PON* cluster transgenic mice	*PON1*, *PON2*, *PON3* overexpression	Enzymatic activity assay, RT-qPCR, Western blot, ELISA		↑PON1 expression, ↓atherosclerosis ↓Icam-1, ↓Mcp-1, ↓TNF-α, ↓IL-6, ↓Mmp-9	PON Tg HDL ameliorated Cu-induced LDL oxidation	She Z.G. et al. [66]
Pon1$^{-/-}$ vs. *Pon1*$^{+/+}$mice, std chow diet	Pon1 deletion	2D-SDS-PAGE gel electrophoresis, MALDI-TOF mass spectrometry	Brain	↓Sod1, ↓DJ-1		[111] Brain
			Liver	↑Prdx2, ↑Ftl, ↑ApoE		[112] Liver
			Kidney	↑Prdx2, ↓ApoA1		[113] Kidney
		Enzymatic activity assay, label-free nanoLC-MS/MS mass spectrometry	Plasma	↓Alb, ↓Blvrb, ↑Ambp, ↑(Hpx, ↑ApoD, ↑ApoM, ↑Hp), ↑Ttr		Sikora M. et al. [23]

Table 3. *Cont.*

Model	Treatment	Gene Expression Assessment		Outcome		References
		Methods	Tissue	In Vivo	In Vitro	
Pon1$^{-/-}$ vs. *Pon1*$^{+/+}$mice, high methionine diet	Pon1 deletion	Enzymatic activity assay, label-free nanoLC-MS/MS mass spectrometry	Plasma	↓**Alb**, ↑Hp, ↑Hpx, ↓Alad, ↑Cp, ↓Gclm, ↓Cat, ↑Ctsb, ↓Gsn, ↑Grn, ↓Prdx2 ↓Prdx6, ↓Txn, ↓Igfbp3, ↓Park7, ↓Pebp1, ↓Ppia, ↓Serpina3k		Sikora M. et al. [114]
PON1-192QQ vs. *PON1-192RR+QR* humans	none	Enzymatic activity assay, label-free nanoLC-MS/MS mass spectrometry	Plasma	APOA1↓, PON1↓, APOD↑, APOM↑, HP↓, GPX3↑		Sikora M. et al. [23]
SR-BI$^{-/-}$ vs *SR-BI*$^{-/-}$ mice	*SR-BI* deletion, probucol treatment	Enzymatic activity assay, 2D-SDS-PAGE gel electrophoresis, LC-MS/MS mass spectrometry, Western blot, RT-qPCR	Plasma, HDL	↓HDL protein, ↓ApoA1, ↓Pon1 protein and activity, ↑Saa, ↑ApoA4, ↑A1AT, ↑Mpo Probucol upregulated Pon1, downregulated Saa, ApoA4, A1AT, and Mpo thereby improving HDL function	↑Mcp1, Tnf-α in oxLDL treated macrophages; *SR-BI*$^{+/+}$ HDL reduced Mcp1, Tnf-α while *SR-BI*$^{-/-}$ HDL had no effect	Cao J. et al. [115]
Pon1^{+}*SR-BI*$^{-/-}$ mice	Pon1 overexpression *SR-BI*$^{-/-}$ mice using lentivirus vector	Enzymatic activity assay, RT-qPCR, Western blot	Kidney	*Pon1*$^{+}$*SR-BI*$^{-/-}$ mice: ↓renal Pon1 expression and plasma activity, ↑ expression of redox (p47phox, Nox1, Nox4) and inflammation related (Il1b, Il6) genes, ↓anti-inflammatory cytokine Il10. *Pon1*$^{+}$*SR-BI*$^{-/-}$ mice fed with a high-fat diet: ↑plasma and renal Pon1 expression and activity, ↓renal redox (p47phox, Nox1, Nox4, Sod) and inflammation related (Tnfα, Il6) genes, ↑anti-inflammatory cytokine Il10		Liu Q. et al. [116]
			Liver	*Pon1*$^{+}$*SR-BI*$^{-/-}$ mice: ↑hepatic/plasma Pon1, ↑ApoE, ↑Lcat, ↓plasma ALT activity, ↓ROS levels and MPO activity, ↓acute-phase and pro-inflammatory plasma proteins (ApoA4, A1AT, Saa), ↑hepatic ApoA1, Ldlr, Lxrα, Abca, Abcg5, Abcg8, ↓Tnf-α, ↓Il6, ↓ atherosclerosis	Macrophages treated with *Pon1*$^{+}$*SR-BI*$^{-/-}$ HDL: ↓mRNA for inflammatory cytokines IL-6, TNFα, NOX1, ↑mRNA for anti-inflammatory cytokines IL-4, IL-10; mRNA for cholesterol transport ↓Scarb1, ↑Abca1	Zhao X.J. et al. [117]

HO1, heme oxidase 1; PPARγ, peroxisome proliferator-activated receptor gamma; MCP1, monocyte chemotactic protein; MPO, myeloperoxidase; *Pon1*$^{+}$*SR-BI*$^{-/-}$ mice, Pon1-overexpressing *SR-BI*$^{-/-}$ mice; Up and down arrows indicate the direction of change in gene expression.

5.1. Low PON1 Activity in Dysfunctional HDL Is Associated with Impaired Nitric Oxide Production in Endothelial Cells

Native HDL possesses anti-inflammatory and anti-oxidative properties [35] and directly influences the vascular endothelium by the activation of nitric oxide (NO) synthesis by eNOS [118,119], thus promoting endothelial repair [120]. Such cardio-protective processes are, at least in part, mediated by the binding of HDL to endothelial scavenger receptor B, type I (SR-BI), and by PON1 [6], carried in the circulation in a minor fraction of HDL [16].

Patients with stable coronary artery disease (CAD) or an acute coronary syndrome carry dysfunctional HDL_{CAD}, which does not promote the endothelial NO synthesis, anti-inflammatory effects, and repair that are characteristic of normal HDL isolated from healthy individuals [6]. This has been shown to be due to activation by HDL_{CAD} of the endothelial lectin-like oxLDL receptor 1 (LOX-1), which induces endothelial PKCβII activation, thereby inhibiting eNOS-dependent NO generation. These newly acquired properties were conferred by elevated MDA, a product of lipid peroxidation, which chemically modified PON1, thereby reducing its activity and generating dysfunctional HDL_{CAD}, which activates PKCβII and lacks the anti-oxidative, anti-inflammatory properties of normal HDL. Moreover, HDL from *Pon1*$^{-/-}$ mice failed to enhance endothelial NO production, while the addition of pure PON1 or HDL from healthy individuals partially ameliorated the stimulating effects of HDL on NO production. Even though PON1 activity in HDL_{CAD} was decreased, PON1 protein content in HDL_{CAD} was elevated compared to HDL from healthy controls, suggesting that the enzymatic activity of PON1 was inactivated in HDL_{CAD}. These findings show that HDL-associated PON1 activity has an important function in maintaining the ability to stimulate endothelial-atheroprotective effects of HDL, i.e., NO production. The impairment of this fundamental role of PON1/HDL by oxidative stress can account for the increased risk of adverse cardiovascular events in CAD patients [28,29]. These findings also show that PON1 regulates the expression of genes involved in endothelial homeostasis and that the dysregulation of these processes leads to CAD or acute coronary syndrome.

5.2. Pon1 Depletion Affects Expression of Genes Involved in Inflammation, Oxidative Stress, and Blood Clotting

Although Pon1 depletion in mice in the absence of hyperlipidemia does not induce atherosclerosis [55], *Pon1*$^{-/-}$ mice fed with a standard normolipidemic chow diet show an altered expression of proteins involved in vascular inflammation, oxidative stress, and thrombogenicity [121]. Specifically, there was a significant 2-fold increase in leukocyte adhesion revealed by intravital microscopy, but no significant change in leukocyte rolling in *Pon1*$^{-/-}$ mice compared to *Pon1*$^{+/+}$ control animals. The increase in adhesion was correlated with significant increases in aortic *P-selectin* and *Icam* mRNA levels (p = 0.016) and a 1.3-fold increase in *Vcam1* mRNA (p =0.096). Aortic Tnf-α mRNA expression was not affected. The rate of aortic superoxide production was significantly increased in *Pon1*$^{-/-}$ vs. *Pon1*$^{+/+}$ mice (3-fold, p = 0.04). *Pon1*$^{-/-}$ mice were also predisposed to thrombosis, as shown by a significant 57% reduction in time to occlusion in a carotid thrombosis assay ($p < 0.001$). Notably, these vascular changes mimic those seen in severely hyperlipidemic *ApoE*$^{-/-}$ mice [121]. These findings also show that *Pon1* interacts with genes involved in inflammation, oxidative stress, and blood clotting.

5.3. Pon1 Depletion Increases Expression of Liver Oxidative Stress Genes and Accelerates Atherosclerosis

In mice fed with a high-fat diet, *Pon1* gene deletion led to increased atherosclerosis and increased lipid peroxides levels in isolated HDL compared to *Pon*$^{+/+}$ animals [55]. In *ApoE*$^{-/-}$ mice, *Pon1* gene deletion also increased atherosclerosis and oxidative stress, manifested by elevated epitopes in plasma-oxidized phospholipid, biologically active oxidized phospholipids in isolated endogenous intermediate-density lipoprotein/LDL. RT-qPCR analyses showed that these changes were accompanied by the upregulated expression of genes involved in oxidative stress-responsive genes in the liver) HO-1, PPARγ, and oxidized LDL-R) [56] (Table 3). These findings show that Pon1 deficiency promotes oxidative stress and atherogenesis. These results also suggest that Pon1 interacts with oxidative stress-responsive genes and that the disruption of these interactions induces oxidative stress and causes atherosclerosis.

5.4. Pon1 Depletion Increases Expression of Oxidative Stress Genes in Liver, Kidney, and Brain

Proteomic analyses of *Pon1*$^{-/-}$ mice show that, in addition to controlling Hcy-thiolactone and *N*-Hcy-protein levels [40], Pon1 is important in maintaining cellular proteostasis. Specifically, in the brains of *Pon1*$^{-/-}$ mice fed with a normal chow diet, the levels of proteins involved in anti-oxidant defenses (Sod1, DJ-1) were significantly reduced compared to *Pon*$^{+/+}$ animals. In the presence of hyperhomocysteinemia (HHcy) induced by feeding with a high-methionine diet, DJ-1 and Prdx2 proteins were significantly upregulated in HHcy *Pon1*$^{-/-}$ mice compared to HHcy *Pon*$^{+/+}$ animals [60]. In the kidneys [113] and livers [112] of *Pon1*$^{-/-}$ mice, the levels of the anti-oxidant protein Prdx2 were significantly elevated compared to *Pon*$^{+/+}$ animals. These findings suggest that Pon1 interacts with oxidative stress-responsive proteins in an organ-specific way and that HHcy modulates these interactions.

5.5. Pon1 Depletion in Scarb1$^{-/-}$ *Mice Is Associated with Upregulated Expression of Oxidative Stress Genes*

Scavenger receptor BI (SR-BI) plays a central role in reverse cholesterol transport (RCT) as the major receptor for HDL cholesterol (HDL-C) [122]. Although elevated plasma HDL-C levels are associated with a lower risk of CVD in humans, a rate mutation in the human *SCARB1* gene encoding SR-BI increases the risk of CVD, suggesting that high concentrations of HDL-C are not causally protective against CVD and that cholesterol flux and HDL function are more important than the steady-state levels [123]. The SR-BI knockout mice (*Scarb1*$^{-/-}$ mice) have dysfunctional HDL characterized by impaired macrophage reverse cholesterol transport (RCT) [124], high plasma HDL-C levels, and impaired anti-oxidative and anti-inflammatory properties, and are susceptible to atherosclerosis [125].

Notably, the dysfunctional HDL is also characterized by reduced PON1 arylesterase and paraoxonase activities and is associated in a tissue-dependent way with indices of oxidative stress such as isoprostane F2α-VI (iPF2α-VI) and protein carbonyls in *Scarb1*$^{-/-}$ mice. The levels of monocyte chemoattractant protein-1 (MCP1) were similar in *Scarb1*$^{-/-}$ and wild-type mice, indicating that SR-BI deletion has no effect on inflammation. A Western diet did not affect MCP1 levels in *Scarb1*$^{-/-}$ mice but increased serum PON1 paraoxonase activity and urinary iPF2α-VI in both *Scarb1*$^{-/-}$ and wild-type mice [126].

The dysfunctional HDL and reduced PON1 activity in *Scarb1*$^{-/-}$ mice were associated with the upregulated expression of genes encoding oxidative stress proteins. Specifically, mRNAs for glutathione peroxidases GPx1 and GPx4, superoxide dismutase SOD1 and SOD2, glutathione S-transferases GSTA2 and GSTA4, which reduce lipid peroxidation products, and HO-1, which removes free prooxidant heme and generates of the anti-oxidant bilirubin, were upregulated in *Scarb1*$^{-/-}$ mice compared to wild-type animals. PAF-AH activity and catalase expression were not affected by *Scarb1* depletion and reduced Pon1 activity [126].

5.6. Pon1 Depletion in Scarb1$^{-/-}$ *Mice Affects Expression of Oxidative Stress and Inflammation-Related Liver Genes*

Lipo-proteomics analysis showed that the protein content of dysfunctional HDL from *SR-BI*$^{-/-}$ mice was decreased by 25%, compared to wild-type *SR-BI*$^{+/+}$ animals [115]. Out of 78 proteins identified in *SR-BI*$^{-/-}$ HDL, 26 were upregulated and 10 were downregulated compared to *SR-BI*$^{+/+}$ HDL. Specifically, ApoA1, ApoA2, ApoC1, ApoC2, ApoM, and PON1 were downregulated, while ApoE, ApoH, Lcat, acute phase proteins ApoA4, Saa, complement C3, proteinase inhibitors such as A1AT, inter alpha-trypsin inhibitor (3 of Itih1-4), and α-2-macroglobulin were upregulated in *SR-BI*$^{-/-}$ HDL compared to *SR-BI*$^{+/+}$ HDL. Interestingly, plasma proteomics showed that these proteins were also affected in the plasma of *Pon1*$^{-/-}$ mice compared to wild-type *Pon1*$^{+/+}$ animals (Table 3) and in *PON1-Q192R* polymorphism in humans [23]. Proteins involved in lipid metabolism were significantly decreased (37.34% vs. 57.98%), as were anti-oxidant proteins (1.94% vs. 7.09%). In contrast, proteins involved in inflammatory/immune response were significantly increased (22.14% vs. 9.19%), as were proteinase-inhibiting proteins (15.67% vs. 8.49%). In in vitro experiments, *SR-BI*$^{+/+}$ HDL significantly reduced Mcp1 and Tnf-α levels in oxLDL-treated macrophages while *SR-BI*$^{-/-}$ HDL had no effect [115].

Probucol is a cholesterol-lowering and anti-oxidant drug [127] that rescues female infertility in *SR-BI*$^{-/-}$ mice [128]. Treatments with probucol lowered plasma total and free cholesterol mainly in the HDL-C fraction, upregulated Pon1 and ApoA1, and downregulated ApoA4, Saa, A1AT, and myeloperoxidase (MPO) activity in *SR-BI*$^{-/-}$mice. These findings indicate that the anti-oxidant properties of HDL were improved by the probucol treatment [115].

5.7. PON1 Regulates the Expression of Hepatic Genes Involved in HDL Metabolism, Oxidative Stress, and Inflammation

Lentivirus-mediated Pon1 overexpression resulted in a significant elevation of PON1 levels in liver and plasma by 63% in *SR-BI*$^{-/-}$ mice [117]. Pon 1 overexpression improved the anti-oxidative and anti-inflammatory properties of dysfunctional HDL and reduced hepatic steatosis and aortic atherosclerosis through its effects on the expression of genes involved in these processes. Specifically, cholesterol transporter *Scarb1*, inflammatory cytokines *Il-6*, *Tnf-α*, and *Nox1* mRNAs were significantly downregulated, while *Abca1* mRNA and the anti-inflammatory cytokines *Il-4* and *Il-10* were upregulated in macrophages treated with plasma from Pon1^{+}*SR-BI*$^{-/-}$ mice. The levels of plasma MPO activity, an oxidative enzyme secreted by activated neutrophils, monocytes, and macrophages, were significantly reduced in *Pon1*$^{+}$*SR-BI*$^{-/-}$ mice. Lecithin-cholesterol acyltransferase (Lcat) (which removes cholesterol from the blood and tissues), ApoA1, and ApoE were significantly upregulated in *Pon1*$^{+}$*SR-BI*$^{-/-}$ plasma. Histological examinations showed that aortic lesions and hepatic lipid depositions were significantly reduced in *Pon1*$^{+}$*SR-BI*$^{-/-}$ mice. Hepatic ApoA1, ApoE, LDLR, LXRα, Abca1, Abcg5/8, and Acat were significantly upregulated, while inflammatory cytokines Il-6 and Tnf-α were downregulated, in *Pon1*$^{+}$*SR-BI*$^{-/-}$ mice. These findings indicate that Pon1 can regulate proteins important for HDL function and ameliorate atherosclerosis and hepatosteatosis [117].

5.8. Pon1 1 Ameliorates Renal Lipotoxicity by Regulating Genes Involved in Activating Lipophagy and Inhibiting Pyroptosis

Excessive lipid accumulation can lead to lipotoxicity due to the generation of toxic lipid intermediates. In the kidney, one of the more vulnerable organs, lipotoxicity causes tissue damage and dysfunction via oxidative stress, inflammation, and autophagy impairment, which lead to renal disease [129]. Pon1 is expressed in the glomerular clusters and the epithelial cells of the proximal tubules in the kidney [130]. *Pon1*$^{-/-}$ mice show increased oxidative stress in the kidney manifested by elevated expression of renal Prdx2 [111]. Renal disease patients show significantly reduced plasma HDL-C, APOA-I, serum PON1 protein concentration, PON1 arylesterase/ paraoxonase activity, and LCAT activity [131], indicating the impaired interactions of PON1 with APOAI and LCAT in dysfunctional HDL in these patients.

Mice deficient in the scavenger receptor class B type I (*SR-BI*$^{-/-}$) fed with a normal diet showed significantly reduced serum PON1 activity and renal PON1 expression, which was accompanied by renal pathology involving oxidative stress, inflammation, and fibrosis [116]. Western blot analysis and qRT-PCR showed that the expression of p47phox protein, a key regulator of NADPH oxidase, was significantly higher in the kidneys of *SR-BI*$^{-/-}$ mice compared with wild type *SR-BI*$^{+/+}$ mice. mRNA levels of NADPH oxidase genes *Nox 1* and *Nox4* were also significantly increased. Levels of inflammation-related Il1b and Il6 mRNAs were significantly increased, while anti-inflammatory cytokine Il10 mRNA tended to decrease. These findings show that the renal oxidative stress and inflammation were significantly upregulated in *SR-BI*$^{-/-}$ mice compared to wild-type *SR-BI*$^{+/+}$ animals.

Overexpression of PON1 (mRNA, 2.03-fold; protein, 3.36-fold) using a lentivirus vector significantly attenuated the pathologic changes in the kidneys of *SR-BI*$^{-/-}$ mice fed with a high-fat diet. Specifically, PON1-overexpressing (Pon1^{+}) *SR-BI*$^{-/-}$ mice showed a significant decrease in the fluorescence intensity of dihydroethidium bromide staining, a significant decrease in the immunohistochemical renal staining for lipid peroxidation indicator 4-hydroxynonenal, a significant decrease in the oxidative stress-related indicators such as renal p47phox protein and Nox1, Nox2, Nox4 mRNAs, and a significant increase in the activity of the anti-oxidant enzyme SOD in the kidney. In addition, PON1-overexpressing mice showed reduced levels of *Tnf-α* and *Il6* mRNAs and elevated levels of anti-inflammatory cytokine Il10. These findings show that PON1 overexpression has beneficial effects on the kidney function in *SR-BI*$^{-/-}$ mice by reducing renal ROS production, improving antioxidant status, and ameliorating renal inflammation. PON1 overexpression also attenuated renal lipid accumulation by upregulating cholesterol ester hydrolysis-related genes (*Nceh1*, *Lipa*) and cholesterol efflux-related receptors (Abca1, Abcag1). Western blot and qRT-PCR analyses showed that fibrosis-related proteins (fibronectin, collagen, type I, a1, and actin a2 in smooth muscle and aorta) were significantly downregulated in PON1-overexpressing mice compared to the control lentivirus-GFP-injected mice; mRNA levels for fibronectin, *Col1a1*, *Ccn2*, and *Lcn2*, a marker of kidney injury, were also significantly reduced, indicating that PON1 overexpression ameliorated fibrosis. Moreover, Pon1 overexpression inhibited mTOR signaling and restored autophagy flux in the mouse kidney [116]. That Pon1 can regulate mTOR signaling and autophagy was also reported in another study that found upregulated mTOR signaling and downregulated autophagy in *Pon1*$^{-/-}$ mice brains and in *Pon1*-silenced mouse neural cells [15].

5.9. PON1-Q192R Polymorphism Influences Oxidative Stress and Inflammation Proteins in Human Plasma

To ascertain how changes in PON1 expression/activity affect the expression of other proteins, plasma proteomes were analyzed in healthy participants recruited from the population of Poznań, Poland [23]. *PON1-Q192R* polymorphism affected serum paraoxonase activity (7-fold reduction in *PON1-192QQ* vs. *PON1-192RR*) and protein (40% reduction *PON1-192QQ* vs. *PON1-192RR*) (Table 4). Label-free nanoLC-MS/MS mass spectrometry analyses showed that there was an overlap in the principal component analysis (PCA) profiles between low-activity *PON1-192QQ*, intermediate-activity *PON1-192QR*, and high-activity *PON1-192RR* genotypes (Figure 6B).

Table 4. *PON1* genotype, activity, and protein levels in humans.

	Human PON1	
Genotype (n)	**Activity** [a]	**Protein** [b]
PON1-192RR (19)	100	100
PON1-192QR (30)	20.6	63.0
PON1-192QQ (51)	14.3	60.0

[a] Relative mean values determined in serum using paraoxon as a substrate. [b] PON1 protein quantified by label-free mass spectrometry. Adapted with permission from ref. [23]. Copyright 2020 by the authors.

The *PON1-Q192R* polymorphism affected the expression of 21 plasma proteins, including six oxidative stress-related proteins (APOA1↓, PON1↓, APOD↑, APOM↑, haptoglobin (HP)↓, and glutathione peroxidase 3 (GPX3)↑), four immune response proteins: CFP↑, IGHG3↑, ↑PGLYRP2, and ↑V2-6 (IGL), four lipoprotein metabolism proteins (APOA1↓, APOB↑, APOC1↓, and PON1↓), two acute phase response protein (TTR ↑ and AMBP↑), and seven blood coagulation protein (F13B↓, PLG↓, SERPINA10↓, VTN↓, ↑C9, ↑V2-17 (IGL), and FETUB↑). Six of those proteins (APOA1, APOB, APOC1, APOD, APOM, and PON1), representing 29% of total number of proteins affected by the *PON1-Q192R* polymorphism, are components of HDL [10,132]. These findings suggest that PON1 regulates the expression of other components of HDL as well as HDL proteins involved in oxidative stress, inflammation, and complement/coagulation in humans. The dysregulation of these processes may account for the pro-oxidant and pro-atherogenic phenotypes associated with attenuated PON1 levels in humans [28] and mice [55].

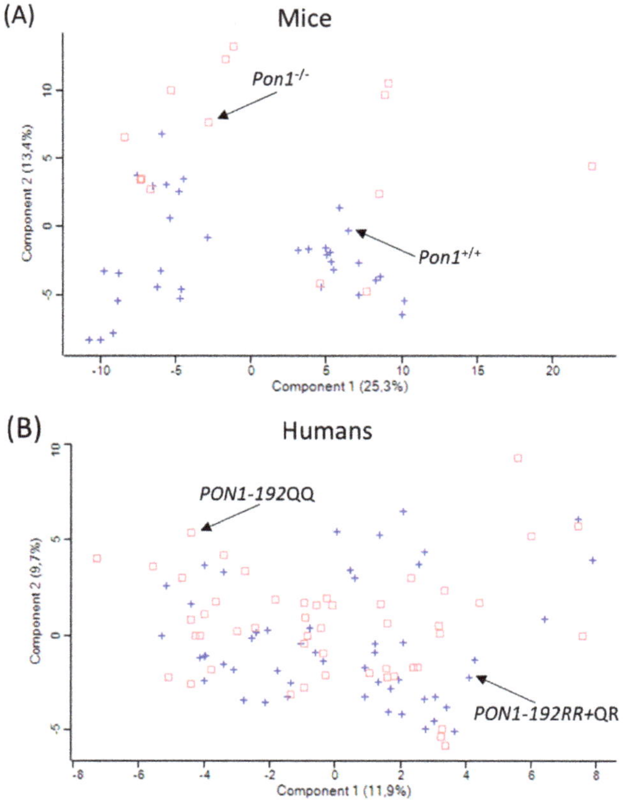

Figure 6. Principal component analysis of the LFQ intensities for plasma proteins. (**A**) *Pon1*$^{-/-}$ mice (*n* = 17; blue cross) and *Pon1*$^{+/+}$ siblings (*n* = 8; red square). (**B**). *PON1*$^{-/-}$*-192QQ* (*n* = 50; blue cross) and *PON1*$^{-/-}$*-192QQ* healthy humans (*n* = 50; red square). Calculations were performed with Perseus. Adapted from ref. [23].

5.10. Pon1$^{-/-}$ *Genotype Influences Oxidative Stress and Inflammation Proteins in Mouse Plasma*

Pon1 activity and protein are absent in *Pon1*$^{-/-}$ mice [55] (Table 5). To determine how Pon1 depletion affects the expression of other proteins, plasma proteomes were analyzed in *Pon1*$^{-/-}$ mice (*n* = 17) and their *Pon1*$^{+/+}$ littermates (*n* = 8) using label-free nanoLC-MS/MS mass spectrometry [23]. PCA profiles differed between *Pon1*$^{-/-}$ vs. *Pon1*$^{+/+}$ siblings (Figure 6A). Pon1 depletion in mice affected the expression of 50 plasma proteins, including seven redox proteins (↓Alb, ↓Blvrb, ↑ Ambp, ↑Hp, ↑Hpx, ↑ApoD, and ↑ApoM), seven lipoprotein metabolism proteins (↓ApoA1, ↑ApoB, ↓ApoC1, ↑ApoD, ↑ApoM, ↓Pon1, and ↑Lcat), four acute phase response proteins (↑Ambp, ↑Hp, ↑Hpx, and ↑Ttr), and 11 complement/coagulation proteins (↑AI182371, ↑Cfh, ↑Clu, ↑F2 (prothrombin), ↓Klkb1, ↓Mbl1, ↓Serpinc1, ↑Fetub, ↓F13B, ↑Hrg, and ↓Itih1) (arrows indicate direction of change). Nine of those proteins (↓Alb, ↓ApoA1, ↓ApoC1, ↑ApoD, ↑ApoM, ↑Clu, ↑Saa1, ↑Saa2, and ↑Lcat), representing 18% of total number of proteins affected by the *Pon1*$^{-/-}$ genotype, are components of HDL [10,16]. Clu (ApoJ) is also involved in amyloid beta (Aβ) transport from plasma to the brain [76].

Table 5. *Pon1* genotype, activity, and protein levels in mice.

	Mouse Pon1	
Genotype (n)	**Activity** [a]	**Protein** [b]
$Pon1^{+/+}$ (17)	100	100
$Pon1^{-/-}$ (8)	0.0	2.0

[a] Relative mean values, determined in serum using paraoxon as a substrate. [b] PON1 protein quantified by label-free mass spectrometry. Adapted from ref. [23].

Nine proteins that were affected by Pon1 genotype in mice (↓ApoA1↓, ↑ApoD↑, ↑ApoM↑, ↓Pon1↓, ↑haptoglobin (Hp)↓, ↓Ighg3↑, ↑Ttr↓, ↓F13B↓, and ↑Fetub↓), were also affected by the *PON1-Q192R* polymorphism in humans (representing 22% and 43% of the total number of differentiating proteins in mice and humans, respectively) (right and left arrows refer to the change in humans and mice, respectively). These findings show that changes in the mouse plasma proteome associated with the $Pon1^{-/-}$ genotype were like those in the human plasma proteome associated with the *PON1-Q192R* polymorphism. These findings also suggest that Pon1 regulates the expression of other protein components of HDL in addition to proteins involved in oxidative stress, inflammation, and complement/coagulation in mice.

Ingenuity pathway analysis identified the "Lipid Metabolism, Molecular Transport, Small Molecule Biochemistry" network, affected by PON1 activity in mice (Figure 7A) and humans (Figure 7B). Proteins in the human network are involved in acute phase/immune response and lipid metabolism and exhibit strong interactions focusing on LDL and HDL, the cytokine IL6, and the transforming growth factor beta 1 (TGFB1). In mice, this network contains oxidative stress proteins such as Alb, Hpx, Hp, Blvrd, Ambp, ApoD, and ApoM.

(A)

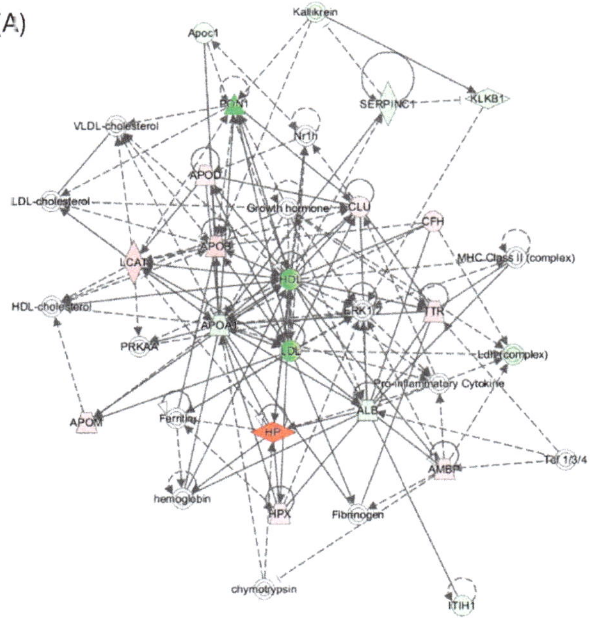

Figure 7. *Cont.*

(B)

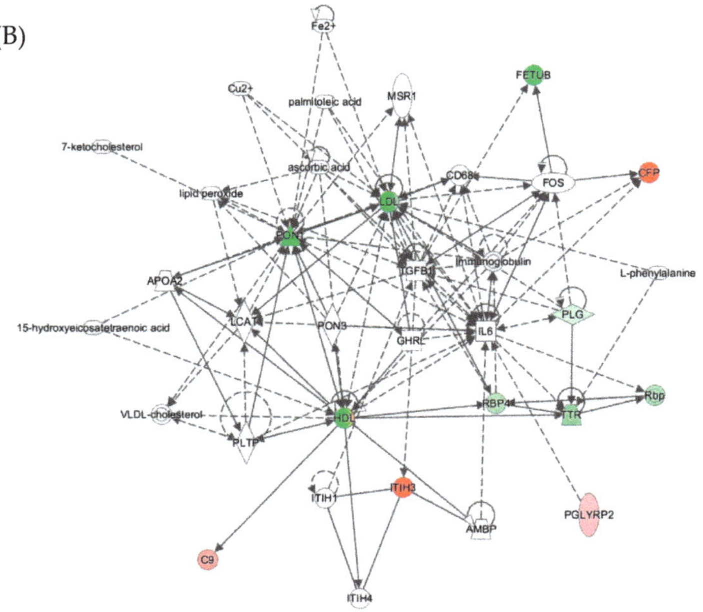

Figure 7. Top molecular network 'Lipid Metabolism, Molecular Transport, Small Molecule Biochemistry' associated with (**A**) *Pon1*$^{-/-}$ genotype in mice and (**B**) *PON1-Q192R* polymorphism in humans. The mouse network (**A**) includes redox-related proteins (Alb, Ambp, Hp, Hpx, ApoD, and ApoM) and inflammation-related proteins (Ambp and Ttr). The human network (**B**) contains inflammation-related AMBP and TTR proteins. Reprinted with permission from ref. [23]. Copyright 2020 by the authors.

These findings suggest that PON1 interacts with molecular pathways involved in oxidative stress, inflammatory response, complement/blood coagulation, and lipoprotein metabolism, processes that are essential for blood homeostasis. The dysregulation of these processes by attenuated PON1 protein/activity levels can account for PON1's association with cardiovascular and neurological diseases and cancer.

5.11. Metabolic Stress Amplifies Pro-Inflammatory, Pro-Oxidative, and Pro-Atherogenic Changes in Mouse Plasma Proteome Induced by Pon1 Depletion

To determine the effects of Pon1 depletion under the condition of metabolic stress on gene expression, plasma proteomes were examined in *Pon1*$^{-/-}$ mice and their wild-type *Pon1*$^{+/+}$ littermates fed with a high-methionine HHcy diet [114]. There was a clear difference in the PCA profiles of LFQ intensities for *Pon1*$^{-/-}$ mice compared to wild-type *Pon1*$^{+/+}$ animals, with a partial overlap between them (seven out of 44, 16%; *Pon1*$^{-/-}$, blue squares □ vs. *Pon1*$^{+/+}$, green triangles Δ) (Figure 8). In mice fed with a standard chow diet, the overlap was greater (28 out of 48, 58%; *Pon1*$^{-/-}$, blue crosses + vs. *Pon1*$^{+/+}$, purple circles ○), indicating that the *Pon1*$^{-/-}$ genotype exerts a stronger influence under the conditions of the metabolic stress of HHcy (Figure 8).

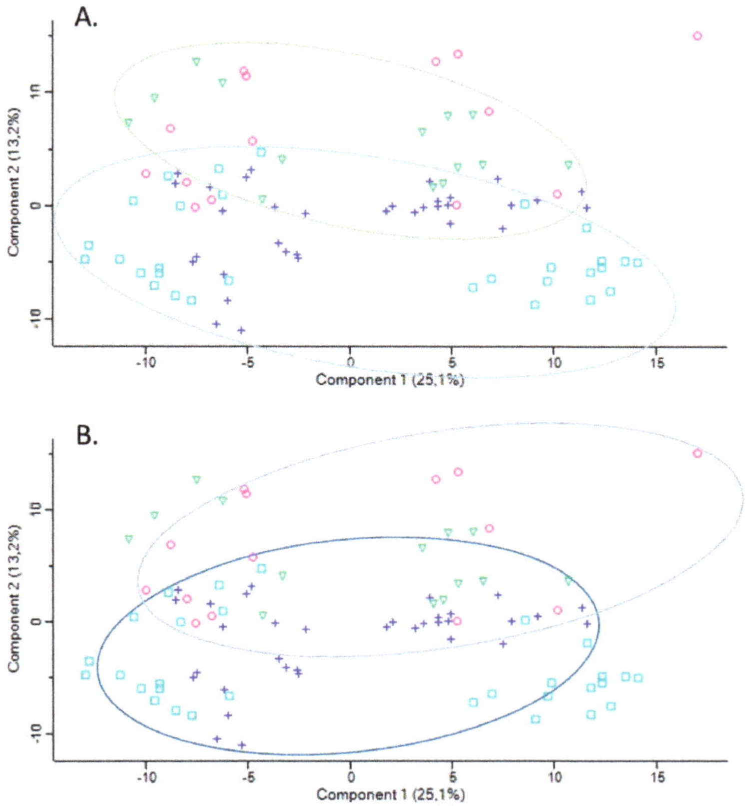

Figure 8. Principal component analysis (PCA) of label-free quantification (LFQ) intensities of mouse plasma proteins: effects of *Pon1* genotype and diet. *Pon1*$^{-/-}$ mice, control diet (n = 17, blue cross); *Pon1*$^{-/-}$ mice, HHcy diet (n = 15, blue square); *Pon1*$^{+/+}$ siblings, control diet (n = 8, purple circle); *Pon1*$^{+/+}$ siblings, HHcy diet (n = 7, green triangle). Calculations were carried out using Perseus. Ovals illustrate a smaller overlap between data points for *Pon1*$^{-/-}$ and *Pon1*$^{+/+}$ mice fed with high-met (**A**) than for mice fed with control diet (**B**). Reprinted with permission from ref. [114]. Copyright 2021 by Elsevier, Inc.

Pon1 depletion in HHcy mice changed the expression of 89 proteins, 1.8-fold more than in chow diet mice, including 18 redox proteins, 24 immune response proteins, six acute phase proteins, 15 complement/blood coagulation proteins, nine lipoprotein/lipid metabolism proteins, protein turnover proteins, and 10 other proteins (Table 6). Eight of those proteins (↓Alb, ↓ApoA1, ↓ApoA2, ↑ApoB, ↓ApoC1, ↓ApoC2, ↑Clu, and ↓Pon1), representing 8% of total number of proteins affected by the *Pon1*$^{-/-}$ genotype, are components of HDL [10,132].

The largest changes in the number of *Pon1*$^{-/-}$ genotype-dependent proteins in HHcy vs. chow diet mice were observed for oxidative stress-related proteins (18 proteins in HHcy diet vs. four proteins in chow diet mice), acute phase proteins (seven vs. two), and protein turnover proteins (six vs. two) (Table 6). Smaller changes between the diets were observed in the number of proteins involved in immune response (24 vs. 19), complement/coagulation (eight vs. seven), blood coagulation (six vs. three), lipoprotein/lipid metabolism (nine vs. eight), and other proteins (10 vs. five) (Table 6). These findings clearly show that the metabolic stress of HHcy greatly amplifies the effects of the *Pon1*$^{-/-}$ genotype on oxidative stress and inflammation.

Table 6. Plasma proteins affected by *Pon1*$^{-/-}$ genotype in mice fed with HHcy or control diet *.

Unique to HHcy-Diet Mice (*n* = 66)	**Unique to Control-Diet Mice (*n* = 27)**	**Proteins Affected Both in HHcy and Control-Diet Mice (*n* = 23)**
Oxidative stress (*n* = 15): ↓Alad, ↑Cp, ↓Gclm, ↓Cat, ↑Ctsb, ↓Gsn, ↑Grn, ↓Prdx2 #, ↓Prdx6, ↓Txn, ↓Igfbp3, ↓Park7 #, ↓Pebp1 #, ↓Ppia, ↓Serpina3k	Oxidative stress (*n* = 1): ↓Blvrb	Oxidative stress (*n* = 3): ↓**Alb** $, ↑Hp, ↑Hpx
Immune response (*n* = 15): ↓Il1rap, Igh (*n* = 10↑, 1↓), ↑Igk (*n* = 3),	Immune response (*n* = 10): ↑**Clu** $, ↑Igh (*n* = 3↑, 1↓), ↑Igk (*n* = 3), ↑Igl, ↑Igm	Immune response (*n* = 9): ↑Igh (*n* = 4), ↑Igj, ↑Igk (*n* = 3), ↑Igl
Acute phase response (*n* = 6): ↑**A2m** $, ↑Ahsg, ↑Orm1, ↑Orm2, ↑**Saa1**, ↑**Saa2**	Acute phase response (*n* = 1): ↑Ttr	Acute phase response (*n* = 1): ↑Ambp
Complement/coagulation (*n* = 5): ↑Apcs, ↓F13a1, ↑C3, ↑Cfb, ↑Cfhr1	Complement/coagulation (*n* = 4): ↑AI182371, ↑F2, ↓F13b, ↓Mbl1	Complement/coagulation (*n* = 3): ↑Cfh, ↓Klkb1, ↓Serpinc1
Blood coagulation (*n* = 6): ↑Serpina10, ↓Gp1ba, ↑Gp5, ↑Itih3, ↑**Pros1** $, ↓Proz	Blood coagulation (*n* = 3): ↓Hgfac, ↑**Hrg** ‡, ↓Itih1	
Lipoprotein/lipid metabolism (*n* = 5): ↓**ApoA2**, ↓**ApoC2**, ↓Azgp1, ↓Pgp, ↑**Pltp**	Lipoprotein metabolism (*n* = 4): ↓Afm, ↑**ApoD**, ↑**ApoM**, ↑**Lcat**	Lipoprotein metabolism (*n* = 4): ↓**ApoA1**, ↑**ApoB**, ↓**ApoC1**, ↓**Pon1**
Protein turnover (*n* = 5): ↓Apeh, ↓Mug2, ↓Serpina3m, ↓Uba1, ↓Uba52	Protein turnover (*n* = 1): ↑Fetub	Protein turnover (*n* = 1): ↓Mug1
Other proteins (*n* = 8): ↓Atic, ↓Nme1, ↓Pnp (purine metabolism), ↓Tpi, ↓Tkt (glucose metabolism), ↓Ran # (nucleoplasmic transport), ↓Rbp4 (retinol transport), ↓Spp2 (bone remodeling)	Other proteins (*n* = 3): ↓Aldoa, ↓Ldha (glucose metabolism), ↓Lifr (tissue regeneration)	Other proteins (*n* = 2): ↓Bpgm (glucose metabolism), ↓Ica (carbonic anhydrase inhibitor)

* Up and down arrows indicate the direction of change in protein levels. # Proteins affected also in mouse brain [58]. $ Enriched in, or ‡ largely excluded from, PON1-containg HDL subfraction of normal human HDL [16]. Bold font indicates proteins identified as components of HDL. Adapted with permission from ref. [114]. Copyright 2021 by Elsevier, Inc.

Eleven of the proteins (12%) affected by the *Pon1*$^{-/-}$ genotype in HHcy mice (ApoA1, ApoA2, ApoC1, ApoC2, Pltp, Saa1, Saa2, Alb, A2m, Pros1, and Pon1) are the components of HDL [10,130], some of which were found to be enriched in the PON1-containg HDL subfraction (Alb, Clu, A2m, and Pros1) [16]. Phospholipid transfer protein (Pltp), found to be upregulated in *Pon1*$^{-/-}$ HHcy mice (Table 6), regulates the size/composition of HDL in the circulation and controls plasma HDL levels [133]. These findings show that Pon1 affects the expression of plasma proteins involved in oxidative stress, inflammation, and other processes linked to CVD. The dysregulation of these processes may account for the pro-oxidant and pro-atherogenic phenotypes associated with attenuated PON1 levels in humans [28] and mice [55].

Nineteen oxidative stress-related proteins such as Parkinson disease protein 7 (Park7, DJ-1), peroxiredoxin-2 (Prdx2), peroxiredoxin-6 (Prdx6), and thioredoxin (Txn) were significantly downregulated, while seven inflammatory response proteins were upregulated in HHcy Pon1-depleted mice (Table 6). The impairment of anti-oxidant and anti-inflammatory defenses caused by changes in the expression of oxidative stress- and inflammation-related proteins can account for the increased oxidative stress and inflammation observed in *Pon1*$^{-/-}$ mice [55] and in humans with low activity of PON1 [28].

6. Conclusions

Transcriptomic and proteomic analyses provided new insights regarding PON1 function by identifying the proteins and molecular pathways influenced by PON1 depletion or PON1 overexpression. Accumulating evidence shows that changes in PON1 expression/activity influence both extracellular and cellular proteostasis by impairing epigenetic regulation, upregulating mTOR signaling, and inhibiting autophagy. Pon1 depletion induces oxidative stress and inflammation by influencing the expression of genes involved in these processes. The changes in gene expression caused by low PON1 expression/activity levels are exacerbated by the metabolic stress of hyperlipidemia or hyperhomocysteinemia. Although these changes are linked to CVD, Alzheimer's disease, and cancer, the molecular mechanisms by which PON1 affects gene expression remain to be elucidated in future studies.

Funding: This research was funded by grants 2018/29/B/NZ4/00771, 2019/33/B/NZ4/01760, and 2021/43/B/NZ4/00339 from the National Science Center, Poland, and 17GRNT32910002 from the American Heart Association.

Conflicts of Interest: No conflicts of interest, financial or otherwise, are declared by the author.

References

1. Libby, P. Inflammation in atherosclerosis. *Nature* **2002**, *420*, 868–874. [CrossRef] [PubMed]
2. Hopkins, P.N. Molecular biology of atherosclerosis. *Physiol. Rev.* **2013**, *93*, 1317–1542. [CrossRef] [PubMed]
3. Witztum, J.L.; Steinberg, D. The oxidative modification hypothesis of atherosclerosis: Does it hold for humans? *Trends Cardiovasc. Med.* **2001**, *11*, 93–102. [CrossRef] [PubMed]
4. Navab, M.; Ananthramaiah, G.M.; Reddy, S.T.; Van Lenten, B.J.; Ansell, B.J.; Fonarow, G.C.; Vahabzadeh, K.; Hama, S.; Hough, G.; Kamranpour, N.; et al. The oxidation hypothesis of atherogenesis: The role of oxidized phospholipids and HDL. *J. Lipid Res.* **2004**, *45*, 993–1007. [CrossRef]
5. Libby, P.; Ridker, P.M.; Hansson, G.K. Progress and challenges in translating the biology of atherosclerosis. *Nature* **2011**, *473*, 317–325. [CrossRef] [PubMed]
6. Besler, C.; Heinrich, K.; Rohrer, L.; Doerries, C.; Riwanto, M.; Shih, D.M.; Chroni, A.; Yonekawa, K.; Stein, S.; Schaefer, N.; et al. Mechanisms underlying adverse effects of HDL on eNOS-activating pathways in patients with coronary artery disease. *J. Clin. Investig.* **2011**, *121*, 2693–2708. [CrossRef]
7. Barter, P.J.; Nicholls, S.; Rye, K.A.; Anantharamaiah, G.M.; Navab, M.; Fogelman, A.M. Antiinflammatory properties of HDL. *Circ. Res.* **2004**, *95*, 764–772. [CrossRef]
8. Zerrad-Saadi, A.; Therond, P.; Chantepie, S.; Couturier, M.; Rye, K.A.; Chapman, M.J.; Kontush, A. HDL3-mediated inactivation of LDL-associated phospholipid hydroperoxides is determined by the redox status of apolipoprotein A-I and HDL particle surface lipid rigidity: Relevance to inflammation and atherogenesis. *Arterioscler. Thromb. Vasc. Biol.* **2009**, *29*, 2169–2175. [CrossRef]
9. Navab, M.; Hama, S.Y.; Anantharamaiah, G.M.; Hassan, K.; Hough, G.P.; Watson, A.D.; Reddy, S.T.; Sevanian, A.; Fonarow, G.C.; Fogelman, A.M. Normal high density lipoprotein inhibits three steps in the formation of mildly oxidized low density lipoprotein: Steps 2 and 3 *J. Lipid Res.* **2000**, *41*, 1495–1508. [CrossRef]
10. Brites, F.; Martin, M.; Guillas, I.; Kontush, A. Antioxidative activity of high-density lipoprotein (HDL): Mechanistic insights into potential clinical benefit. *BBA Clin.* **2017**, *8*, 66–77. [CrossRef]
11. Soran, H.; Schofield, J.D.; Liu, Y.; Durrington, P.N. How HDL protects LDL against atherogenic modification: Paraoxonase 1 and other dramatis personae. *Curr. Opin. Lipidol.* **2015**, *26*, 247–256. [CrossRef] [PubMed]
12. Mackness, B.; Beltran-Debon, R.; Aragones, G.; Joven, J.; Camps, J.; Mackness, M. Human tissue distribution of paraoxonases 1 and 2 mRNA. *IUBMB Life* **2010**, *62*, 480–482. [CrossRef]
13. Marsillach, J. Mackness, B.; Mackness, M.; Riu, F.; Beltran, R.; Joven, J.; Camps, J. Immunohistochemical analysis of paraoxonases-1, 2, and 3 expression in normal mouse tissues. *Free. Radic. Biol. Med.* **2008**, *45*, 146–157. [CrossRef]
14. Leduc, V.; Legault, V.; Dea, D.; Poirier, J. Normalization of gene expression using SYBR green qPCR: A case for paraoxonase 1 and 2 in Alzheimer's disease brains. *J. Neurosci. Methods* **2011**, *200*, 14–19. [CrossRef] [PubMed]
15. Witucki, L.; Jakubowski, H. Depletion of Paraoxonase 1 (Pon1) Dysregulates mTOR, Autophagy, and Accelerates Amyloid Beta Accumulation in Mice. *Cells* **2023**, *12*, 746. [CrossRef]
16. Moren, X.; Lhomme, M.; Bulla, A.; Sanchez, J.C.; Kontush, A.; James, R.W. Proteomic and lipidomic analyses of paraoxonase defined high density lipoprotein particles: Association of paraoxonase with the anti-coagulant, protein S. *Proteom. Clin. Appl.* **2016**, *10*, 230–238. [CrossRef] [PubMed]
17. Humbert, R.; Adler, D.A.; Disteche, C.M.; Hassett, C.; Omiecinski, C.J.; Furlong, C.E. The molecular basis of the human serum paraoxonase activity polymorphism. *Nat. Genet.* **1993**, *3*, 73–76. [CrossRef]
18. Gan, K.N.; Smolen, A.; Eckerson, H.W.; La Du, B.N. Purification of human serum paraoxonase/arylesterase. Evidence for one esterase catalyzing both activities. *Drug Metab. Dispos.* **1991**, *19*, 100–106.
19. Jakubowski, H. Calcium-dependent human serum homocysteine thiolactone hydrolase. A protective mechanism against protein N-homocysteinylation. *J. Biol. Chem.* **2000**, *275*, 3957–3962. [CrossRef]
20. Jakubowski, H.; Goldman, E. Synthesis of homocysteine thiolactone by methionyl-tRNA synthetase in cultured mammalian cells. *FEBS Lett.* **1993**, *317*, 237–240. [CrossRef]
21. Jakubowski, H. Quality control in tRNA charging. *Wiley Interdiscip. Rev. RNA* **2012**, *3*, 295–310. [CrossRef] [PubMed]

22. Jakubowski, H. Homocysteine Modification in Protein Structure/Function and Human Disease. *Physiol. Rev.* **2019**, *99*, 555–604. [CrossRef] [PubMed]
23. Sikora, M.; Bretes, E.; Perla-Kajan, J.; Lewandowska, I.; Marczak, L.; Jakubowski, H. Genetic Attenuation of Paraoxonase 1 Activity Induces Proatherogenic Changes in Plasma Proteomes of Mice and Humans. *Antioxidants* **2020**, *9*, 1198. [CrossRef] [PubMed]
24. Jakubowski, H.; Ambrosius, W.T.; Pratt, J.H. Genetic determinants of homocysteine thiolactonase activity in humans: Implications for atherosclerosis. *FEBS Lett.* **2001**, *491*, 35–39. [CrossRef]
25. Jakubowski, H. Homocysteine thiolactone: Metabolic origin and protein homocysteinylation in humans. *J. Nutr.* **2000**, *130*, 377S–381S. [CrossRef]
26. Perla-Kajan, J.; Borowczyk, K.; Glowacki, R.; Nygard, O.; Jakubowski, H. Paraoxonase 1 Q192R genotype and activity affect homocysteine thiolactone levels in humans. *FASEB J.* **2018**, *32*, fj201800346R.
27. Costa, L.G.; Cole, T.B.; Jarvik, G.P.; Furlong, C.E. Functional genomic of the paraoxonase (PON1) polymorphisms: Effects on pesticide sensitivity, cardiovascular disease, and drug metabolism. *Annu. Rev. Med.* **2003**, *54*, 371–392. [CrossRef]
28. Bhattacharyya, T.; Nicholls, S.J.; Topol, E.J.; Zhang, R.; Yang, X.; Schmitt, D.; Fu, X.; Shao, M.; Brennan, D.M.; Ellis, S.G.; et al. Relationship of paraoxonase 1 (PON1) gene polymorphisms and functional activity with systemic oxidative stress and cardiovascular risk. *JAMA* **2008**, *299*, 1265–1276. [CrossRef]
29. Tang, W.H.; Hartiala, J.; Fan, Y.; Wu, Y.; Stewart, A.F.; Erdmann, J.; Kathiresan, S.; Consortium, C.A.; Roberts, R.; McPherson, R.; et al. Clinical and genetic association of serum paraoxonase and arylesterase activities with cardiovascular risk. *Arterioscler. Thromb. Vasc. Biol.* **2012**, *32*, 2803–2812. [CrossRef]
30. Mackness, B.; Durrington, P.; McElduff, P.; Yarnell, J.; Azam, N.; Watt, M.; Mackness, M. Low paraoxonase activity predicts coronary events in the Caerphilly Prospective Study. *Circulation* **2003**, *107*, 2775–2779. [CrossRef]
31. Dube, P.; Khalaf, F.K.; DeRiso, A.; Mohammed, C.J.; Connolly, J.A.; Battepati, D.; Lad, A.; Breidenbach, J.D.; Kleinhenz, A.L.; Khatib-Shahidi, B.; et al. Cardioprotective Role for Paraoxonase-1 in Chronic Kidney Disease. *Biomedicines* **2022**, *10*, 2301. [CrossRef] [PubMed]
32. Meneses, M.J.; Silvestre, R.; Sousa-Lima, I.; Macedo, M.P. Paraoxonase-1 as a Regulator of Glucose and Lipid Homeostasis: Impact on the Onset and Progression of Metabolic Disorders. *Int. J. Mol. Sci.* **2019**, *20*, 4049. [CrossRef] [PubMed]
33. Cervellati, C.; Trentini, A.; Romani, A.; Bellini, T.; Bosi, C.; Ortolani, B.; Zurlo, A.; Passaro, A.; Seripa, D.; Zuliani, G. Serum paraoxonase and arylesterase activities of paraoxonase-1 (PON-1), mild cognitive impairment, and 2-year conversion to dementia: A pilot study. *J. Neurochem.* **2015**, *135*, 395–401. [CrossRef] [PubMed]
34. Dong, L.; Dong, C.; Yu, Y.; Jiao, X.; Zhang, X.; Zhang, X.; Li, Z. Transcriptomic analysis of Paraoxonase 1 expression in hepatocellular carcinoma and its potential impact on tumor immunity. *Clin. Transl. Oncol.* **2024**. *Online ahead of print*. [CrossRef]
35. Zhang, Q.; Jiang, Z.; Xu, Y. HDL and Oxidation. *Adv. Exp. Med. Biol.* **2022**, *1377*, 63–77.
36. Marsillach, J.; Adorni, M.P.; Zimetti, F.; Papotti, B.; Zuliani, G.; Cervellati, C. HDL Proteome and Alzheimer's Disease: Evidence of a Link. *Antioxidants* **2020**, *9*, 1224. [CrossRef]
37. Davidson, W.S.; Silva, R.A.; Chantepie, S.; Lagor, W.R.; Chapman, M.J.; Kontush, A. Proteomic analysis of defined HDL subpopulations reveals particle-specific protein clusters: Relevance to antioxidative function. *Arterioscler. Thromb. Vasc. Biol.* **2009**, *29*, 870–876. [CrossRef]
38. de Souza, J.A.; Vindis, C.; Negre-Salvayre, A.; Rye, K.A.; Couturier, M.; Therond, P.; Chantepie, S.; Salvayre, R.; Chapman, M.J.; Kontush, A. Small, dense HDL 3 particles attenuate apoptosis in endothelial cells: Pivotal role of apolipoprotein A-I. *J. Cell. Mol. Med.* **2010**, *14*, 608–620. [CrossRef]
39. Jakubowski, H. Proteomic Exploration of Paraoxonase 1 Function in Health and Disease. *Int. J. Mol. Sci.* **2023**, *24*, 7764. [CrossRef]
40. Borowczyk, K.; Shih, D.M.; Jakubowski, H. Metabolism and neurotoxicity of homocysteine thiolactone in mice: Evidence for a protective role of paraoxonase 1. *J. Alzheimer's Dis. JAD* **2012**, *30*, 225–231. [CrossRef]
41. Borowczyk, K.; Piechocka, J.; Glowacki, R.; Dhar, I.; Midtun, O.; Tell, G.S.; Ueland, P.M.; Nygard, O.; Jakubowski, H. Urinary excretion of homocysteine thiolactone and the risk of acute myocardial infarction in coronary artery disease patients: The WENBIT trial. *J. Intern. Med.* **2019**, *285*, 232–244. [CrossRef] [PubMed]
42. Sauls, D.L.; Lockhart, E.; Warren, M.E.; Lenkowski, A.; Wilhelm, S.E.; Hoffman, M. Modification of fibrinogen by homocysteine thiolactone increases resistance to fibrinolysis: A potential mechanism of the thrombotic tendency in hyperhomocysteinemia. *Biochemistry* **2006**, *45*, 2480–2487. [CrossRef] [PubMed]
43. Sikora, M.; Skrzydlewski, P.; Perla-Kajan, J.; Jakubowski, H. Homocysteine thiolactone contributes to the prognostic value of fibrin clot structure/function in coronary artery disease. *PLoS ONE* **2022**, *17*, e0275956. [CrossRef] [PubMed]
44. Khersonsky, O.; Tawfik, D.S. Structure-reactivity studies of serum paraoxonase PON1 suggest that its native activity is lactonase. *Biochemistry* **2005**, *44*, 6371–6382. [CrossRef] [PubMed]
45. Draganov, D.I.; Teiber, J.F.; Speelman, A.; Osawa, Y.; Sunahara, R.; La Du, B.N. Human paraoxonases (PON1, PON2, and PON3) are lactonases with overlapping and distinct substrate specificities. *J. Lipid Res.* **2005**, *46*, 1239–1247. [CrossRef]
46. Mohammed, C.J.; Lamichhane, S.; Connolly, J.A.; Soehnlen, S.M.; Khalaf, F.K.; Malhotra, D.; Haller, S.T.; Isailovic, D.; Kennedy, D.J. A PON for All Seasons: Comparing Paraoxonase Enzyme Substrates, Activity and Action including the Role of PON3 in Health and Disease. *Antioxidants* **2022**, *11*, 590. [CrossRef]

47. Slutsky Smith, E.A.; Khatib, S.; Szuchman-Sapir, A. Fishing for lipid lactones using selective reaction and characteristic fragmentation pattern. *J. Chromatogr. B Anal. Technol. Biomed. Life Sci.* **2022**, *1197*, 123201. [CrossRef]
48. Momma, T.Y.; Kuhnle, G.G.C.; Fong, R.Y.; Ensunsa, J.L.; Crozier, A.; Schroeter, H.; Ottaviani, J.I. 5-(3′,4′-Dihydroxyphenyl)-gamma-Valerolactone Is a Substrate for Human Paraoxonase: A Novel Pathway in Flavan-3-ol Metabolism. *Mol. Nutr. Food Res.* **2023**, *67*, e2300281. [CrossRef]
49. Sesso, H.D.; Manson, J.E.; Aragaki, A.K.; Rist, P.M.; Johnson, L.G.; Friedenberg, G.; Copeland, T.; Clar, A.; Mora, S.; Moorthy, M.V.; et al. Effect of cocoa flavanol supplementation for the prevention of cardiovascular disease events: The COcoa Supplement and Multivitamin Outcomes Study (COSMOS) randomized clinical trial. *Am. J. Clin. Nutr.* **2022**, *115*, 1490–1500. [CrossRef]
50. Baker, L.D.; Manson, J.E.; Rapp, S.R.; Sesso, H.D.; Gaussoin, S.A.; Shumaker, S.A.; Espeland, M.A. Effects of cocoa extract and a multivitamin on cognitive function: A randomized clinical trial. *Alzheimer's Dement.* **2023**, *19*, 1308–1319. [CrossRef]
51. Mena, P.; Bresciani, L.; Brindani, N.; Ludwig, I.A.; Pereira-Caro, G.; Angelino, D.; Llorach, R.; Calani, L.; Brighenti, F.; Clifford, M.N.; et al. Phenyl-gamma-valerolactones and phenylvaleric acids, the main colonic metabolites of flavan-3-ols: Synthesis, analysis, bioavailability, and bioactivity. *Nat. Prod. Rep.* **2019**, *36*, 714–752. [CrossRef] [PubMed]
52. Angelino, D.; Carregosa, D.; Domenech-Coca, C.; Savi, M.; Figueira, I.; Brindani, N.; Jang, S.; Lakshman, S.; Molokin, A.; Urban, J.F., Jr.; et al. 5-(Hydroxyphenyl)-gamma-Valerolactone-Sulfate, a Key Microbial Metabolite of Flavan-3-ols, Is Able to Reach the Brain: Evidence from Different in Silico, In Vitro and In Vivo Experimental Models. *Nutrients* **2019**, *11*, 2678. [CrossRef] [PubMed]
53. Corral-Jara, K.F.; Nuthikattu, S.; Rutledge, J.; Villablanca, A.; Morand, C.; Schroeter, H.; Milenkovic, D. Integrated Multi-Omic Analyses of the Genomic Modifications by Gut Microbiome-Derived Metabolites of Epicatechin, 5-(4′-Hydroxyphenyl)-gamma-Valerolactone, in TNFalpha-Stimulated Primary Human Brain Microvascular Endothelial Cells. *Front. Neurosci.* **2021**, *15*, 622640. [CrossRef] [PubMed]
54. Costa, L.G.; Giordano, G.; Cole, T.B.; Marsillach, J.; Furlong, C.E. Paraoxonase 1 (PON1) as a genetic determinant of susceptibility to organophosphate toxicity. *Toxicology* **2013**, *307*, 115–122. [CrossRef] [PubMed]
55. Shih, D.M.; Gu, L.; Xia, Y.R.; Navab, M.; Li, W.F.; Hama, S.; Castellani, L.W.; Furlong, C.E.; Costa, L.G.; Fogelman, A.M.; et al. Mice lacking serum paraoxonase are susceptible to organophosphate toxicity and atherosclerosis. *Nature* **1998**, *394*, 284–287. [CrossRef]
56. Shih, D.M.; Xia, Y.R.; Wang, X.P.; Miller, E.; Castellani, L.W.; Subbanagounder, G.; Cheroutre, H.; Faull, K.F.; Berliner, J.A.; Witztum, J.L.; et al. Combined serum paraoxonase knockout/apolipoprotein E knockout mice exhibit increased lipoprotein oxidation and atherosclerosis. *J. Biol. Chem.* **2000**, *275*, 17527–17535. [CrossRef]
57. Hong, C.G.; Florida, E.; Li, H.; Parel, P.M.; Mehta, N.N.; Sorokin, A.V. Oxidized low-density lipoprotein associates with cardiovascular disease by a vicious cycle of atherosclerosis and inflammation: A systematic review and meta-analysis. *Front. Cardiovasc. Med.* **2022**, *9*, 1023651. [CrossRef]
58. Kotani, K.; Watanabe, Y.; Miura, K.; Gugliucci, A. Paraoxonase 1 and Non-Alcoholic Fatty Liver Disease: A Meta-Analysis. *Biomolecules* **2021**, *26*, 2323. [CrossRef]
59. Suszynska-Zajczyk, J.; Luczak, M.; Marczak, L.; Jakubowski, H. Inactivation of the paraoxonase 1 gene affects the expression of mouse brain proteins involved in neurodegeneration. *J. Alzheimer's Dis.* **2014**, *42*, 247–260. [CrossRef]
60. Bednarz-Misa, I.; Berdowska, I.; Zboch, M.; Misiak, B.; Zielinski, B.; Placzkowska, S.; Fleszar, M.; Wisniewski, J.; Gamian, A.; Krzystek-Korpacka, M. Paraoxonase 1 decline and lipid peroxidation rise reflect a degree of brain atrophy and vascular impairment in dementia. *Adv. Clin. Exp. Med.* **2020**, *29*, 71–78. [CrossRef]
61. Bade, J.D.; Veeramalla, V.; Naidu, M.B.R.; Lalitha, D.L.; Ponnada, S.C.; Kandi, V. Serum Activities of Paraoxonase 1 (PON1) in Predicting Liver Damage Among Patients Diagnosed With Hepatocellular Carcinoma: A Case-Control Study. *Cureus* **2023**, *15*, e46234. [CrossRef] [PubMed]
62. Bacchetti, T.; Vignini, A.; Giulietti, A.; Nanetti, L.; Provinciali, L.; Luzzi, S.; Mazzanti, L.; Ferretti, G. Higher Levels of Oxidized Low Density Lipoproteins in Alzheimer's Disease Patients: Roles for Platelet Activating Factor Acetyl Hydrolase and Paraoxonase-1. *J. Alzheimers Dis.* **2015**, *46*, 179–186. [CrossRef] [PubMed]
63. Tward, A.; Xia, Y.R.; Wang, X.P.; Shi, Y.S.; Park, C.; Castellani, L.W.; Lusis, A.J.; Shih, D.M. Decreased atherosclerotic lesion formation in human serum paraoxonase transgenic mice. *Circulation* **2002**, *106*, 484–490. [CrossRef] [PubMed]
64. Mackness, B.; Quarck, R.; Verreth, W.; Mackness, M.; Holvoet, P. Human paraoxonase-1 overexpression inhibits atherosclerosis in a mouse model of metabolic syndrome. *Arterioscler. Thromb. Vasc. Biol.* **2006**, *26*, 1545–1550. [CrossRef] [PubMed]
65. She, Z.G.; Zheng, W.; Wei, Y.S.; Chen, H.Z.; Wang, A.B.; Li, H.L.; Liu, G.; Zhang, R.; Liu, J.J.; Stallcup, W.B.; et al. Human paraoxonase gene cluster transgenic overexpression represses atherogenesis and promotes atherosclerotic plaque stability in ApoE-null mice. *Circ. Res.* **2009**, *104*, 1160–1168. [CrossRef] [PubMed]
66. Brophy, V.H.; Jampsa, R.L.; Clendenning, J.B.; McKinstry, L.A.; Jarvik, G.P.; Furlong, C.E. Effects of 5′ regulatory-region polymorphisms on paraoxonase-gene (PON1) expression. *Am. J. Hum. Genet.* **2001**, *68*, 1428–1436. [CrossRef] [PubMed]
67. Kresanov, P.; Vasankari, T.; Ahotupa, M.; Kaikkonen, J.; Hutri-Kahonen, N.; Juonala, M.; Kahonen, M.; Lehtimaki, T.; Viikari, J.; Raitakari, O.T. Paraoxonase-1 and oxidized lipoprotein lipids. The Cardiovascular Risk in Young Finns Study. *Atherosclerosis* **2015**, *241*, 502–506. [CrossRef] [PubMed]
68. Ahotupa, M.; Marniemi, J.; Lehtimaki, T.; Talvinen, K.; Raitakari, O.T.; Vasankari, T.; Viikari, J.; Luoma, J.; Yla-Herttuala, S. Baseline diene conjugation in LDL lipids as a direct measure of in vivo LDL oxidation. *Clin. Biochem.* **1998**, *31*, 257–261. [CrossRef]

69. Esterbauer, H.; Striegl, G.; Puhl, H.; Rotheneder, M. Continuous monitoring of in vitro oxidation of human low density lipoprotein. *Free Radic. Res. Commun.* **1989**, *6*, 67–75. [CrossRef]
70. Kuchta, A.; Strzelecki, A.; Cwiklinska, A.; Toton, M.; Gruchala, M.; Zdrojewski, Z.; Kortas-Stempak, B.; Gliwinska, A.; Dabkowski, K.; Jankowski, M. PON-1 Activity and Plasma 8-Isoprostane Concentration in Patients with Angiographically Proven Coronary Artery Disease. *Oxid. Med. Cell. Longev.* **2015**, *2015*, 5136937. [CrossRef] [PubMed]
71. Carlson, C.S.; Heagerty, P.J.; Hatsukami, T.S.; Richter, R.J.; Ranchalis, J.; Lewis, J.; Bacus, T.J.; McKinstry, L.A.; Schellenberg, G.D.; Rieder, M.; et al. TagSNP analyses of the PON gene cluster: Effects on PON1 activity, LDL oxidative susceptibility, and vascular disease. *J. Lipid Res.* **2006**, *47*, 1014–1024. [CrossRef] [PubMed]
72. Dias, I.H.; Mistry, J.; Fell, S.; Reis, A.; Spickett, C.M.; Polidori, M.C.; Lip, G.Y.; Griffiths, H.R. Oxidized LDL lipids increase beta-amyloid production by SH-SY5Y cells through glutathione depletion and lipid raft formation. *Free Radic Biol Med* **2014**, *75*, 48–59. [CrossRef] [PubMed]
73. Schulz, B.; Liebisch, G.; Grandl, M.; Werner, T.; Barlage, S.; Schmitz, G. Beta-amyloid (Abeta40, Abeta42) binding to modified LDL accelerates macrophage foam cell formation. *Biochim. Biophys. Acta* **2007**, *1771*, 1335–1344. [CrossRef] [PubMed]
74. Hayden, K.M.; Norton, M.C.; Darcey, D.; Ostbye, T.; Zandi, P.P.; Breitner, J.C.; Welsh-Bohmer, K.A.; Cache County Study, I. Occupational exposure to pesticides increases the risk of incident AD: The Cache County study. *Neurology* **2010**, *74*, 1524–1530. [CrossRef]
75. Jones, N. Alzheimer disease: Risk of dementia and Alzheimer disease increases with occupational pesticide exposure. *Nat. Rev. Neurol.* **2010**, *6*, 353. [CrossRef]
76. Tanzi, R.E. The genetics of Alzheimer disease. *Cold Spring Harb. Perspect. Med.* **2012**, *2*, a006296. [CrossRef]
77. Blatter, M.C.; James, R.W.; Messmer, S.; Barja, F.; Pometta, D. Identification of a distinct human high-density lipoprotein subspecies defined by a lipoprotein-associated protein, K-45. Identity of K-45 with paraoxonase. *Eur. J. Biochem.* **1993**, *211*, 871–879. [CrossRef]
78. Oakley, H.; Cole, S.L.; Logan, S.; Maus, E.; Shao, P.; Craft, J.; Guillozet-Bongaarts, A.; Ohno, M.; Disterhoft, J.; Van Eldik, L.; et al. Intraneuronal beta-amyloid aggregates, neurodegeneration, and neuron loss in transgenic mice with five familial Alzheimer's disease mutations: Potential factors in amyloid plaque formation. *J. Neurosci.* **2006**, *26*, 10129–10140. [CrossRef]
79. Khayati, K.; Antikainen, H.; Bonder, E.M.; Weber, G.F.; Kruger, W.D.; Jakubowski, H.; Dobrowolski, R. The amino acid metabolite homocysteine activates mTORC1 to inhibit autophagy and form abnormal proteins in human neurons and mice. *FASEB J.* **2017**, *31*, 598–609. [CrossRef]
80. Yates, S.C.; Zafar, A.; Hubbard, P.; Nagy, S.; Durant, S.; Bicknell, R.; Wilcock, G.; Christie, S.; Esiri, M.M.; Smith, A.D.; et al. Dysfunction of the mTOR pathway is a risk factor for Alzheimer's disease. *Acta Neuropathol. Commun.* **2013**, *1*, 3. [CrossRef]
81. Chen, X.; Wang, S.; Zhou, Y.; Han, Y.; Li, S.; Xu, Q.; Xu, L.; Zhu, Z.; Deng, Y.; Yu, L.; et al. Phf8 histone demethylase deficiency causes cognitive impairments through the mTOR pathway. *Nat. Commun.* **2018**, *9*, 114. [CrossRef] [PubMed]
82. Witucki, L.; Jakubowski, H. Homocysteine metabolites inhibit autophagy, elevate amyloid beta, and induce neuropathy by impairing Phf8/H4K20me1-dependent epigenetic regulation of mTOR in cystathionine β-synthase-deficient mice. *J. Inherit. Metab. Dis.* **2023**, *46*, 1114–1130. [CrossRef] [PubMed]
83. Jakubowski, H. Homocysteine Thiolactone Detoxifying Enzymes and Alzheimer's Disease. *Int. J. Mol. Sci.* **2024**, *25*, 8095. [CrossRef] [PubMed]
84. Perla-Kajan, J.; Jakubowski, H. Paraoxonase 1 protects against protein N-homocysteinylation in humans. *FASEB J.* **2010**, *24*, 931–936. [CrossRef]
85. Jakubowski, H.; Perla-Kajan, J.; Finnell, R.H.; Cabrera, R.M.; Wang, H.; Gupta, S.; Kruger, W.D.; Kraus, J.P.; Shih, D.M. Genetic or nutritional disorders in homocysteine or folate metabolism increase protein N-homocysteinylation in mice. *FASEB J.* **2009**, *23*, 1721–1727. [CrossRef]
86. Smith, A.D.; Refsum, H. Homocysteine—From disease biomarker to disease prevention. *J. Intern. Med.* **2021**, *290*, 826–854. [CrossRef]
87. Cagnin, A.; Leon, A.; Vianello, D.; Colavito, D.; Favaretto, S.; Zarantonello, G.; Stecca, A.; Ermani, M.; Zambon, A. LDL density and oxidation are modulated by PON1 promoter genotype in patients with Alzheimer's disease. *J. Alzheimer's Dis.* **2013**, *34*, 377–385. [CrossRef]
88. Forner, A.; Reig, M.; Bruix, J. Hepatocellular carcinoma. *Lancet* **2018**, *391*, 1301–1314. [CrossRef]
89. Mackness, M.I.; Durrington, P.N.; Mackness, B. The role of paraoxonase 1 activity in cardiovascular disease: Potential for therapeutic intervention. *Am. J. Cardiovasc. Drugs* **2004**, *4*, 211–217. [CrossRef]
90. Mackness, M.I.; Arrol, S.; Durrington, P.N. Paraoxonase prevents accumulation of lipoperoxides in low-density lipoprotein. *FEBS Lett.* **1991**, *286*, 152–154. [CrossRef]
91. Watson, A.D.; Berliner, J.A.; Hama, S.Y.; La Du, B.N.; Faull, K.F.; Fogelman, A.M.; Navab, M. Protective effect of high density lipoprotein associated paraoxonase. Inhibition of the biological activity of minimally oxidized low density lipoprotein. *J. Clin. Investig.* **1995**, *96*, 2882–2891. [CrossRef] [PubMed]
92. Aviram, M.; Rosenblat, M.; Bisgaier, C.L.; Newton, R.S.; Primo-Parmo, S.L.; La Du, B.N. Paraoxonase inhibits high-density lipoprotein oxidation and preserves its functions. A possible peroxidative role for paraoxonase. *J. Clin. Investig.* **1998**, *101*, 1581–1590. [CrossRef] [PubMed]

93. Aviram, M.; Billecke, S.; Sorenson, R.; Bisgaier, C.; Newton, R.; Rosenblat, M.; Erogul, J.; Hsu, C.; Dunlop, C.; La Du, B. Paraoxonase active site required for protection against LDL oxidation involves its free sulfhydryl group and is different from that required for its arylesterase/paraoxonase activities: Selective action of human paraoxonase allozymes Q and R. *Arterioscler. Thromb. Vasc. Biol.* **1998**, *18*, 1617–1624. [CrossRef] [PubMed]
94. Bayrak, A.; Bayrak, T.; Bodur, E.; Kilinc, K.; Demirpence, E. The effect of HDL-bound and free PON1 on copper-induced LDL oxidation. *Chem. Biol. Interact.* **2016**, *257*, 141–146. [CrossRef]
95. Aviram, M.; Rosenblat, M. Paraoxonases 1, 2, and 3, oxidative stress, and macrophage foam cell formation during atherosclerosis development. *Free Radic. Biol. Med.* **2004**, *37*, 1304–1316. [CrossRef]
96. Liu, Y.; Mackness, B.; Mackness, M. Comparison of the ability of paraoxonases 1 and 3 to attenuate the in vitro oxidation of low-density lipoprotein and reduce macrophage oxidative stress. *Free Radic. Biol. Med.* **2008**, *45*, 743–748. [CrossRef]
97. Kornberg, A. Ten commandments of enzymology, amended. *Trends Biochem. Sci.* **2003**, *28*, 515–517. [CrossRef]
98. Kresge, N.; Simoni, R.D.; Hill, R.L. Unraveling the Enzymology of Oxidative Phosphorylation: The Work of Efraim Racker. *J. Biol. Chem.* **2006**, *281*, e4–e6. [CrossRef]
99. Marathe, G.K.; Zimmerman, G.A.; McIntyre, T.M. Platelet-activating factor acetylhydrolase, and not paraoxonase-1, is the oxidized phospholipid hydrolase of high density lipoprotein particles. *J. Biol. Chem.* **2003**, *278*, 3937–3947. [CrossRef]
100. Ahmed, Z.; Ravandi, A.; Maguire, G.F.; Emili, A.; Draganov, D.; La Du, B.N.; Kuksis, A.; Connelly, P.W. Apolipoprotein A-I promotes the formation of phosphatidylcholine core aldehydes that are hydrolyzed by paraoxonase (PON-1) during high density lipoprotein oxidation with a peroxynitrite donor. *J. Biol. Chem.* **2001**, *276*, 24473–24481. [CrossRef]
101. Ahmed, Z.; Ravandi, A.; Maguire, G.F.; Emili, A.; Draganov, D.; La Du, B.N.; Kuksis, A.; Connelly, P.W. Multiple substrates for paraoxonase-1 during oxidation of phosphatidylcholine by peroxynitrite. *Biochem. Biophys. Res. Commun.* **2002**, *290*, 391–396. [CrossRef] [PubMed]
102. Ahmed, Z.; Babaei, S.; Maguire, G.F.; Draganov, D.; Kuksis, A.; La Du, B.N.; Connelly, P.W. Paraoxonase-1 reduces monocyte chemotaxis and adhesion to endothelial cells due to oxidation of palmitoyl, linoleoyl glycerophosphorylcholine. *Cardiovasc. Res.* **2003**, *57*, 225–231. [CrossRef] [PubMed]
103. Teiber, J.F.; Draganov, D.I.; La Du, B.N. Purified human serum PON1 does not protect LDL against oxidation in the in vitro assays initiated with copper or AAPH. *J. Lipid Res.* **2004**, *45*, 2260–2268. [CrossRef] [PubMed]
104. Connelly, P.W.; Draganov, D.; Maguire, G.F. Paraoxonase-1 does not reduce or modify oxidation of phospholipids by peroxynitrite. *Free Radic. Biol. Med.* **2005**, *38*, 164–174. [CrossRef] [PubMed]
105. Rodrigo, L.; Mackness, B.; Durrington, P.N.; Hernandez, A.; Mackness, M.I. Hydrolysis of platelet-activating factor by human serum paraoxonase. *Biochem. J.* **2001**, *354 Pt 1*, 1–7. [CrossRef]
106. Mashima, R.; Yamamoto, Y.; Yoshimura, S. Reduction of phosphatidylcholine hydroperoxide by apolipoprotein A-I: Purification of the hydroperoxide-reducing proteins from human blood plasma. *J. Lipid Res.* **1998**, *39*, 1133–1140. [CrossRef]
107. Rye, K.A.; Barter, P.J. Cardioprotective functions of HDLs. *J. Lipid Res.* **2014**, *55*, 168–179. [CrossRef]
108. Garner, B.; Waldeck, A.R.; Witting, P.K.; Rye, K.A.; Stocker, R. Oxidation of high density lipoproteins. II. Evidence for direct reduction of lipid hydroperoxides by methionine residues of apolipoproteins AI and AII. *J. Biol. Chem.* **1998**, *273*, 6088–6095. [CrossRef] [PubMed]
109. Panzenbock, U.; Stocker, R. Formation of methionine sulfoxide-containing specific forms of oxidized high-density lipoproteins. *Biochim. Biophys. Acta* **2005**, *1703*, 171–181. [CrossRef]
110. Graham, A.; Hassall, D.G.; Rafique, S.; Owen, J.S. Evidence for a paraoxonase-independent inhibition of low-density lipoprotein oxidation by high-density lipoprotein. *Atherosclerosis* **1997**, *135*, 193–204. [CrossRef]
111. Suszynska-Zajczyk, J.; Luczak, M.; Marczak, L.; Jakubowski, H. Hyperhomocysteinemia and bleomycin hydrolase modulate the expression of mouse brain proteins involved in neurodegeneration. *J. Alzheimer's Dis.* **2014**, *40*, 713–726. [CrossRef] [PubMed]
112. Suszynska-Zajczyk, J.; Jakubowski, H. Paraoxonase 1 and dietary hyperhomocysteinemia modulate the expression of mouse proteins involved in liver homeostasis. *Acta Biochim. Pol.* **2014**, *61*, 815–823. [CrossRef] [PubMed]
113. Suszynska-Zajczyk, J.; Sikora, M.; Jakubowski, H. Paraoxonase 1 deficiency and hyperhomocysteinemia alter the expression of mouse kidney proteins involved in renal disease. *Mol. Genet. Metab.* **2014**, *113*, 200–206. [CrossRef]
114. Sikora, M.; Jakubowski, H. Changes in redox plasma proteome of Pon1-/- mice are exacerbated by a hyperhomocysteinemic diet. *Free Radic. Biol. Med.* **2021**, *169*, 169–180. [CrossRef] [PubMed]
115. Cao, J.; Xu, Y.; Li, F.; Shang, L.; Fan, D.; Yu, H. Protein markers of dysfunctional HDL in scavenger receptor class B type I deficient mice. *J. Transl. Med.* **2018**, *16*, 155. [CrossRef] [PubMed]
116. Liu, Q.; Xiao, J.J.; Wang, S.; Li, Y.; Yang, L.J.; Lu, Q.Y.; Wu, X.Y.; Cao, J.; Yu, H.; Zhang, B.F. Paraoxonase 1 Ameliorates Renal Lipotoxicity by Activating Lipophagy and Inhibiting Pyroptosis. *Am. J. Pathol.* **2022**, *192*, 1531–1545. [CrossRef]
117. Zhao, X.J.; Liu, L.C.; Guo, C.; Shen, W.W.; Cao, J.; Du, F.; Wu, D.F.; Yu, H. Hepatic paraoxonase 1 ameliorates dysfunctional high-density lipoprotein and atherosclerosis in scavenger receptor class B type I deficient mice. *Ann. Transl. Med.* **2021**, *9*, 1063. [CrossRef]
118. Yuhanna, I.S.; Zhu, Y.; Cox, B.E.; Hahner, L.D.; Osborne-Lawrence, S.; Lu, P.; Marcel, Y.L.; Anderson, R.G.; Mendelsohn, M.E.; Hobbs, H.H.; et al. High-density lipoprotein binding to scavenger receptor-BI activates endothelial nitric oxide synthase. *Nat. Med.* **2001**, *7*, 853–857. [CrossRef] [PubMed]

119. Trigatti, B.L.; Fuller, M. HDL signaling and protection against coronary artery atherosclerosis in mice. *J. Biomed. Res.* **2016**, *30*, 94–100.
120. Seetharam, D.; Mineo, C.; Gormley, A.K.; Gibson, L.L.; Vongpatanasin, W.; Chambliss, K.L.; Hahner, L.D.; Cummings, M.L.; Kitchens, R.L.; Marcel, Y.L.; et al. High-density lipoprotein promotes endothelial cell migration and reendothelialization via scavenger receptor-B type I. *Circ. Res.* **2006**, *98*, 63–72. [CrossRef]
121. Ng, D.S.; Chu, T.; Esposito, B.; Hui, P.; Connelly, P.W.; Gross, P.L. Paraoxonase-1 deficiency in mice predisposes to vascular inflammation, oxidative stress, and thrombogenicity in the absence of hyperlipidemia. *Cardiovasc. Pathol.* **2008**, *17*, 226–232. [CrossRef]
122. Acton, S.; Rigotti, A.; Landschulz, K.T.; Xu, S.; Hobbs, H.H.; Krieger, M. Identification of scavenger receptor SR-BI as a high density lipoprotein receptor. *Science* **1996**, *271*, 518–520. [CrossRef]
123. Zanoni, P.; Khetarpal, S.A.; Larach, D.B.; Hancock-Cerutti, W.F.; Millar, J.S.; Cuchel, M.; DerOhannessian, S.; Kontush, A.; Surendran, P.; Saleheen, D.; et al. Rare variant in scavenger receptor BI raises HDL cholesterol and increases risk of coronary heart disease. *Science* **2016**, *351*, 1166–1171. [CrossRef] [PubMed]
124. Zhang, Y.; Da Silva, J.R.; Reilly, M.; Billheimer, J.T.; Rothblat, G.H.; Rader, D.J. Hepatic expression of scavenger receptor class B type I (SR-BI) is a positive regulator of macrophage reverse cholesterol transport in vivo. *J. Clin. Investig.* **2005**, *115*, 2870–2874. [CrossRef] [PubMed]
125. Leiva, A.; Verdejo, H.; Benitez, M.L.; Martinez, A.; Busso, D.; Rigotti, A. Mechanisms regulating hepatic SR-BI expression and their impact on HDL metabolism. *Atherosclerosis* **2011**, *217*, 299–307. [CrossRef]
126. Van Eck, M.; Hoekstra, M.; Hildebrand, R.B.; Yaong, Y.; Stengel, D.; Kruijt, J.K.; Sattler, W.; Tietge, U.J.; Ninio, E.; Van Berkel, T.J.; et al. Increased oxidative stress in scavenger receptor BI knockout mice with dysfunctional HDL. *Arterioscler. Thromb. Vasc. Biol.* **2007**, *27*, 2413–2419. [CrossRef] [PubMed]
127. Chester, J.; Johnston, E.; Walker, D.; Jones, M.; Ionescu, C.M.; Wagle, S.R.; Kovacevic, B.; Brown, D.; Mikov, M.; Mooranian, A.; et al. A Review on Recent Advancement on Age-Related Hearing Loss: The Applications of Nanotechnology, Drug Pharmacology, and Biotechnology. *Pharmaceutics* **2021**, *13*, 1041. [CrossRef]
128. Miettinen, H.E.; Rayburn, H.; Krieger, M. Abnormal lipoprotein metabolism and reversible female infertility in HDL receptor (SR-BI)-deficient mice. *J. Clin. Investig.* **2001**, *108*, 1717–1722. [CrossRef]
129. Ruan, X.Z.; Varghese, Z.; Moorhead, J.F. An update on the lipid nephrotoxicity hypothesis. *Nat. Rev. Nephrol.* **2009**, *5*, 713–721. [CrossRef]
130. Rodrigo, L.; Hernandez, A.F.; Lopez-Caballero, J.J.; Gil, F.; Pla, A. Immunohistochemical evidence for the expression and induction of paraoxonase in rat liver, kidney, lung and brain tissue. Implications for its physiological role. *Chem. Biol. Interact.* **2001**, *137*, 123–137. [CrossRef]
131. Miljkovic, M.; Stefanovic, A.; Vekic, J.; Zeljkovic, A.; Gojkovic, T.; Simic-Ogrizovic, S.; Bogavac-Stanojevic, N.; Cerne, D.; Ilic, J.; Stefanovic, I.; et al. Activity of paraoxonase 1 (PON1) on HDL(2) and HDL(3) subclasses in renal disease. *Clin. Biochem.* **2018**, *60*, 52–58. [CrossRef] [PubMed]
132. Kontush, A.; Lindahl, M.; Lhomme, M.; Calabresi, L.; Chapman, M.J.; Davidson, W.S. Structure of HDL: Particle subclasses and molecular components. *Handb. Exp. Pharmacol.* **2015**, *224*, 3–51. [PubMed]
133. Huuskonen, J.; Olkkonen, V.M.; Jauhiainen, M.; Ehnholm, C. The impact of phospholipid transfer protein (PLTP) on HDL metabolism. *Atherosclerosis* **2001**, *155*, 269–281. [CrossRef] [PubMed]

antioxidants

MDPI

Article

Healthier Lipid Profiles of Japanese Adults, Especially in Women with Elevated High-Density Lipoprotein Cholesterol (HDL-C), Are Associated with Low HDL-C Peroxide Content

Loni Berkowitz-Fiebich [1], Shelby M. Flaherty [2], Shinobu Kitayama [3], Mayumi Karasawa [4], Norito Kawakami [5], Attilio Rigotti [1] and Christopher L. Coe [6,*]

1 Departamento de Nutricion Diabetes y Metabolismo, Potificia Universidad Catolica de Chile, Santiago 8320165, Chile; lberkowi@uc.cl (L.B.-F.); arigotti@med.puc.cl (A.R.)
2 Department of Surgery, Duke University, Durham, NC 27708, USA; shelby.flaherty@duke.edu
3 Department of Psychology, University of Michigan, Ann Arbor, MI 48109, USA; kitayama@umich.edu
4 Department of Comparative Psychology, Tokyo Woman's Christian University, Tokyo 167-004, Japan; mayumik@lab.twcu.ac.jp
5 Department of Mental Health, University of Tokyo, Tokyo 113-8654, Japan; norito@m.u-tokyo.ac.jp
6 Department of Psychology, University of Wisconsin-Madison, 1202 West Johnson Street, Madison, WI 53706, USA
* Correspondence: ccoe@wisc.edu

Abstract: Japanese adults typically have healthier lipid profiles than American and European adults and a lower prevalence and later onset of atherosclerotic cardiovascular disease (ASCVD). Many Japanese also have uniquely elevated levels of high-density lipoprotein cholesterol (HDL-C). The following analysis examined the relationship between HDL-C level and HDL-C peroxide content, a bioindicator of unhealthy lipid metabolism in Japanese adults. Blood samples were collected from 463 participants, 31–84 years of age, who lived in Tokyo. A second blood sample was collected 5 years later from 241 of the participants, allowing us to evaluate the temporal stability of the inverse correlation between HDL-C level and HDL-C peroxide content. Glucoregulation and inflammatory activity were assessed because both can be associated with dyslipidemia and HDL-C dysfunction. Obesity and central adiposity were also considered. Overall, women had healthier HDL-C profiles than men. Elevated HDL-C (>90 mg/dL) was common (16.6%) and found more often in women. Higher HDL-C peroxide content was associated with older age and central adiposity and incremented further when HA1c and CRP were higher. When assessed 5 years later, lower HDL-C peroxide content continued to be evident in adults with higher HDL-C. While similar associations have been described for other populations, most Japanese adults typically had healthier levels of HDL-C with lower HDL-C peroxide content than previously reported for American adults.

Keywords: Japan; high-density lipoprotein cholesterol; HDL peroxide content; aging; sex; obesity; lipid peroxidation

1. Introduction

Ever since the seven countries study was initiated in the 1950s, it has been known that there is a lower prevalence of atherosclerotic cardiovascular disease (ASCVD) in Japan than in many other countries, and that most Japanese adults typically have healthier lipid profiles than found in other populations [1–3]. Some health benefits can be attributed to the Japanese diet and the relatively low occurrence of obesity [4–6]. In addition, there are national programs that encourage engagement in physical activity, including walking, and an effective universal health care delivery system. However, there is also evidence for a genetic basis for some population-level differences in lipid physiology. Many studies have documented that lipid profiles are already distinct in young Japanese children [7,8]. Similarly, while cholesterol levels change when Japanese adults reside in other countries and eat the local cuisine, their cholesterol values and disease risks continue to differ from the indigenous populations [9–13]. Historically, elevated levels of low-density lipoprotein cholesterol (LDL-C) were considered the primary risk factor for the pathogenesis of ASCVD [14,15]. However, there is now an increased awareness of the importance of the atheroprotective benefits of HDL-C and the deleterious consequences of having low levels of HDL-C [16]. Many Japanese adults have higher levels of HDL-C than typically seen in other populations [17–19]. The following analysis was designed to further characterize the lipid profiles of middle-aged and older adult residents of Tokyo with a focus on HDL-C. This assessment provided an opportunity to examine whether the benefits of higher HDL-C would increase in a linear and progressive manner or if there would be a biphasic association with health and HDL-C peroxide content when HDL-C levels were very elevated [20–22]. Studies of European and American adults have indicated that elevated HDL-C levels may be associated with an increased hazard risk for all-cause mortality, suggestive of dysfunctional HDL-C, although the specific link to ASCVD is usually more evident when HDL-C is low [23,24].

The anti-atherogenic benefits of HDL-C are due primarily to its involvement in the efflux of cholesterol from peripheral tissues and the reverse transport of this excess cholesterol to the liver for excretion by the gut, which limits deposition on the vasculature and reduces lipid accumulation in activated macrophages. HDL-C also has additional anti-oxidative and anti-inflammatory functions, moderating the oxidation of LDL-C [25]. HDL-C can become dysfunctional with the onset of Type 2 diabetes and fatty liver disease, and its beneficial actions can be undermined by unhealthy lifestyles, such as excessive alcohol consumption, and by increased inflammatory activity [26–28]. The health-promoting actions of HDL-C are associated with its particle size and composition, which can be impacted by oxidative stress, leading to lipid peroxidation and a build-up of reactive oxygen species, hydrogen peroxides, and superoxides [29–31]. One novel feature of the biomarker panel employed in our analyses was the inclusion of an assay to index lipid peroxidation by determining the peroxide content of HDL-C. This cell-free, fluorometric method was developed originally to evaluate the side effects of anti-viral treatments on cholesterol structures and levels in HIV-infected patients [32]. It was also shown to sensitively reflect improvements in lipid metabolism in obese patients after bariatric surgery and weight loss [33]. The protocol was then adapted for high throughput processing of sera to examine the peroxide content of HDL-C in a survey of middle-aged and older Americans [34]. That study showed that HDL-C peroxide content was associated with the adverse effects of obesity, diabetes, and aging on lipid metabolism.

The primary aim of the following analysis was to evaluate the lipid and health profiles of adult Japanese residents of Tokyo and to investigate the influence of age and sex. The effects of adiposity, poor glycemic control and increased inflammatory activity were also examined as possible mediators of the variation in lipid profiles. In addition, a further goal was to explore the potentially distinctive aspects of lipid physiology in Japanese adults who had particularly high HDL-C levels. There have been many prior reports on Japanese adults with HDL-C elevated above 80–90 mg/dL [35,36], which were linked to the actions of genes associated with cholesteryl ester transfer protein (CETP). CETP transfers cholesterol from HDL-C to apolipoprotein-B, containing lipoproteins (i.e., VLDL and LDL) [36]. Patients with CETP deficiency were first identified in Japan in 1985 when examining individuals who had extremely high HDL-C [37]. Several studies have indicated that some CETP polymorphisms convey a risk for poor health, but the findings specifically on hypertension and ASCVD are inconsistent. Our analyses compared adults with HDL-C levels above 90 mg/dL to participants with HDL-C in the more typical range, specifically to assess the possible association with HDL-C peroxide content.

2. Methods

2.1. Participants

The 463 participants (247 female and 216 male) were a subset of 1684 middle-aged and older adults in the Midlife in Japan (MIDJA) study. They were recruited with random survey methods in 2008 and 2013 to represent the age and sex composition of the 23 residential wards of Tokyo (Table 1). Demographic variables and information about psychological measures and the use of prescription medications were obtained from all respondents by a questionnaire [38]. Individuals who consented to participate in the biomarker subproject provided blood samples at either a medical clinic or a laboratory at the University of Tokyo. The mean age of adults in this lipid profile analysis was 56.4 years (S.D. = 13.9 years, range: 31–84 years). Blood samples were also obtained 5 years later from 241 of the adults recruited in 2008, providing an opportunity to assess the stability of their lipid profiles. All procedures were approved by the Health Sciences Institutional Review Board at the University of Wisconsin as well as re-reviewed and approved by the Ethics Committee at the University of Tokyo (see IRB Statement and Informed Consent Statement for details).

Table 1. Number of female and male participants at the first biomarker assessment and the longitudinal follow-up 5 years later. Number of individuals who reported taking prescription medications or supplements that could have cholesterol-lowering effects is also shown.

	Baseline			Follow-Up		
	Female	Male	Total	Female	Male	Total
Participant Number	247	216	463	138	103	241
No/Yes Meds *	30/217	18/198	48/415	16/172	8/95	41/217

* Medicine and supplement use was considered as a covariate in the regression modeling.

2.2. Demographic Information and Prescription Medications

Age, sex, marital status, and educational attainment were determined for all participants. The average age and sex distribution in the biomarker subproject did not differ from that of the participants in the general survey. The statistical modeling of biological predictors of HDL-C peroxide content included a covariate for prescription medication use, based on the self-reporting of drugs and/or supplements that might have lipid-lowering actions (e.g., antihyperlipidemic agents, cholesterol absorption inhibitors, HMC-CoA reductase inhibitors, bile acid sequestrants, fibrates, niacin, and omega-3). Forty-eight of the 463 participants reported taking one or more of these medications and supplements.

2.3. Sample Collection

Blood was obtained from 247 women and 216 men for the biomarker assessments. Because many participants worked, it was not possible to obtain samples in the very early morning following an overnight fast. However, recent studies have shown that fasting has only a modest effect on total cholesterol and HDL-C test results, with the consumption of a recent meal primarily affecting triglyceride levels [39,40]. Over 95% of the samples were collected between 0900 and 1145, with most of the remainder by 1330. Only 8 samples were collected in the afternoon, all before 1530. During the visit, height and weight were measured and used to calculate body mass index (BMI, weight/height, kg/m^2). Waist circumference was determined as an indicator of central adiposity. Systolic and diastolic blood pressure was also recorded during the visit.

2.4. Lipid Panel and HDL-C Peroxide Content

A traditional lipid panel, including total cholesterol, HDL-C, LDL-C, and triglyceride levels (mg/dL), was obtained at the clinical laboratory of the Showa University School of Medicine (Tokyo, Japan). In addition, frozen sera were stored in an ultracold freezer and shipped using an overnight courier on dry ice for analysis in the United States. One hundred lipid panels were ordered from a CLIA-certified clinical laboratory (Unity Health-

Meriter Laboratory, Madison, WI, USA) to confirm that the lipid values determined in Tokyo were comparable to diagnostic testing in the U.S. (Figures S1 and S2).

The assays to determine HDL-C peroxide content were all conducted at one laboratory (Biomarker Core, Madison, WI, USA). The methods for generating this measure of lipid peroxidation have been published previously [32]. Briefly, a fixed volume protocol was adapted from the fluorescence assay used to assess HDL-C composition in patients, both lipid dysfunction in HIV-infected individuals on anti-viral medications, as well as the beneficial changes in obese adolescents after bariatric surgeries and weight loss [32,33]. Adaptations to optimize procedures for high throughput processing included the use of 96-well, Greiner polypropylene round bottom plates (Sigma-Aldrich, Milwaukee, WI, USA), and the inclusion of a positive control with purified HDL-C on each plate (Lee Biosolutions, Maryland Heights, MO, USA). The control HDL-C was maintained at a stock concentration of 2070 mg/dL and diluted to working concentrations of 300 mg/dL using 0.15 NaCl for each assay. Participant samples were assayed in triplicate on the same plate (CV < 0.5%). Sera were prepared by depleting apoB-containing particles via precipitation using dextran sulfate and magnesium chloride at concentrations of 2 μM and 50 mM, respectively (Millipore Sigma, Burlington, MA, USA). Fluorescence was measured with a Biotek Synergy H1 fluorimeter (Agilent, Santa Clara, CA, USA) at 530 nm and 590 nm wavelengths, and fluorescence at 2 h was used in the analysis. Quantification of HDL-C for the HDL-C positive control and ensuring HDL-C levels in the serum aliquots were concordant with the clinical laboratory value were performed with a WAKO Cholesterol E kit (Fujifilm Pure Chemical Corp., Tokyo, Japan), using a MRX^e DYNEX microplate reader (Magellan Biosciences, Chantilly, VA, USA). HDL peroxide content values were generated with the following calculations:

1. Fluorescence in sample minus fluorescence in blank = peroxidized HDL-C in participant sera, quantified in fluorescence units (FU).
2. FU/ HDL-C in sample = normalized peroxidized HDL-C per 1 mg/dL HDL-C (FU/mg HDL-C), the primary unit of quantification.
3. HDL-C peroxide content = normalized, peroxidized HDL-C per 1 mg/dL HDL-C in sera (FU per mg/dL HDL-C)/ standardized HDL-C peroxide content in a purified reference control. Steps 2 and 3 were performed with respect to the HDL-C level in the sera. The same pool of purified HDL-C was included in every assay as a common reference point for harmonizing values across assays given the large number of samples.

2.5. Additional Biomarkers

Glycosylated hemoglobin (HA1c) was determined from fresh, whole blood on the day of collection at the clinical laboratory of the Showa University School of Medicine (Tokyo, Japan). To ensure comparability with the diagnostic values generated by clinical laboratories in the U.S., aliquots from 10 blood samples were shipped overnight on cold refrigerant blocks and tested on arrival at the Unity Health-Meriter Laboratory (Madison, WI, USA). HA1c was determined by using a turbidimetric immunoinhibition assay. The test results from the two laboratories were highly correlated ($r = 0.85$, $p < 0.01$), but because the assay calibration scales were different, an algorithm was generated to calibrate the values to match HA1c testing in U.S. clinical studies (Figure S3). This adjustment did not change the relative ranking of HA1c values, nor alter the position on the continuum from low to high. A cutoff of 6.5% was used to identify individuals showing signs of insulin resistance and poor glycemic control [41].

Serum IL-6 levels were determined by a high-sensitivity enzyme-linked immunosorbent assay (Quantikine ELISA, R&D Systems, Minneapolis, MN, USA), with a lower sensitivity of detection at 0.16 pg/mL. All values were quantified in duplicate; values over 10 pg/mL were re-run in diluted sera to fall on the standard curve. The intra-assay coefficient of variance (CV) was 4.1%, and the inter-assay CV was 12.9%. High-sensitivity CRP was assessed with a particle-enhanced immunonephelometric assay at the Laboratory of Clinical Biochemistry Research (University of Vermont, Burlington, VT, USA). Briefly, polystyrene particles were coated with monoclonal antibodies to CRP, which resulted in an antigen agglutinate in the presence of CRP and increased light intensity, which was quantified with a BNII nephelometer (Seimans Healthcare Diagnostics, Deerfield, IL, USA). The assay range was 0.16–1100 mg/L; the intra-assay CV range was 2.3–4.4%, and the inter-assay CV ranged from 2.1 to 5.7%.

2.6. Statistical Analysis

Descriptive statistics, including means and variance indices, were generated for all variables and examined for outliers. Predictors and endpoints evincing skewness were log-transformed to normalize the distribution. Data from all participants were retained to include the continuum from healthy to unhealthy and to ensure the findings were representative of the adult residents in Tokyo. Sex and age differences in predictor and endpoint variables were examined initially with two-way analyses of variance (ANOVA: female vs. male in 3 age categories, <50, 51–64, >65 years, respectively). To interrogate the primary predictors of HDL-C peroxide content, a series of six hierarchical regression models were run, sequentially adding in the following predictors: sex (male as reference), age, HA1c, CRP, waist circumference, and non-HDL-C. The possible influence of lipid-lowering medications and supplements that could affect HDL-C level and compositions was considered by including a binary covariate in the modeling (i.e., Yes/No for use of antihyperlipidemic agents, cholesterol absorption inhibitors, HMC-CoA reductase inhibitors, bile acid sequestrants, fibrates, niacin, omega-3, etc.). Differences in HDL-C peroxide content between adults with extremely high HDL-C and those with HDL-C in a more typical range were then compared by a 3-way ANOVA, including HDL-C level (<89 and >90 mg/dL), gender (female vs male) and age (3 levels: <50, 51–64, >65 years), as the between factors. For the participants who provided a second blood sample at follow-up 5 years later, variations in HDL-C and HDL-C peroxide content over time were evaluated with a repeated measures ANOVA. The lipid profiles and HDL-C peroxide content at the two time points were compared in the adults with lower and elevated levels of HDL-C. Pairwise comparisons were conducted with the Pearson's r test. The alpha value for attaining statistical significance was set at <0.05.

3. Results

3.1. Descriptive Statistics

As shown in Table 2, the mean age of the participants at the initial recruitment was 56.4 years, with a range of 31–84 years. The adiposity measurements indicated that obesity with a BMI over 30, or even 25, was not common, but the assessment of waist circumference conveyed that central adiposity increased with age and was more evident in men than women. Mean systolic and diastolic blood pressures were also higher in males and evinced a similar trend to increase with age. Glycemic control, as reflected by glycosylated hemoglobin levels (HA1c), was considered as one of the biological predictors in the statistical modeling of HDL-C peroxide content. Based on HA1c values over 6.5% (>48 mmol/mol), and participant reports of physician-diagnosed diabetes, the prevalence of poor glycemic control was 7%. However, only seven female participants met these criteria, and they were older adults with a mean age of 66.9 years. Forty-eight of the 458 participants reported using prescription drugs and/or supplements that could have lipid-lowering effects. For that reason, medication use was included as a covariate in the regression models that examined predictors of HDL-C peroxide content. Participants taking medications were more likely to be older. Their mean age was 66.6 years as compared to 55.4 years for those not taking medications. It is also noteworthy that the HDL-C peroxide content was higher in the participants who reported taking lipid-lowering and/or hypertensive drugs (9.27 +/−0.63 vs. 7.83 +/−0.17, $p < 0.007$). Thus, these medications did not account for a reduction in the HDL-C peroxide content when HDL-C levels were high. Instead, the results suggested that higher HDL-C peroxide content was associated with poorer health.

Table 2. Descriptive summary of demographic and biomarker variables.

	Female (n = 247)	Male (216)	*p* Values Sex	Age **
Age (yr)	55.1 (0.9) *	58.0 (0.9)	0.025	-
BMI (kg/M^2)	21.7 (0.2)	23.8 (0.2)	0.002	0.0001
WC (cm)	70.9 (0.5)	82.0 (0.6)	0.001	0.0001
HA1c	5.7 (0.03)	5.9 (0.01)	NS	NS
CRP (nmol) ***	5.3 (0.7)	14.1 (2.2)	0.04	NS
IL-6 (pg/mL)	1.5 (0.1)	1.9 (0.2)	0.05	NS
Total Chol (mg/dL)	209.4 (2.3)	202.8 (8.7)	NS	0.0003
HDL-C (mg/dL)	79.0 (1.2)	61.7 (1.2)	0.0001	0.0001
LDL-C (mg/dL)	119.7 (2.3)	118.9 (2.5)	NS	NS
Non-HDL-C (mg/dL)	130.4 (2.3)	143.9 (2.9)	NS	0.004
Triglyceride (mg/dL) ****	109.5 (3.5)	164.0 (7.9)	0.0008	0.05
HDL-C peroxide (FU) *****	7.4 (0.2)	8.7 (0.3)	NS	0.0001
Systolic (mmHg)	120.5 (1.2)	130.3 (1.32)	0.0001	0.0001
Diastolic (mmHg)	74.8 (0.7)	80.3 (0.7)	0.0001	0.0001

* Mean (+S.E.) values. ** Significant effects of Age are shown; the extent of some age effects differed by Sex. *** Mean CRP in metric units was 0.56 (0.07) and 1.48 (0.23) mg/L, respectively). **** TG values may have been influenced by the collection of non-fasted samples. ***** HDL-C peroxide content was quantified in fluorescence units (FU) and calibrated with respect to the level of HDL-C in the sera.

The two inflammatory proteins, CRP and IL-6, were typically low, but the circulating levels of both were significantly higher in men than women (Table 2). Because CRP and IL-6 levels were highly correlated ($r = 0.57$, $p < 0.001$), only CRP was included in the prediction modeling of HDL-C peroxide content. The lipid values of the MIDJA participants were generally in keeping with previous publications on middle-aged and older Japanese adults. Total cholesterol levels were high, often above 200 mg/dL, but HDL-C was a relatively large contributor. High levels of HDL-C moderated the proportion accounted for by non-HDL cholesterol. Although LDL-C values tended to be above norms reported for some other countries, they did not differ between women and men, nor did the level of LDL-C increase significantly with age. In contrast, the triglyceride levels were significantly higher in men than women and did increase with age.

3.2. Effects of Sex and Age on HDL-C and HDL-C Peroxide Content

As shown in Figure 1, women had significantly higher levels of HDL-C than men, especially among the female participants younger than 50 years of age. There was also a significant effect of sex on HDL-C peroxide content, which was more pronounced in the women younger than 64 years of age. HDL-C levels tended to decline with age whereas the HDL-C peroxide content increased with age.

3.3. Predictors of HDL-C Peroxide Content

A hierarchical regression analysis was performed to further explore the influence of age and sex on HDL-C peroxide content, and to probe the additional effects of other factors on this measure of oxidized HDL-C (Table 3). An initial bivariate analysis affirmed the significant effect of sex: being female was associated with lower HDL-C peroxide content (Model 1). When age, which was associated with higher HDL-C peroxide content, was added, the model fit improved (Model 2). The previously detected beneficial effect of being female remained significant. HA1c and CRP, two biomarkers associated with dyslipidemia and HDL-C dysfunction, were then added sequentially to the model. The inclusion of biomarkers indicative of poor glycemic control and inflammatory activity improved the R^2 value without significantly affecting the *p*-value of the overall model (Models 3 and 4, respectively). They did not lessen the influence of sex on HDL-C peroxide content but reduced the amount of variance accounted for by age. Upon adding waist circumference, which was highly correlated with HDL-C peroxide content, the association between sex and

HDL-C peroxide content no longer retained significance (Model 5). However, the overall model's R^2 improved. Moreover, this effect was enhanced further by adding non-HDL cholesterol to the model (Model 6). The level of non-HDL cholesterol was directly associated with HDL-C peroxide content, and its inclusion improved the model fit, independent of the effects of gender on HDL-C peroxide content.

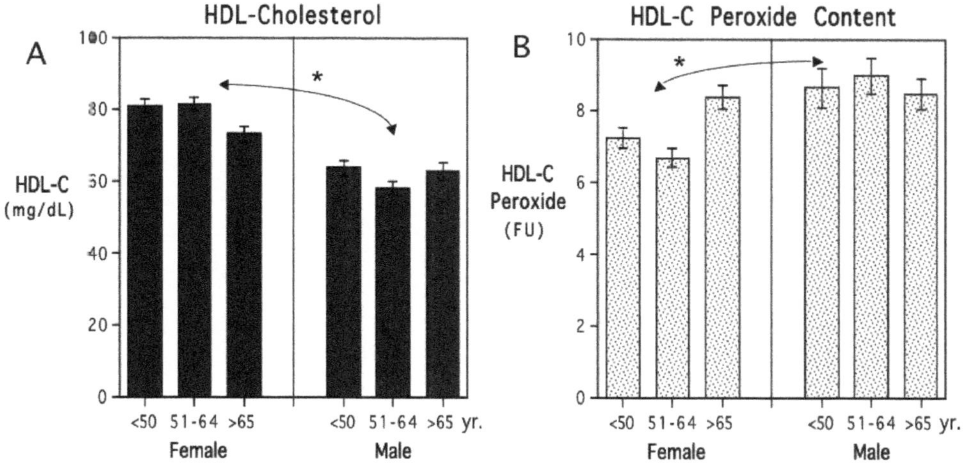

Figure 1. Mean (+/− S.E.) HDL-C and HDL-C peroxide content in female and male adults stratified by age (n = 247 and 216, respectively). Women had significantly higher levels of HDL-C and lower HDL-C peroxide content than men ((**A**,**B**), respectively). Information on other lipids in the panel is provided in Table 2. Participant ages are shown in three categories (<50, 51–64, and >65 years) to illustrate the influence of age, but age was treated as a continuous, parametric variable in the regression models. Asterisk (*) indicates the significant difference between females and males.

Table 3. Hierarchical regression models assessing 6 predictors of HDL-C peroxide content in middle-aged and older Japanese adults.

$HDL\text{-}C_{perox}$		Sex (*Male Ref*)	Age	HA1c	CRP	Waist Circum.	Non-HDL-C	Model *p*-Value	Adjusted R^2
Model 1	Coeff	−0.141						8.9×10^{-5}	0.031
	P	8.9×10^{-5}							
Model 2	Coeff	−0.133	0.003					5.7×10^{-5}	0.037
	P	2.1×10^{-4}	0.041						
Model 3	Coeff	−0.127	0.002	0.365				4.0×10^{-5}	0.043
	P	4×10^{-4}	0.201	0.062					
Model 4	Coeff	−0.108	0.001	0.358	0.027			3.0×10^{-5}	0.047
	P	3.6×10^{-4}	0.330	0.067	0.085				
Model 5	Coeff	0.004	0.007	0.202	0.009	0.011		1.2×10^{-8}	0.085
	P	0.927	0.618	0.301	0.558	1.2×10^{-5}			
Model 6	Coeff	−0.003	0.000	0.106	0.012	0.009	0.002	8.7×10^{-11}	0.109
	P	0.941	0.852	0.584	0.447	5.3×10^{-4}	2.9×10^{-4}		

3.4. Prevalence of Elevated HDL-C and Its Effect on HDL-Peroxide Content

Many Japanese adults had particularly high levels of HLD-C. Values over 90 mg/dL were categorized as elevated, and the potential influence on HDL-C peroxide content was examined. As shown in Table 4, this categorization yielded two dichotomous subgroups with significantly different mean levels of HDL-C (64.4 vs. 103.6 mg/dL, $p < 0.0001$). In addition, the 77 participants (16.6%) with elevated HDL-C also had significantly lower levels of HDL-C peroxide content (5.8 vs. 8.4 FU, $p < 0.0001$). The individuals with elevated HDL-C did not show overt signs of poor health or hypertension, nor did their circulating levels of CRP and IL-6 differ (Table 4). They also had smaller BMIs and waist circumferences, and lower HA1c levels than did the adults with HDL-C levels below 89 mg/dL.

Table 4. Biomarker values in Japanese adults with HDL-C in the typical range (<89 mg/dL) compared to participants who had elevated HDL-C (>90 mg/dL).

	<89 mg/dL	**>90 mg/dL**	
	(n = 386)	**(n = 77)**	*p*
Total Chol (mg/dL)	203.4 (1.9) *	224.7 (3.9)	0.003
HDL-C (mg/dL)	**64.4 (0.8)**	**103.6 (1.4)**	0.0001
LDL-C (mg/dL)	119.3 (1.7)	115.1 (3.6)	NS
Non-HDL (mg/dL)	138.9 (2.0)	121.1 (4.2)	0.004
Trig (mg/dL)	141.3 (5.0)	102.2 (5.6)	0.05
HDL-C peroxide (FU) **	**8.4 (0.2)**	**5.8 (0.2)**	0.0001
BMI (kg/M^2)	23.1 (0.2)	20.5 (0.2)	0.0001
WC (cm)	78.0 (2.5)	69.2 (0.8)	0.0001
HA1c (%)	5.9 (0.04)	5.7 (0.04)	0.0019
CRP (nmol)	9.9 (1.3)	7.1 (2.2)	NS
IL-6 (pg/mL)	1.8 (0.1)	1.4 (0.1)	NS
Systolic BP (mmHg)	125.9 (1.0)	120.5 (2.3)	NS
Diastolic BP (mmHg)	78.1 (0.6)	73.8 (1.3)	NS

* Mean +S.E. values are shown. HDL-C and HDL-C peroxide content highlighted in Bold font. ** HDL-C peroxide content was quantified in fluorescence units (FU) and calibrated with respect to the level of HDL-C in the serum sample. HDL-C peroxide content was significantly lower in adults with very high levels of HDL-C.

Differences between the participants with elevated HDL-C, compared to adults with HDL-C in more typical ranges, are illustrated in Figure 2. The graphs also show the influence of sex and age on the association between the HDL-C level and HDL-C peroxide content. Although an influence of being female on HDL-C peroxide content is evident, the large effect of elevated HDL-C is predominant. There was some synergism with the effect of sex because participants with elevated HDL-C were more likely to be female (25.1% of the females versus 6.9% of the males had HDL-C over 90 mg/dL). When the participants were subdivided into three age categories from youngest to oldest adults, the pervasive relationship between very high levels of HDL-C and lower HDL-C peroxide content was still evident in both women and men. Delineating the lipid data by both sex and age highlighted that low levels of HDL-C peroxide content were most prominent in younger women. It also revealed that the age-related increases in HDL-C peroxide content were clearer in women than men, a maturational trend that was evident in both the women with lower and with elevated HDL-C level.

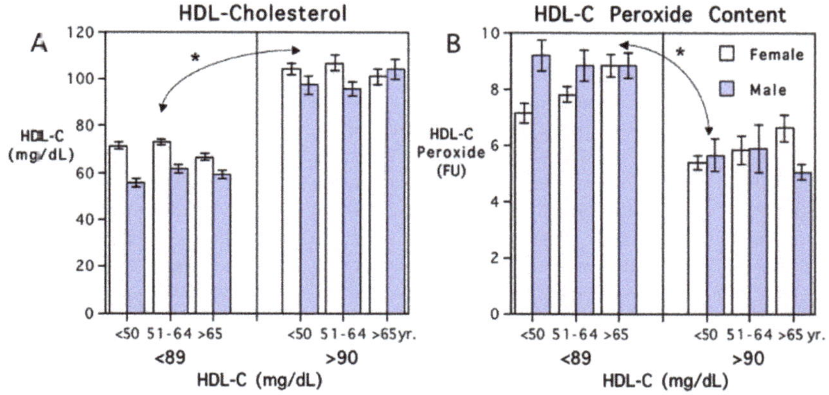

Figure 2. Average levels of HDL-C and HDL-C peroxide content in Japanese adults with HDL-C below 89 mg/dL and with elevated above 90 mg/dL, stratified by age ((**A**,**B**), respectively). Means and S.E. are shown for three age categories. Women had significantly higher levels of HDL-C than men, and a higher percent of the adults with elevated HDL-C were female. Higher HDL-C levels were associated with lower HDL-C peroxide content, and middle-aged women had significantly lower levels of HDL-C peroxide content than men. Asterisk (*) indicates significant difference between participants with HDL-C levels below 89 mg/dL and above 90 mg/dL.

3.5. Stability of Elevated HDL-C and Lower HDL-C Peroxide Content over Time

The persistence of individual differences in HDL-C levels and HDL-C peroxide content was assessed further in the 241 adults who participated in the follow-up analysis. Their mean age at the initial recruitment in 2008 was 55.8 (0.9) years, and they were 60.5 (0.9) years of age at follow-up. Figure 3 shows that their levels of total cholesterol and HDL-C remained similar and were consistent at the two assessments ($r = 0.59$, $p < 0.001$; $r = 0.77$, $p < 0.001$, respectively). Their HDL-C peroxide content values were also significantly correlated at the two assessments ($r = 0.47$, $p < 0.001$). The 43 participants with follow-up samples who had elevated HDL-C (>90 mg/dL) at the first collection also continued to have higher total cholesterol and HDL-C levels and lower HDL-C peroxide content at the second assessment than did the 198 adults with HDL-C values below 89 mg/dL when the first blood was collected ($p < 0.0001$).

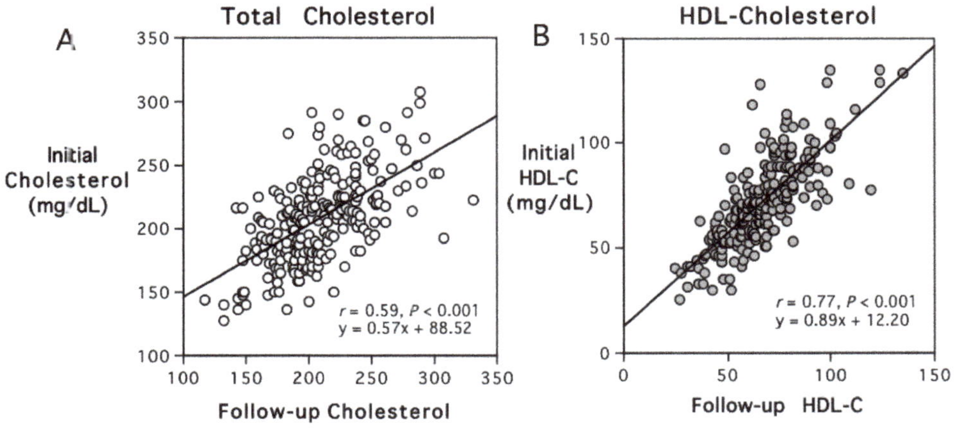

Figure 3. Scatterplots showing the stability of total cholesterol (**A**) and HDL-cholesterol levels (**B**) in the 241 participants evaluated during the initial recruitment phase in 2008 and then at follow-up 5 years later. HDL-C levels are conveyed with gray-fill in the circles.

4. Discussion

Our findings on cholesterol levels in middle-aged and older Tokyo residents align with many previous studies, which showed that the lipid profiles of Japanese adults are generally healthier than those of European populations as well as other East and South Asian countries [42–44]. In particular, the prevalence of high levels of HDL-C in Japan is distinctive and contributes to a comparatively high total cholesterol level that is often above 200 mg/dL [45]. Total cholesterol test results in this range are typically considered unhealthy in other populations due to elevated levels of LDL-C and triglycerides. Given the occurrence of so many high total cholesterol and HDL-C values, we verified that the cholesterol values generated by the clinical laboratory in Tokyo were comparable to test results when the sera were tested again at a CLIA-certified clinical laboratory in the United States (Figures S1 and S2).

In keeping with expectations, women had healthier lipid profiles than men [45,46]. Sex differences in lipid values were associated with the two measures of adiposity, which highlighted the low BMIs and smaller waist circumferences of most Japanese women [47]. In addition, there were sex differences in the levels of the two protein measures of inflammatory activity, CRP and IL-6, as well as in the levels of HA1c, the bioindicator of glycemic control, which can adversely impact lipid metabolism [48–52]. However, it should be reiterated that CRP and IL-6 levels generally tend to be low in both Japanese women and men, and the prevalence of Type 2 diabetes in the MIDJA participants was only 7% [41].

Higher levels of HDL-C were associated with lower HDL-C peroxide content. But it should be acknowledged that there have been mixed findings on whether extremely elevated levels of HDL-C are associated with an increase in ASCVD morbidity and mortality [20–24]. For example, one study of patients with ASCVD found that elevated HDL-C was associated with an increased hazard risk for all-cause mortality, but the association between HDL-C levels and cardiovascular disease was linear, with an increased risk evident only in patients with low HDL-C [24]. Within our study population, comprised primarily of healthy adults, we did not detect the clinical conditions evident in some patients with a hyperalphaliproteinemia diagnosis (HALP) [53]. However, we did not use genotypes to identify the participants with CETP alleles that underlie the elevated HDL-C levels that often occur in many HALP patients. It has been estimated that CETP mutations and the resulting deficiency of CETP may be present in over 30% of Japanese adults who have HDL-C elevated above 80 mg/dL [54,55]. We did not detect any negative consequences of maintaining elevated HDL-C over time among the adults who provided a second blood sample 5 years later. In fact, the adults in the follow-up who had elevated HDL-C above 90 mg/dL had lower blood pressures and HA1c levels. They also had lower BMIs and smaller waist circumferences and tended to have lower CRP and IL-6 levels.

This follow-up assessment demonstrated the stability of the association between higher levels of HDL-C and lower HDL-C peroxide content. However, it should be noted that in the MIDJA participants, very high HDL-C levels occurred more commonly in women than men. HDL-C levels above 90 mg/dL were found in 25.1% of the women versus 6.9% of the men, a sex difference found by others [56]. There was also a pronounced sex difference in the HDL-C peroxide content, which was most evident in the Japanese women younger than 50 years of age. Given that higher HDL-C levels and low HDL-C peroxide were prominent in the younger women, it may reflect the health-promoting effects of estrogen in premenopausal women [48,49]. The healthier lipid profiles of the younger women contributed to clearer age-related trends in HDL-C and HDL-C peroxide content in the female participants, although the rise in central adiposity among many older Japanese men was associated with their higher HDL-C peroxide content.

4.1. Limitations

While our findings on the predictors of HDL-C level and HDL-C peroxide content are in keeping with the common risk factors for ASCVD, including age, sex, obesity, diabetes, and inflammatory activity [42–45], we should acknowledge several limitations. First, we did not obtain detailed dietary records. It is known that nutrition, as well as exercise, can have strong effects on lipid metabolism [57–59]. In addition, we had reported previously that adherence to more traditional diets and lifestyle practices, including drinking green tea, eating seafood regularly, and partaking in relaxing hot baths, reduced the inflammatory physiology of participants in the MIDJA [60]. The current analysis also did not consider the many psychosocial and economic factors that can influence cholesterol levels and risk for ASCVD [61]. The prevalence of ASCVD and diabetes is also known to vary across cities and to differ between urban and rural areas of Japan, reflecting the important effects of socioeconomic factors. Social processes associated with psychological well-being and stress were a major focus of the MIDJA, so these variables can be integrated into future analyses. We consider the current findings to be formative and foundational to further investigation.

Importantly, we should also acknowledge another limitation, which is that we did not include paraoxonase-1 (PON-1) in the biomarker panel. Many constituents of HDL are responsible for its role in preventing atherosclerosis, but PON-1 is among the most important of the lipid-modifying features, accounting for its antioxidant activity, anti-inflammatory, anti-thrombotic, and anti-adhesion properties [62]. Several different PON-1 polymorphisms have been identified in the Japanese population and have been linked to a differential risk for atherogenic dyslipidemia, diabetes, diabetic microvascular complications, stroke, and osteoporosis [63–69]. In addition, PON-1 polymorphisms are associated with a differential sensitivity to salt, which is high in Japanese cuisine, and salt intake contributes to hypertension and risk for stroke [70]. The vulnerability of older Japanese adults to cerebral infarction has also been linked to high triglyceride levels [71,72]. While triglyceride values were determined and were in the typical range for Japanese adults, we did not incorporate them into the current analysis because the levels may have been influenced by not being able to collect blood after an overnight fast.

4.2. Conclusions

Notwithstanding these caveats and the need for additional research, to our knowledge, this study is the first to investigate lipid peroxidation of HDL-C among Japanese adults in a large-scale and representative manner. The ability to employ the HDL-C peroxide assay on cryopreserved serum samples made it a useful test for interrogating how HDL-C may respond to and contribute to metabolic disorders, inflammatory conditions, and ASCVD. Because the same assay of HDL-C-peroxide content was also used in a survey of middle-aged and older American adults [34], it provides a unique opportunity to compare HDL-C levels and HDL-C peroxide content in two countries. As shown in Figure S4, Japanese adults typically had higher levels of HDL-C and lower HDL-C peroxide content, suggestive of population-level differences in lipid peroxidation and antioxidant activity. It is also of interest that women in both countries had lower HDL-C peroxide content, a sex difference that was particularly evident in both Japanese and African American women. Furthermore, it was of value to document the cholesterol profiles of adult residents of Tokyo during the period from 2008 to 2013, proximal to when national health surveys were conducted [73]. Several investigators have reported that the continuation of dietary changes in Japan, including the inclusion of more Westernized foods, along with the adiposity that accompanies the sedentary inactivity of modern life, have led to temporal changes in the lipid values seen in Japanese adults across the last several decades [74–76]. While our findings need to be confirmed with tests of in vivo function and an assessment of long-term clinical outcomes, and the ex vivo determination of HDL-C peroxide content provides only an indirect measure of HDL-C's anti-oxidative potential, the findings offer some insight into how HDL-C will respond and function.

4.3. Clinical Implications

The findings on HDL-C in Japanese adults also affirm the value of considering race and sex when establishing diagnostic norms and the importance of patient diversity when conducting clinical trials. Elevated levels of HDL-C were found more often among Japanese women, typically without overt clinical symptoms, including hypertension. In addition, while extreme obesity was uncommon, the results conveyed that a negative influence of adiposity on lipid metabolism becomes evident in East Asian adults with a lower BMI and smaller waist circumference than for most European and American adults.

Supplementary Materials: The following supporting information can be downloaded at: https://www.mdpi.com/article/10.3390/antiox13121434/s1, Figure S1: Total Cholesterol Comparison; Figure S2: HDL-C Assay Validation; Figure S3: Glycosylated Hemoglobin (HA1c%) validation; Figure S4: Comparison of HDL-C and HDL-C peroxide content in Japanese and American adults (MIDJA and MIDUS, respectively).

Author Contributions: Conceptualization, C.L.C.; Methodology, S.M.F. and L.B.-F.; Validation and Formal Analysis, C.L.C., S.M.F., L.B.-F. and A.R.; Investigation, C.L.C., S.K., M.K. and N.K.; Resources, C.L.C., S.K., M.K. and N.K.; Data Curation, C.L.C., S.M.F. and L.B.-F.; Initial Draft, C.L.C. and L.B.-F.; Writing, C.L.C., L.B.-F., S.M.F., S.K., M.K. and N.K.; Graphic Visualization, C.L.C.; Supervision, C.L.C. and N.K.; Project Administration, C.L.C., S.K., M.K. and N.K.; Funding, C.L.C. and S.K. All authors have read and agreed to the published version of the manuscript.

Funding: This research was supported by an award from the National Institute on Aging, R37 AG027343. The Principal Investigator was C. Ryff; CLC and SK were co-investigators.

Institutional Review Board Statement: All procedures were approved by the Health Sciences Institutional Review Board at the University of Wisconsin (H-2005-0415, 2005-2010; and 1022-0458, 07/01/2011-08/23/2021 Midlife health in Japan, MIDJA, and the US, MIDUS). In addition, the MIDJA protocol was approved by the Ethics Committee at the University of Tokyo (Assessment Number: 3515, 08/012011, Principal Investigator, Dr. N. Kawakami).

Informed Consent Statement: Participants provided informed consent twice; both for the survey phase and the specimen collection in the biomarker project.

Data Availability Statement: Demographic and biological data from the MIDJA project are publicly available at the Inter-university Consortium for Political and Social Research (ICPSR) as part of the MIDUS collection. This public portal provides researchers access to searchable variable-level metadata and longitudinal harmonization information, which can be downloaded as customized datasets and codebooks. For more information about data availability and the MIDJA and MIDUS projects see: http://midus.wisc.edu/data/index.php, accessed on 17 November 2024.

Acknowledgments: The invaluable assistance of C. Kan and H. Haruko in sample collection, D. Brar in sample processing, and G. Love in data compilation, especially the identification of medications prescribed in Japan, is acknowledged.

Conflicts of Interest: All authors declare there are no conflicts or competing interests.

References

1. Menotti, A.; Lanti, M.; Kromhout, D.; Blackburn, H.; Jacobs, D.; Nissinen, A.; Dontas, A.; Kafatos, A.; Nedeljkovic, S.; Adachi, H. Homogeneity in the relationship of serum cholesterol to coronary deaths across different cultures: 40-year follow-up of the Seven Countries Study. *Eur. J. Cardiovasc. Prev. Rehab.* **2008**, *15*, 719–725. [CrossRef] [PubMed]
2. Martin, S.S.; Niles, J.K.; Kaufman, H.W.; Awan, Z.; Elgaddar, O.; Choi, R.; Ahn, S.; Verma, R.; Nagarajan, M.; Don-Wauchope, A.; et al. Lipid distributions in the Global Diagnostics Network across five continents. *Eur. Heart J.* **2023**, *44*, 2305–2318. [CrossRef] [PubMed]
3. Ueshima, H.; Sekikawa, A.; Miura, K.; Turin, T.C.; Takashima, N.; Kita, Y.; Watanabe, M.; Kadota, A.; Okuda, N.; Kadowaki, T.; et al. Cardiovascular disease and risk factors in Asia: A selected review. *Circulation* **2008**, *118*, 2702–2709. [CrossRef]
4. Htun, N.C.; Suga, H.; Imai, S.; Shimizu, W.; Takimoto, H. Food intake patterns and cardiovascular risk factors in Japanese adults: Analyses from the 2012 National Health and Nutrition Survey, Japan. *Nutr. J.* **2017**, *16*, 61. [CrossRef]
5. Tsugane, S. Why has Japan become the world's most long-lived country: Insights from a food and nutrition perspective. *Eur. J. Clin. Nutr.* **2021**, *75*, 921–928. [CrossRef]
6. Okami, Y.; Chan, Q.; Miura, K.; Kadota, A.; Elliott, P.; Masaki, K.; Okayama, A.; Okuda, N.; Yoshita, K.; Miyagawa, N.; et al. Small high-density lipoprotein and omega-3 fatty acid intake differentiates Japanese and Japanese-Americans: The INTERLIPID Study. *J. Atheroscler. Thromb.* **2023**, *30*, 884–906. [CrossRef]

7. Dwyer, T.; Iwane, H.; Dean, K.; Odagiri, Y.; Shimomitsu, T.; Blizzard, L.; Srinivasan, S.; Nicklas, T.; Wattigney, W.; Riley, M.; et al. Differences in HDL cholesterol concentrations in Japanese, American, and Australian children. *Circulation* **1997**, *96*, 2830–2836. [CrossRef] [PubMed]
8. Kouda, K.; Nakamura, H.; Nishio, N.; Fujita, Y.; Takeuchi, H.; Iki, M. Trends in body mass index, blood pressure, and serum lipids in Japanese children: Iwata population-based annual screening (1993–2008). *J. Epidemiol.* **2010**, *20*, 212–218. [CrossRef]
9. Katsuhiko, Y.; Willcox, B.; Chen, R.; Grove, J.S.; Rodriguez, B.L.; Curb, J.D. The impact of westernization on the risk of atherosclerotic vascular disease among Japanese Americans in Hawaii. *Int. Congr. Ser. Atheroscler.* **2004**, *1262*, 180–183. [CrossRef]
10. Yoneda, M.; Kubota, M.; Watanabe, H.; Egusa, G. Westernization of lifestyle and atherosclerosis in the Japanese: Lessons from the Hawaii—Los Angeles—Hiroshima Study. *J. Atheroscler. Thromb.* **2021**, *28*, 214–222. [CrossRef]
11. Namekata, T.; Moore, D.; Knopp, R.; Marcovina, S.; Perrin, E.; Hughes, D.; Suzuki, K.; Mori, M.; Sempos, C.; Hatano, S.; et al. Cholesterol levels among Japanese Americans and other populations: Seattle Nikkei Health Study. *J. Atheroscler. Thromb.* **1996**, *3*, 105–113. [CrossRef] [PubMed]
12. Schwingel, A.; Nakata, Y.; Ito, L.S.; Chodzko-Zajko, W.J.; Shigematsu, R.; Erb, C.; Souza, S.M.; Oba-Shinjo, S.M.; Matsuo, T.; Marie, S.K.; et al. Lower HDL-cholesterol among healthy middle-aged Japanese-Brazilians in São Paulo compared to Natives and Japanese-Brazilians in Japan. *Eur. J. Epidemiol.* **2007**, *22*, 33–42. [CrossRef] [PubMed]
13. Kwan, T.W.; Wong, S.S.; Hong, Y.; Kanaya, A.M.; Khan, S.S.; Hayman, L.L.; Shah, S.H.; Welty, F.K.; Deedwania, P.C.; Khaliq, A.; et al. Epidemiology of diabetes and atherosclerotic cardiovascular disease among Asian American adults: Implications, management, and future directions: A scientific statement from the American Heart Association. *Circulation* **2023**, *148*, 74–94. [CrossRef] [PubMed]
14. Higashi, Y. Endothelial function in dyslipidemia: Roles of LDL-cholesterol, HDL-cholesterol and triglycerides. *Cells* **2023**, *12*, 1293. [CrossRef]
15. Voros, S.; Bansal, A.T.; Barnes, M.R.; Narula, J.; Maurovich-Horvat, P.; Vazquez, G.; Marvasty, I.B.; Brown, B.O.; Voros, I.D.L.; Harris, W.; et al. Bayesian network analysis of panomic biological big data identifies the importance of triglyceride-rich LDL in atherosclerosis development. *Front. Cardiovasc. Med.* **2023**, *9*, 960419. [CrossRef]
16. Kjeldsen, E.W.; Thomassen, J.Q.; Frikke-Schmidt, R. HDL cholesterol concentrations and risk of atherosclerotic cardiovascular disease—Insights from randomized clinical trials and human genetics. *Biochim. Biophys. Acta Mol. Cell Biol. Lipids* **2022**, *867*, 159063. [CrossRef]
17. Liu, C.; Dhindsa, D.; Almuwaqqat, Z.; Sun, Y.V.; Quyyum, A.A. Very high high-density lipoprotein cholesterol levels and cardiovascular mortality. *Am. J. Cardiol.* **2022**, *167*, 43–53. [CrossRef]
18. Oda, E.; Kawai, R. High-density lipoprotein cholesterol is positively associated with hypertension in apparently healthy Japanese men and women. *Brit. J. Biomed. Sci.* **2011**, *68*, 29–33. [CrossRef]
19. Yokoyama, S. Unique features of high-density lipoproteins in the Japanese: In population and in genetic factors. *Nutrients* **2015**, *7*, 2359–2381. [CrossRef]
20. Moriyama, K.; Takahashi, E.; Negami, M.; Otsuka, H.; Mitsuhashi, T.; Tsurugano, S.; Inabe, F.; Hiratsuka, N. Evaluation of high-density lipoprotein cholesterol levels in Japanese women. *Tokai J. Exp. Clin. Med.* **2012**, *37*, 77–83. [PubMed]
21. Ko, D.T.; Alter, D.A.; Guo, H.; Koh, M.; Lau, G.; Austin, P.C.; Booth, G.L.; Hogg, W.; Jackevicius, C.A.; Lee, D.S.; et al. High-density lipoprotein cholesterol and cause-specific mortality in individuals without previous cardiovascular conditions: The CANHEART study. *J. Am. Coll. Cardiol.* **2016**, *68*, 2073–2083. [CrossRef] [PubMed]
22. Yang, Y.; Han, K.; Park, S.H.; Kim, M.K.; Yoon, K.H.; Lee, S.H. High-density lipoprotein cholesterol and the risk of myocardial infarction, stroke, and cause-specific mortality: A nationwide cohort study in Korea. *J. Lipid Atheroscler.* **2021**, *10*, 74–87. [CrossRef] [PubMed]
23. Liu, C.; Dhindsa, D.; Almuwaqqa, Z.; Ko, Y.A.; Mehta, A.; Alkhoder, A.A.; Alras, Z.; Desai, S.R.; Patel, K.J.; Hooda, A.; et al. Association between high-density lipoprotein cholesterol levels and adverse cardiovascular outcomes in high-risk populations. *JAMA Cardiol.* **2022**, *7*, 672–680. [CrossRef] [PubMed]
24. Hamer, M.; O'Donovan, G.; Stamatakis, E. High-density lipoprotein cholesterol and mortality: Too much of a good thing? *Arterioscler. Thromb. Vasc. Biol.* **2018**, *38*, 669–672. [CrossRef]
25. Soran, H.; Schofield, J.D.; Durrington, P.N. Antioxidant properties of HDL. *Front. Pharmacol.* **2015**, *6*, 222. [CrossRef]
26. Srivastava, R.A.K. Dysfunctional HDL in diabetes mellitus and its role in the pathogenesis of cardiovascular disease. *Mol. Cell Biochem.* **2018**, *440*, 167–187. [CrossRef]
27. Rosenson, R.S.; Brewer, H.B.; Ansell, B.J.; Barter, P.; Chapman, M.J.; Heinecke, J.W.; Kontash, A.; Tall, A.R.; Webb, N.R. Dysfunctional HDL and atherosclerotic cardiovascular disease. *Nat. Rev. Cardiol.* **2016**, *13*, 48–60. [CrossRef]
28. Van Lenten, B.J.; Hama, S.Y.; Beer, F.C.; Stafforini, D.M.; Mcintyre, T.M.; Prescott, S.M.; La Du, B.N.; Fogelman, A.M.; Navab, M. Anti-inflammatory HDL becomes pro-inflammatory during the acute phase response. *J. Clin. Investig.* **1995**, *96*, 2758–2767. [CrossRef]
29. Ito, F.; Sono, Y.; Ito, T. Measurement and clinical significance of lipid peroxidation as a biomarker of oxidative stress: Oxidative stress in diabetes, atherosclerosis, and chronic inflammation. *Antioxidants* **2019**, *8*, 72. [CrossRef]
30. Jayaraman, S.; Gantz, D.L.; Gursky, O. Effects of protein oxidation on the structure and stability of model discoidal high-density lipoproteins. *Biochem.* **2008**, *47*, 3875–3882. [CrossRef]

31. Samadi, S.; Mehramiz, M.; Kelesidis, T.; Mobarhan, M.G.; Sahebkar, A.H.; Esmaily, H.; Moohebati, M.; Farjami, Z.; Ferns, G.A.; Mohammadpour, A.; et al. High-density lipoprotein lipid peroxidation as a molecular signature of the risk for developing cardiovascular disease: Results from MASHAD cohort. *J. Cell Physiol.* **2019**, *234*, 16168–16177. [CrossRef] [PubMed]
32. Kelesidis, T.; Roberts, C.K.; Huynh, D.; Martínez-Maza, O.; Currier, J.S. A high throughput biochemical fluorometric method for measuring lipid peroxidation in HDL. *PLoS ONE* **2014**, *9*, e111716. [CrossRef] [PubMed]
33. Sen Roy, S.; Nguyen, H.C.X.; Angelovich, T.A.; Hearps, A.C.; Huynh, D.; Jaworowski, A.; Kelesidis, T. Cell-free biochemical fluorometric enzymatic assay for high-throughput measurement of lipid peroxidation in high density lipoprotein. *J. Vis. Exp.* **2017**, *128*, e56325. [CrossRef]
34. Flaherty, S.M.; Wood, E.K.; Ryff, C.D.; Love, G.D.; Kelesidis, T.; Berkowitz, L.; Echeverría, G.; Rivera, K.; Rigotti, A.; Coe, C.L. Race and sex differences in HDL peroxide content among American adults with and without type 2 diabetes. *Lipids Health Dis.* **2022**, *21*, 18. [CrossRef]
35. Hiratsuka, N.; Yamada, C.; Mitsuhashi, T.; Inabe, F.; Araida, N.; Takahash, E. Significance of high HDL cholesterol levels in Japanese men with metabolic syndrome. *Intern. Med.* **2011**, *50*, 2113–2120. [CrossRef] [PubMed]
36. Maruyama, T.; Sakai, N.; Ishigami, M.; Hirano, K.; Arai, T.; Okada, S.; Okuda, E.; Ohya, A.; Nakajima, N.; Kadowaki, K.; et al. Prevalence and phenotypic spectrum of cholesteryl ester transfer protein gene mutations in Japanese hyperalphalipoproteinemia. *Atherosclerosis* **2003**, *166*, 177–185. [CrossRef]
37. Koizumi, J.; Mabuchi, H.; Yoshimura, A.; Michishita, I.; Takeda, M.; Itoh, H.; Sakai, Y.; Sakai, T.; Ueda, K.; Takeda, R. Deficiency of serum cholesteryl-ester transfer activity in patients with familial hyperalphalipoproteinaemia. *Atherosclerosis* **1985**, *58*, 175–186. [CrossRef]
38. Kapoulea, E.A.; Ready, R.E.; Ginn, J.C. Loneliness and risk for cardiovascular disease in the United States and Japan: The effects of nationality, collectivism, and gender. *Soc. Sci. Med.* **2023**, *337*, 116299. [CrossRef]
39. Grant, L.K.; Czeisler, C.A.; Lockley, S.W.; Rahman, S.A. Time-of-day and meal size effects on clinical lipid markers. *J. Clin. Endocrinol. Metab.* **2021**, *106*, e1373–e1379. [CrossRef]
40. Driver, S.L.; Martin, S.S.; Gluckman, T.J.; Clary, J.M.; Blumenthal, R.S.; Stone, N.J. Fasting or non-fasting lipid measurements: It depends on the question. *J. Am. Coll. Cardiol.* **2016**, *10*, 1227–1234. [CrossRef]
41. Coe, C.L.; Tsenkova, V.; Love, G.D.; Kawakami, N.; Karasawa, M.; Kitayama, S.; Markus, H.R.; Ryff, C.D. Age-related trends in the prevalence of Type 2 Diabetes among Japanese and white and black American adults. *Arch. Epidemiol.* **2020**, *4*, 142. [CrossRef] [PubMed]
42. Mutlu, A.S.; Duffy, J.; Wang, M.C. Lipid metabolism and lipid signals in aging and longevity. *Dev. Cell* **2021**, *56*, 1394–1407. [CrossRef] [PubMed]
43. Félix-Redondo, F.J.; Grau, M.; Fernández-Bergés, D. Cholesterol and cardiovascular disease in the elderly. Facts and gaps. *Aging Dis.* **2013**, *4*, 154–169. [PubMed] [PubMed Central]
44. Yamada, T.; Kimura-Koyanagi, M.; Sakaguchi, K.; Ogawa, W.; Tamori, Y. Obesity and risk for its comorbidities diabetes, hypertension, and dyslipidemia in Japanese individuals aged 65 years. *Sci. Rep.* **2023**, *3*, 2346. [CrossRef]
45. Takaeko, Y.; Matsui, S.; Kajikawa, M.; Maruhashi, T.; Yamaji, T.; Harada, T.; Han, Y.; Hashimoto, H.; Kihara, Y.; Hida, E.; et al. Relationship between high-density lipoprotein cholesterol levels and endothelial function in women: A cross-sectional study. *BMJ Open* **2020**, *10*, e038121. [CrossRef]
46. Schaefer, E.J. Clinical, biochemical, and genetic features in familial disorders of high density lipoprotein deficiency. *Arterioscler.* **1984**, *4*, 303–322. [CrossRef]
47. Saijo, Y.; Kiyota, N.; Kawasaki, Y.; Miyazaki, Y.; Kashimura, J.; Fukuda, M.; Kishi, R. Relationship between C-reactive protein and visceral adipose tissue in healthy Japanese subjects. *Diabetes Obes. Metab.* **2004**, *6*, 249–258. [CrossRef]
48. Palmisano, B.T.; Zhu, L.; Eckel, R.H.; Stafford, J.M. Sex differences in lipid and lipoprotein metabolism. *Mol. Metab.* **2018**, *15*, 45–55. [CrossRef] [PubMed]
49. Wang, X.; Magkos, F.; Mittendorfer, B. Sex differences in lipid and lipoprotein metabolism: It's not just about sex hormones. *J. Clin. Endocrinol. Metab.* **2011**, *96*, 885–893. [CrossRef]
50. Lee, G.; Jeon, H.K.; Yoo, H.Y. Sex-related differences in single nucleotide polymorphisms associated with dyslipidemia in a Korean population. *Lipids Health Dis.* **2022**, *21*, 124. [CrossRef]
51. Conlon, D.M.; Welty, F.K.; Reyes-Soffer, G.; Amengual, J. Sex-specific differences in lipoprotein production and clearance. *Arterioscler. Thromb. Vasc. Biol.* **2023**, *43*, 1617–1625. [CrossRef] [PubMed]
52. Yu, H.; Armstrong, N.; Pavela, G.; Kaiser, K. Sex and race differences in obesity-related genetic susceptibility and risk of cardiometabolic disease in older US adults. *JAMA Netw. Open.* **2023**, *6*, e2347171. [CrossRef] [PubMed]
53. Giammanco, A.; Noto, D.; Barbagallo, C.M.; Nardi, E.; Caldarella, R.; Ciaccio, M.; Averna, M.R.; Cefalù, A.B. Hyperalphalipoproteinemia and beyond: The role of HDL in cardiovascular diseases. *Life* **2021**, *11*, 581. [CrossRef]
54. Hirano, K.; Yamashita, S.; Nakajima, N.; Arai, T.; Maruyama, T.; Yoshida, Y.; Ishigami, M.; Sakai, N.; Kameda-Takemura, K.; Matsuzawa, Y. Genetic cholesteryl ester transfer protein deficiency is extremely frequent in the Omagari area of Japan. Marked hyperalphalipoproteinemia caused by CETP gene mutation is not associated with longevity. *Arterioscler. Thromb. Vasc. Biol.* **1997**, *17*, 1053–1059. [CrossRef] [PubMed]

55. Inazu, A.; Jiang, X.C.; Haraki, T.; Yagi, K.; Kamon, N.; Koizumi, J.; Mabuchi, H.; Takeda, R.; Takata, K.; Moriyama, Y.; et al. Genetic cholesteryl ester transfer protein deficiency caused by two prevalent mutations as a major determinant of increased levels of high-density lipoprotein cholesterol. *J. Clin. Investig.* **1994**, *94*, 1872–1882. [CrossRef]
56. Papp, A.C.; Pinsonneault, J.K.; Wang, D.; Newman, L.C.; Gong, Y.; Johnson, J.A.; Pepine, C.J.; Kumari, M.; Hingorani, A.D.; Talmud, P.J.; et al. Cholesteryl ester transfer protein (CETP) polymorphisms affect mRNA splicing, HDL levels, and sex-dependent cardiovascular risk. *PLoS ONE* **2012**, *7*, e31930. [CrossRef]
57. Karimi, E.; Dehghan, P.; Azizi-Soleiman, F.; Mohamadizadeh, M. Date seed (Phoenix dactylifera) supplementation modulates oxidative DNA damage, lipid peroxidation, and cardiometabolic risk factors in type 2 diabetes: A triple-blinded randomized placebo-controlled trial. *J. Funct. Food* **2024**, *117*, 106226. [CrossRef]
58. Kotemori, A.; Sawada, N.; Iwasaki, M.; Yamaji, T.; Shivappa, N.; Hebert, J.R.; Ishihara, J.; Inoue, M.; Tsugane, S.; JPHC FFQ Validation Study Group. Validating the dietary inflammatory index using inflammatory biomarkers in a Japanese population: A cross-sectional study of the JPHC-FFQ validation study. *Nutrition* **2020**, *69*, 110569. [CrossRef]
59. Ni, C.; Ji, Y.; Hu, K.; Xing, K.; Xu, Y.; Gao, Y. Effect of exercise and antioxidant supplementation on cellular lipid peroxidation in elderly individuals: Systematic review and network meta-analysis. *Front. Physiol.* **2023**, *14*, 1113270. [CrossRef]
60. Coe, C.L.; Miyamoto, Y.; Love, G.D.; Karasawa, M.; Kawakami, N.; Kitayama, S.; Ryff, C.D. Cultural and lifestyle practices associated with low inflammatory physiology in Japanese adults. *Brain Behav. Immun.* **2020**, *90*, 385–392. [CrossRef]
61. Ando, E.; Kachi, Y.; Kawakami, N.; Fukuda, Y.; Kawada, T. Associations of non-standard employment with cardiovascular risk factors: Findings from nationwide cross-sectional studies in Japan. *Ind. Health* **2018**, *56*, 336–345. [CrossRef]
62. Garin, M.-C.B.; Moren, X.; James, R.W. Paraoxonase-1 and serum concentrations of HDL-cholesterol and apoA-I. *J. Lipid Res.* **2006**, *47*, 515–520. [CrossRef] [PubMed]
63. Suehiro, T.; Nakauchi, Y.; Yamamoto, M.; Arii, K.; Itoh, H.; Hamashige, N.; Hashimoto, K. Paraoxonase gene polymorphism in Japanese subjects with coronary heart disease. *Int. J. Cardiol.* **1996**, *57*, 69–73. [CrossRef]
64. Yamada, Y.; Ando, F.; Niino, N.; Miki, T.; Shimokata, H. Association of polymorphisms of paraoxonase 1 and 2 genes, alone or in combination, with bone mineral density in community-dwelling Japanese. *J. Hum. Genet.* **2003**, *48*, 469–475. [CrossRef]
65. Ichikawa, K.; Konta, T.; Emi, M.; Toriyama, S.; Takasaki, S.; Ikeda, A.; Shibata, Y.; Takabatake, N.; Takeishi, Y.; Kato, T.; et al. Genetic polymorphisms of paraoxonase-1 are associated with chronic kidney disease in Japanese women. *Kidney Int.* **2009**, *76*, 183–189. [CrossRef]
66. Ikeda, Y.; Suehiro, T.; Itahara, T.; Inui, Y.; Chikazawa, H.; Inoue, M.; Arii, K.; Hashimoto, K. Human serum paraoxonase concentration predicts cardiovascular mortality in hemodialysis patients. *Clin. Nephrol.* **2007**, *67*, 358–365. [CrossRef]
67. Ikeda, Y.; Inoue, M.; Suehiro, T.; Arii, K.; Kumon, Y.; Hashimoto, K. Low human paraoxonase predicts cardiovascular events in Japanese patients with type 2 diabetes. *Acta Diabetol.* **2009**, *46*, 239–242. [CrossRef]
68. Sumi, A.; Nakamura, U.; Iwase, M.; Fujii, H.; Ohkuma, T.; Ide, H.; Jodai-Kitamura, T.; Komorita, Y.; Yoshinari, M.; Hirakawa, Y.; et al. The gene–treatment interaction of paraoxonase-1 gene polymorphism and statin therapy on insulin secretion in Japanese patients with type 2 diabetes: Fukuoka diabetes registry. *BMC Med Genet.* **2017**, *18*, 146. [CrossRef]
69. Ueno, T.; Shimazaki, E.; Matsumoto, T.; Watanabe, H.; Tsunemi, A.; Takahashi, Y.; Mori, M.; Hamano, R.; Fujioka, T.; Soma, M.; et al. Paraoxonase-1 polymorphism Leu-Met55 is associated with cerebral infarction in Japanese population. *Med. Sci. Monit.* **2003**, *9*, CR208-12. [PubMed]
70. Eckerson, H.W.; Romson, J.; Wyte, C.; La Du, B.N. The human serum paraoxonase polymorphism: Identification of phenotypes by their response to salts. *Am. J. Hum. Genet.* **1983**, *35*, 214–227. [PubMed] [PubMed Central]
71. Shimizu, Y.; Nakazato, M.; Sekita, T.; Kadota, K.; Yamasaki, H.; Takamura, N.; Aoyagi, K.; Maeda, T. Association of arterial stiffness and diabetes with triglycerides-to-HDL cholesterol ratio for Japanese men: The Nagasaki Islands Study. *Atherosclerosis* **2013**, *228*, 491–495. [CrossRef]
72. Sone, H.; Tanaka, S.; Tanaka, S.; Iimuro, S.; Oida, K.; Yamasaki, Y.; Oikawa, S.; Ishibashi, S.; Katayama, S.; Ohashi, Y.; et al. Japan Diabetes Complications Study Group. Serum level of triglycerides is a potent risk factor comparable to LDL cholesterol for coronary heart disease in Japanese patients with type 2 diabetes: Subanalysis of the Japan Diabetes Complications Study (JDCS). *J. Clin. Endocrinol. Metab.* **2011**, *96*, 3448–3456. [CrossRef]
73. NIPPON DATA80 Research Group. Risk assessment chart for death from cardiovascular disease based on a 19-year follow-up study of a Japanese representative population. *Circ. J.* **2006**, *70*, 1249–1255. [CrossRef] [PubMed]
74. Iso, H. Changes in coronary heart disease risk among Japanese. *Circulation* **2008**, *118*, 2725–2729. [CrossRef] [PubMed]
75. Yokoyama, S. Continuous and marked increase of Japanese HDL associates paradoxically with their nutritional shift. *J. Atheroscler. Thromb.* **2023**, *30*, 1288, Erratum in *J. Atheroscler Thromb.* **2023**, *30*, 919–933. [CrossRef]
76. Sahashi, Y.; Goto, A.; Takachi, R.; Ishihara, J.; Kito, K.; Kanehara, R.; Yamaji, T.; Iwasaki, M.; Inoue, M.; Shoichiro, T.; et al. Inverse association between fruit and vegetable intake and all-cause mortality: Japan Public Health Center-based prospective study. *J. Nutr.* **2022**, *152*, 2245–2254. [CrossRef]

antioxidants

MDPI

Article

The Role of Paraoxonase-1 Activity, Apolipoprotein B Levels, and Apolipoprotein B/Apolipoprotein A-I Ratio as Risk Markers for Aortic Stenosis in Patients with a Bicuspid Aortic Valve

Maria Kwiatkowska [1], Agnieszka Mickiewicz [1,*], Aleksandra Krzesińska [2], Agnieszka Kuchta [2], Maciej Jankowski [2], Marcin Gruchała [1] and Marcin Fijałkowski [1]

[1] 1st Department of Cardiology, Medical University of Gdańsk, 80-211 Gdańsk, Poland; marianowak@gumed.edu.pl (M.K.); mgruch@gumed.edu.pl (M.G.); marcin.fijalkowski@gumed.edu.pl (M.F.)

[2] Department of Clinical Chemistry, Medical University of Gdańsk, 80-211 Gdańsk, Poland; aleksandra.krzesinska@gumed.edu.pl (A.K.); agnieszka.kuchta@gumed.edu.pl (A.K.); majank@gumed.edu.pl (M.J.)

* Correspondence: amickiewicz@gumed.edu.pl

Abstract: The bicuspid aortic valve (BAV) is commonly associated with the early degeneration of the aortic valve. Up to 45% of BAV patients over the age of 50 develop aortic stenosis (AS). Although published data indicate a robust interplay between lipids and calcific AS in tricuspid aortic valve patients, the studies on the BAV population are lacking. We aimed to evaluate the association between selected lipid markers and the occurrence of AS in BAV patients. Methods: The study included 76 adults (21 female) with a BAV diagnosed by echocardiography, divided by age and AS diagnosis. Biochemical parameters concentrations in serum were measured: high density lipoprotein cholesterol (HDL-C) levels by standard enzymatic colorimetric tests, low density lipoprotein cholesterol (LDL-C) levels by the Friedewald formula, apolipoprotein A-I (Apo AI) and apolipoprotein B (Apo B) serum concentration by the nephelometric method, and paraoxonase-1 activity (PON-1 ASE) and arylesterase activity (PON-1 ARE) based on paraoxon and phenyl acetate hydrolysis. Results: A total of 54 patients (15 female) were more than 45 years old and 22 (6 female) were 45 or less years old. BAV patients with AS aged ≤45 had higher levels of Apo B, compared to those without AS [110.5 (102–132) vs. 95.6 (77–101) mg/d; *p* 0.044]. Similarly, Apo B/Apo AI ratio was higher in BAV patients with AS aged ≤45, compared to those without AS [(0.8 (0.7–1) vs. 0.6 (0.5–0.7); *p* 0.029]. In the group aged ≤45, Apo B showed a positive correlation with the aortic valve peak transvalvular velocity (AV Vmax) measurement (R Spearman 0.6, *p* 0.004). We found also that, among young BAV patients, those with AS had a lower level of PON-1 ARE compared to the cohort without AS [63.4 (52–80) vs. 85.3 (70–102); *p* 0.012]. We did not find any differences in lipid parameters in patients aged >45. Conclusions The metabolic link between Apo B level and Apo B/AI ratio with AS presence in BAV patients under 45 years of age suggests a significant impact of these parameters on the earlier development of AS in the BAV population. Molecules associated with high density lipoprotein and its antioxidant function, such as PON1, are valuable markers for AS development, compared to HDL-C and LDL-C levels.

Keywords: bicuspid aortic valve; aortic stenosis; apolipoprotein B; apolipoprotein A-I; paraoxonase-1

1. Introduction

Bicuspid aortic valve (BAV) is a congenital valvular defect that affects approximately 0.5–2% of the general adult population [1]. The abnormal structure of the leaflets leads to the development of aortic valve dysfunction, both in the form of regurgitation and stenosis. Furthermore, an aortic aneurysm often accompanies this condition [2]. As a consequence, patients with a BAV frequently and at a young age require qualification for cardiac surgery. In the registry from Olmsted County in Minnesota, observing over 200 individuals with a BAV, the mean age at the time of cardiac surgery was 40 ± 20 years compared to 67 ± 16 years for patients with a tricuspid aortic valve [3,4]. Overall, up to 50 percent of BAV individuals undergo aortic valve replacement (AVR) [5]. Aortic stenosis (AS) is a frequent cause of surgery in this group. Calcification of the cusps often occurs by the age of 40 [4]. The BAV is associated with the occurrence of degenerative AS at a significantly younger age compared to the population with a tricuspid aortic valve [5,6].

On the other hand, the BAV population remains a heterogenous group, and the occurrence and course of valve defects in these patients remain unpredictable. While a BAV may lead to advanced calcification of the aortic valve, we do not observe this process in all BAV individuals. Therefore, among the BAV population, factors that may be predictors for the calcified AS have been investigated. Studies evaluating the association between the morphological type of BAV and the occurrence of valve stenosis have not yielded consistent results [6,7]. In a meta-analysis involving over 4000 patients, Zhenzhen Mai indicated that a type of BAV with right-coronary and non-coronary cusps fusion most frequent predisposes to AS [8]. However, earlier registries did not demonstrate similar results [9]. Uncertainties in the relationship between aortic valve cusps fusion morphology and the development of AS highlight the need to focus on modifiable risk factors for valve calcification.

The impact of lipid metabolism disorders on the progression of calcified AS has been demonstrated in tricuspid aortic valve populations [10,11]. High levels of lipids, especially low density lipoprotein cholesterol (LDL-C), stimulate a chronic inflammation of the endothelium resulting in progressive fibrosis and further reduction in the aortic valve area. It has been shown that apolipoprotein B (Apo B), the main and only essential structural protein component of low density lipoprotein (LDL), is a more precise marker for assessing cardiovascular risk than LDL-C levels. Plasma concentration of apo B is a reliable indicator of the number of atherogenic particles that contribute to the development of atherosclerosis. Serum Apo B concentrations are also associated with the AS development [12].

The role of high density lipoprotein cholesterol (HDL-C) levels in preventing atherosclerosis and endothelial dysfunction has been investigated [13]. Recent studies conducted in patients with tricuspid aortic valve suggest that HDL-C may also play a significant protective role in the pathogenesis of AS [14]. This connection underscores broader cardiovascular benefits of high density lipoprotein (HDL) beyond its traditional anti-atherosclerotic mechanisms. HDL has a multifaceted range of protective functions, including neutralizing free radicals and oxidized lipoproteins, facilitating reverse cholesterol transport, and demonstrating potent anti-inflammatory properties [15]. These mechanisms not only inhibit vascular damage but also halt the processes of degeneration and calcification in the aortic valve [16]. Traditionally, serum HDL-C levels have served as a readily accessible biomarker for cardiovascular risk assessment. However, elevated HDL-C levels do not always correlate with its protective function [17]. Moreover, high HDL-C levels may paradoxically exhibit a pro-inflammatory effect [18]. Increasingly, the evaluation of HDL antioxidant properties is recognized as a more precise indicator of cardiovascular risk.

A biomarker associated with HDL, paraoxonase-1 (PON-1), an enzyme exhibiting antioxidant properties and reducing the oxidation of LDL-C, have been studied among patients with AS. Several different activities of PON-1 were described with research mainly focusing on PON-1 paraoxonase (PON-1 ASE) and arylesterase activity (PON-1 ARE), and their role in the development of cardiovascular disease [19] Z. Wang has demonstrated, on over hundred patients who underwent AVR, that a lower PON-1 level in aortic valve tissue may be associated with the progression of calcification in AS [20].

Another marker linked to HDL is apolipoprotein A-I (Apo AI), the main protein component of HDL. Apo AI plays a key role in cholesterol's transport, facilitates the efflux of cholesterol from macrophages in the arterial endothelium, supports antioxidant processes and regulation of inflammatory reactions, and has been shown an important indicator of the risk of AS occurrence [21,22].

The Apo B/Apo AI ratio represents the proportion between atherogenic and antiatherogenic lipoproteins in plasma. Thus, it constitutes an accurate marker of cardiovascular risk [23]. A correlation between this ratio and the occurrence of AS was also demonstrated. In a study involving the EPIC-Norfolk cohort, Kang H Zheng's et al. demonstrated a correlation between the Apo B/Apo AI ratio and the incidence of AS [24].

Patients with a bicuspid and tricuspid aortic valve may differ in terms of their lipid parameters [25,26]. Moreover, BAV patients may be at higher risk of atherosclerosis and coronary artery disease occurrence [27]. Finally, BAV patients are not a homogenous group. The studies profiling the BAV population based on aortic valve function and lipid markers are lacking.

Therefore, we aimed to assess the relationship between the serum concentration of selected lipid markers and the occurrence of AS among BAV patients in different age groups.

2. Material and Methods

2.1. Group Characteritics

Adult patients with a BAV, diagnosed by echocardiography and admitted to the First Clinic of Cardiology of Medical University of Gdansk, were enrolled into the study. Exclusion criteria included active inflammatory process, autoimmune diseases, active oncological disease, hyperthyroidism, pregnancy, unstable clinical condition (clinical features of circulatory or respiratory failure), and familial hypercholesterolemia. Patients were divided into two age groups with an age burden of 45 years. Due to the assessment of the atherogenic markers impact on the occurrence of AS, this division into age groups was established based on the age burden defining young coronary artery disease [28,29]. Subsequently, each age group was divided into two subgroups depending on AS occurrence. Clinical data including age, anthropometric data (weight and height), chronic diseases (such as hypertension, diabetes mellitus, coronary artery disease), smoking habit, and statin therapy were collected during the medical interview. The study protocol was approved by the Local Bioethics Committee at the Medical University of Gdansk (protocol no. NKBBN/487-517/2019). Written informed consent was obtained from each patient prior to their inclusion in the study.

2.2. Echocardiographic Examination

Transthoracic examination was performed in each case and included following parameters: left ventricle ejection fraction (LVEF), aortic valve area (AVA), aortic valve peak transvalvular velocity (AV Vmax), mean transvalvular pressure gradient (PGmean); aortic regurgitation evaluation, aortic complex diameters. AS and aortic regurgitation were defined according to European Society of Cardiology Guidelines from 2021 [30]. Aortopathy was defined by an aortic root or ascending aorta diameter more than 40 mm. Patients with at least a mild stage of AS were included in the AS subgroups.

2.3. Biochemical Analysis

Peripheral blood samples were drawn from each patient between 7 and 8 a.m. following the overnight fast. The serum was separated by centrifugation at 1000× *g* for 15 min and was stored at −80 °C pending analysis. Total cholesterol (TC), HDL-C, and triglycerides (TG) were measured in serum using standard enzymatic colorimetric tests (Wiener Lab, Warsaw, Poland). LDL-C was calculated using the Friedewald formula (there were no cases of TG elevation above 400 mg/dL) [31,32]. The apolipoprotein (Apo AI and Apo B) serum concentrations were determined using the nephelometric method with antibodies obtained from Siemens Healthcare Diagnostics (Eschborn, Germany) on a Behring laser nephelometer. The PON-1 ASE and PON-1 ARE activities were analyzed in serum based on paraoxon and phenyl acetate hydrolysis, respectively, according to the procedure described earlier [33].

2.4. Statistic Analysis

All data were collected and computed in MS Excel and a standard statistical package. Variables with normal distribution were compared with the Student's *t*-test; non-normally distributed data were compared with the U Mann–Whitney test. Dichotomous variables were compared with Chi-squared test with Yates's correction for continuity. Correlation for data with non-normally distribution was calculated by the Spearman correlation. For selected biomarkers, the area under the curve (AUC) was calculated using receiver operating characteristic (ROC) analysis, and the optimal cut-off values corresponding to the minimal false positive and false negative parameters were determined. The continuous variables were expressed as medians with 25th and 75th percentiles. *p*-value less than 0.05 was considered valid for all tests.

3. Results

A total of 76 patients (21 female) were enrolled into the study. Clinical characteristics of the studied group are presented in Tables 1 and 2. The average age of observed patients was 53.7 ± 13 years. A total of 54 patients (15 female) were in the age category of more than 45 years. A total of 22 patients (6 female) were aged 45 or younger. In the group aged >45, there were 35 patients (65%) with AS, and in the group aged ≤45, there were 9 patients (41%) with AS. The group aged >45 had significantly more frequent arterial hypertension (67% vs. 14% of patients; $p < 0.001$), coronary artery disease (35% vs. 5% of patients; *p* 0.014), and frequently required statins therapy (50% vs. 18% of patients; *p* 0.021) compared to patients aged ≤45 (Table 1).

Table 1. Clinical characteristics of BAV patients age ≤ 45 and age > 45.

	Age ≤ 45	Age > 45	*p* Value
No (female)	22 (6)	54(15)	0.812 *
Age	39.5 (33–42)	60.5 (52–68)	<0.001 **
BMI [kg/m^2]	26.6 (23–29)	27.8 (25–31)	0.145 **
Smoking	5 (23%)	19 (35%)	0.431 *
Hypertension	3 (14%)	36 (67%)	<0.001 *
Diabetes mellitus	1 (5%)	8 (15%)	0.387 *
Coronary artery disease	1 (5%)	19 (35%)	0.014 *
Statin therapy	4 (18%)	27 (50%)	0.021 *

Abbreviations: BMI—body mass index. * Chi-squared test with Yates's correction, ** Mann–Whitney U test.

In the group aged ≤45, there were no significant differences in terms of sex, age, body mass index, statin use, and the prevalence of hypertension, smoking, coronary artery disease, or diabetes mellitus depending on the presence of AS. On the contrary, in the cohort aged >45, patients with AS were characterized by their older age and more frequently requiring statins compared to patients without AS (Table 2).

Table 2. Comparison of clinical characteristics of patients in two age groups based on the AS presence.

	Age ≤ 45			**Age > 45**		
	No AS	**AS**	***p* Value**	**No AS**	**AS**	***p* Value**
No (female)	13 (2)	9 (4)	0.309 *	19 (3)	35 (12)	0.258 *
Age	39 (31–41)	40 (34–43)	0.378 ***	55 (49–61)	65 (59–69)	0.002 **
BMI [kg/m^2]	27 (24–32)	25 (23–27)	0.190 ***	27 (25–30)	28 (26–31)	0.340 ***
Smoking	3 (23%)	2 (22%)	0.638 *	7 (37%)	12 (34%)	0.912 *
Hypertension	2 (15%)	1 (11%)	0.730 *	13 (68%)	23 (66%)	0.920 *
Diabetes mellitus	1(8%)	0	0.845 *	2 (10%)	6 (17%)	0.801 *
Coronary artery disease	0	1(11%)	0.845 *	6 (32%)	13 (37%)	0.912 *
Statin therapy	3 (2%)	1(11%)	0.878 *	5 (26%)	22 (63%)	0.023 *

Abbreviations: BMI—body mass index. * Chi-squared test with Yates's correction, ** Mann–Whitney U test, *** Student's *t*-test.

3.1. Echocardiographic Characteristics of Groups

The prevalence of AS and aortopathy was similar in both age groups. Moderate to severe aortic regurgitation was more frequently observed in patients aged ≤45. Function of the left ventricle calculated by LVEF was in a similar range for both age groups (Table 3).

Table 3. Echocardiographic assessment of BAV complications and LVEF according to age.

	Age ≤ 45	**Age > 45**	***p* Value**
LVEF [%]	60 (35–65)	60 (55–64)	0.951 **
AS	9 (41%)	35 (65%)	0.097 *
AR	13 (59%)	14 (26%)	0.013 *
Aortopathy	13 (59%)	37 (69%)	0.604 *

Abbreviations: LVEF—left ventricular ejection fraction, AS—aortic stenosis, AR—moderate to severe aortic regurgitation. * Chi-squared test with Yates's correction, ** Mann–Whitney U test.

In the group aged >45, patients with AS and without AS differed in the frequency of aortic regurgitation occurrence. In the group aged ≤45, there was no significant difference in terms of LVEF, aortic regurgitation, and aortopathy prevalence depending on AS diagnosis (Table 4).

Table 4. Echocardiographic assessment of BAV complications and LVEF in two age groups based on the AS presence.

	Age ≤ 45			**Age > 45**		
	No AS	**AS**	***p* Value**	**No AS**	**AS**	***p* Value**
LEVF [%]	60 (40–64)	60 (32–70)	1.000 **	60 (55–64)	60 (51–64)	0.926 **
AR	7 (54%)	6 (67%)	0.873 *	9 (47%)	5 (14%)	0.020 *
Aortopathy	8 (61%)	5 (56%)	0.873 *	17 (89%)	27 (77%)	0.455 *

Abbreviations: LVEF—left ventricular ejection fraction, AS—aortic stenosis, AR—moderate to severe aortic regurgitation. * Chi-squared test with Yates's correction, ** Mann–Whitney U test.

Among patients with AS, older patients aged >45 had lower AVA compared to those aged ≤45 [AVA 0.9 (0.8–1.2) cm^2 vs. 1.3 (0.9–1.4) cm^2; *p* 0.023]. We found no differences in AV Vmax and PGmean measurements (Table 5).

Table 5. Echocardiographic characteristics of patients with aortic stenosis according to age.

	Age ≤ 45 + AS	Age > 45 + AS	*p* Value
AVA	1.3 (0.9–1.4)	0.9 (0.8–1.2)	0.023 **
AV Vmax	3.5 (2.8–4.1)	3.9 (3.4–4.4)	0.161 *
AV PGmean	32 (16–46)	40 (25–46)	0.457 *

Abbreviations: AVA—aortic valve area, AV Vmax—aortic valve peak transvalvular velocity, AV PGmean—mean transvalvular pressure gradient. * Student's *t*-test, ** Mann–Whitney U test.

3.2. Biochemical Analysis

Patients aged ≤45 with AS in comparison to those without AS had significantly higher levels of Apo B [110.5 (102–132) vs. 95.6 (77–101) mg/dL; *p* 0.044] and Apo B/Apo AI ratio [(0.8 (0.7–1) vs. 0.6 (0.5–0.7); *p* 0.029]. We found no differences in the level of TC, HDL-C, LDL-C, and TG. Moreover, in the group aged ≤45, Apo B level and Apo B/Apo AI ratio showed a positive correlation with AV Vmax measurement (R Spearman was 0.6 for Apo B and AV Vmax, and 0.5 for Apo B/Apo AI and AV Vmax, $p < 0.05$ for both analyses) (Figures 1 and 2). Furthermore, in the group aged ≤45, patients with AS had significantly lower activity of PON-1 ARE compared to those without AS [63.4 (52–80) vs. 85.3 (70–102) U/L; *p* 0.0124].

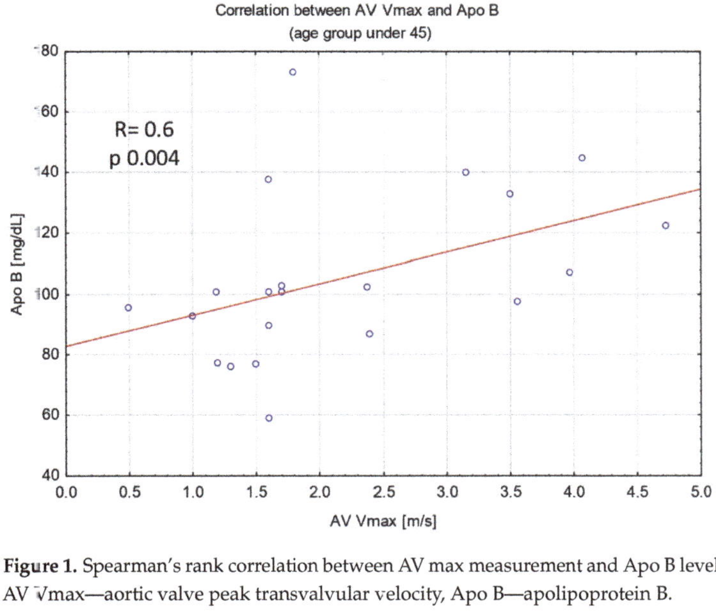

Figure 1. Spearman's rank correlation between AV max measurement and Apo B level. Abbreviations: AV Vmax—aortic valve peak transvalvular velocity, Apo B—apolipoprotein B.

Among patients aged ≤45, the analysis for Apo B levels, Apo B/Apo AI ratio, and PON-1 ARE activity was extended to ROC analysis. AUC for Apo B was 0.761 [95% confidence interval (CI): 0.533 to 0.914; *p* 0.018], for Apo B/Apo AI ratio 0.782 (95% CI: 0.557 to 0.927; *p* 0.007), indicating a moderate to good ability to discriminate between patients with and without AS. PON-1 ARE activity demonstrated the highest AUC of 0.786 (95% CI: 0.561 to 0.930; *p* 0.004), indicating the best discriminatory power among the biomarkers tested (Figure 3).

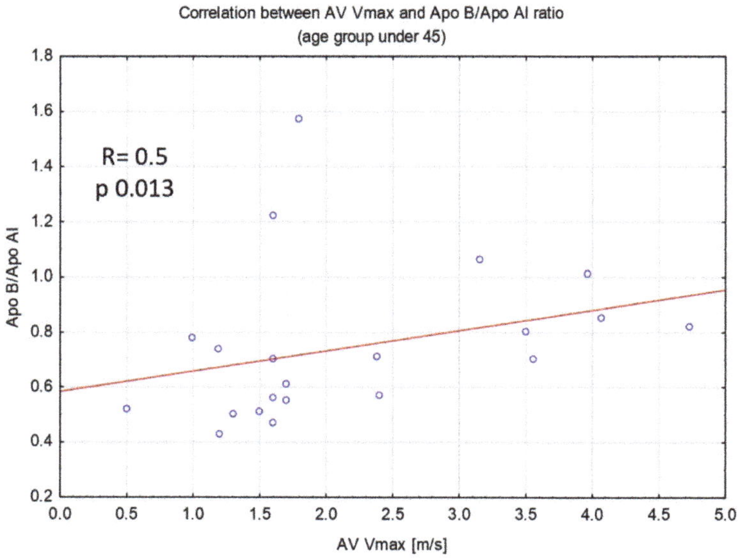

Figure 2. Spearman's rank correlation between AV max measurement and Apo B/Apo AI ratio. Abbreviations: AV Vmax—aortic valve peak transvalvular velocity, Apo B/Apo AI—apolipoprotein B/apolipoprotein A-I ratio.

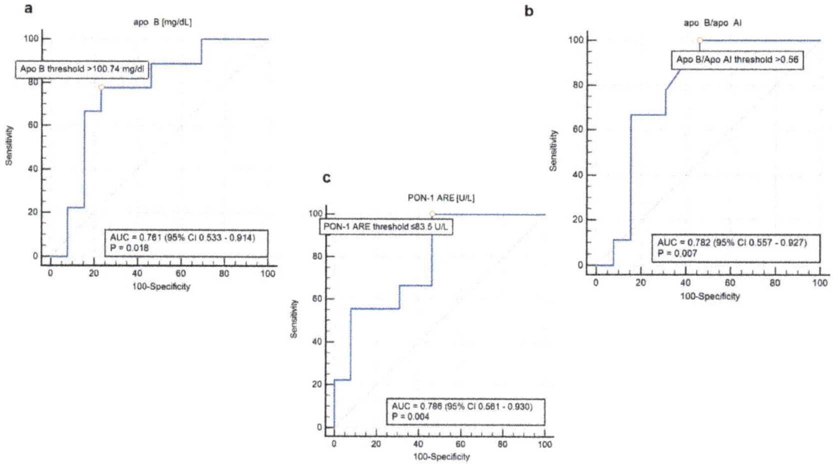

Figure 3. ROC curves of Apo B levels (**a**), Apo B/Apo AI ratio (**b**), PON-1 ARE (**c**) activity and the presence of AS for patients aged ≤45. Abbreviations: AUC—Area Under the Curve; CI—Confidence Interval; Apo B—apolipoprotein B; Apo AI—apolipoprotein AI; PON-1 ARE—arylesterase activity.

Among patients aged >45, there were no differences in analyzed parameters depending on AS prevalence.

All results from the biochemical analysis were presented in Table 6.

Table 6. Lipid parameters in BAV patients according to age and AS diagnosis.

	Age ≤45			Age > 45		
	No AS	**AS**	***p* Value**	**No AS**	**AS**	***p* Value**
Apo AI [mg/dL]	150 (126–168)	144 (131–151)	0.371 *	167 (139–184)	156 (146–173)	0.306 *
Apo B [mg/dL]	95 (77–101)	110 (102–132)	0.044 **	100 (93–114)	83 (77–106)	0.144 *
Apo B/Apo AI	0.6 (0.5–0.7)	0.8 (0.7–1)	0.029 **	0.6 (0.5–0.7)	0.6 (0.5–0.7)	0.096 *
TC [mg/dL]	153 (139–166)	150 (126–164)	0.640 **	144 (124–167)	128 (113–147)	0.065 **
HDL-C [mg/dL]	51 (47–54)	48 (45–52)	0.344 *	51 (47–61)	50 (42–58)	0.492 *
LDL-C [mg/dL]	101 (98–114)	107 (94–111)	0.358 **	99 (91–120)	86 (80–106)	0.056 **
LDL-C/HDL-C	2.1 (1.7–2.3)	2.2 (1.9–2.3)	0.860 *	1.9 (1.7–2.2)	1.8 (1.5–2.2)	0.322 **
non HDL-C/HDL-C	2.1 (1.6–2.4)	2.0 (1.9–2.4)	0.874 *	1.7 (1.4–2.2)	1.6 (1.4–2)	0.259 *
TG [mg/dL]	98 (47–113)	63 (52–108)	0.738 **	105 (69–138)	87 (68–113)	0.269 *
PON-1 ASE [U/L]	70 (55–151)	127 (39–163)	0.894 **	89 (53–154)	59 (47–147)	0.484 **
PON-1 ARE [U/L]	85 (70–102)	63 (52–80)	0.012 *	82 (71–99)	79 (59–88)	0.126 **

Abbreviations: Apo AI—apolipoprotein A-I; Apo B—apolipoprotein B; Apo B/Apo AI—apolipoprotein B/Apolipoprotein A-I ratio; TC—total cholesterol; HDL-C—high density lipoprotein cholesterol; LDL-C—low density lipoprotein cholesterol; non HDL-C—non-HDL cholesterol, TG—triglycerides; PON-1 ASE—paraoxonase activity; PON-1 ARE-arylesterase activity. * Student's *t*-test, ** Mann–Whitney U test.

4. Discussion

The findings of our study showed an association between AS and molecules associated with lipid metabolism, such as Apo B, Apo B/Apo AI ratio, and PON1-ARE in BAV patients at age ≤45. Moreover, the Apo B level and Apo B/Apo AI ratio correlated with the echocardiographic parameter of AS severity such as AV Vmax.

Our results suggest that lipid metabolism may play a significant role in the early development of calcific AS among patients with a BAV, which is a frequent BAV complication, affecting up to 45% of patients over the age of 50 [34]. It is also the most common cause of qualifying for aortic valve replacement in the BAV adult population [35]. Furthermore, patients with a BAV required surgery due to AS at a significantly younger age than patients with a tricuspid aortic valve [36]. In the study of a large Australian cohort by Michelle S Lim's team, the mean age of BAV patients referred to AVR due to AS was 55 ± 17 years (22 years earlier than patients with tricuspid aortic valve) [37]. The exact origin of early calcification and accelerated development of AS in patients with BAV remains unclear. One possible hypothesis considers mechanical factors, such as endothelial damage of valve cusps caused by abnormal blood flow dynamics [38]. However, this anatomical aspect does not fully explain why only a subset of the BAV population experience progression to significant valve calcification, while some individuals remain without a valvular dysfunction throughout their life.

Consequently, attention has also been directed towards a risk factor for calcific AS that overlaps with those for atherosclerosis, including hyperlipidemia, hypertension, and diabetes mellitus [39]. Studies suggest that patients with a BAV constitute a heterogeneous group regarding their lipid profiles. For instance, Elena Sticch et al. showed that an elevated level of lipoprotein (a) in patients with BAV was associated with the degree of aortic valve calcification [40]. Additionally, it has been shown that LDL-C and Apo B levels may significantly affect the progression of BAV in case of aortopathy. [41] These findings underline the need for further investigation into the role of specific lipid markers in the early manifestation of BAV complications.

The second observation derived from our results highlights the need for a broader analysis of lipid markers. To date, the relationship between LDL-C levels and the risk of both atherosclerosis and AS has been well demonstrated [42,43]. The beneficial effect of high HDL-C on the occurrence of calcific AS or cardiac events is less clear [44,45]. Nevertheless, HDL-C and LDL-C levels are the most commonly used markers of cardiovascular risk assessment, though they do not always adequately reflect lipid balance [18,46].

Apo B is a protein found in all atherogenic lipoproteins. Studies have shown that Apo B levels may be a more precise marker of cardiovascular risk than LDL-C [47]. It should be noted that the measurement of Apo B is less dependent on triglyceride (TG) levels and fasting status, making it a more stable parameter than LDL-C [48]. The assessment of HDL properties, including its associated molecules, appears to better explain its role in both the development of atherosclerosis and AS. The main protein component of HDL is Apo AI [49]. The Apo B/Apo AI ratio enables the assessment of the balance between atherogenic and protective lipoproteins, making it an important marker for evaluating cardiovascular risk [50]. Ivert et al. proved an association between elevated Apo B/Apo AI ratio and increased appearance of AS among patients with tricuspid aortic valve [10]. Our findings demonstrate a similar observation among young individuals with BAV. Patients aged $\leq$45 with AS had increased concentrations of Apo B and Apo B/Apo AI ratio. We did not observe any differences in the levels of LDL-C and HDL-C. In our study, the cut-off value for Apo B obtained from the ROC analysis was 100.74 mg/dl, a value that corresponds to an increased cardiovascular risk [51]. The cut-off value for Apo B/Apo AI ratio was 0.56. For comparison, in the AMORIS and INTERHEART studies, the Apo B/Apo AI ratio below 0.7 for men and 0.6 for women was associated with low cardiovascular risk. Nevertheless, it should be noted that there are no clearly established cut-off values for Apo B levels and the Apo B/Apo AI ratio in the context of AS, and further research is needed in this area.

Another marker associated with HDL is PON-1, which demonstrates antioxidant properties. Although the relationship of its different activities and the occurrence of AS is less well understood, some studies have shown a correlation between low activity of PON-1 and the severity of AS [52]. In our study, patients with a BAV and AS at $\leq$45 years of age showed significantly lower activity of PON-1 ARE compared to those without AS, with the cut-off value below 83.5 U/L. The difference was observed despite the fact that the level of Apo AI did not differ between these groups. This relationship underscores the potential significance of the marker in various manifestations of BAV complications and emphasizes the need for further research to determine PON-1 activity values associated with the risk of AS development. By analyzing the antioxidant components of HDL and its associated biomarkers, we can gain a deeper understanding of HDL quality and functionality, which may provide a more accurate assessment of its cardiovascular protective capacity [17,53].

Interestingly, we did not observe similar relationships among patients above 45 years of age. However, it should be noted that in this group, the etiology of AS may be more multifactorial, considering the influence of age. Additionally, these patients more frequently had diagnosed hypertension and chronic coronary syndrome. It should be noted that in the group aged >45, patients with AS more often required statin treatment, which could have significantly affected the obtained results.

The main limitation of the current study is relatively small sample size, drawn from a single-center population, which may have reduced the statistical power of the analysis. Additionally, a longer follow-up period is required to assess the impact of Apo B levels, Apo B/Apo A1 ratio, and PON1 activity on the progression of AS in the BAV population. The study did not consider dietary habits or the dosage of lipid-lowering medications, which also may have affected the evaluated markers. However, the cohort aged $\leq$45 was homogeneous in terms of age, sex, and the chronic conditions included in the study; the older group exhibited greater heterogeneity. Patients aged >45 with AS were significantly older and more frequently used statins compared to those without AS. However, we would like to highlight that, to the best of our knowledge, this is the first prospective study in BAV patients which indicated that Apo B levels, Apo B/Apo A1 ratio, and PON-1 activity are associated with AS appearance. Our results require further prospective studies in larger cohorts.

5. Conclusions

In summary, the AS occurrence among the BAV population has complex etiology and is challenging to predict. Our results suggest a potential metabolic link between Apo B level and Apo B/Apo AI ratio and the occurrence of AS in patients with a BAV. Notably, this association was observed only in patients up to 45 years of age. Furthermore, our findings underscore the value of investigating molecules associated with HDL and its antioxidant function, such as PON1, as a useful marker for AS development, compared to traditionally measured HDL-C and LDL-C levels.

Supplementary Materials: The following supporting information can be downloaded at: https://www.mdpi.com/article/10.3390/antiox14020167/s1, Table S1: Receiver operating characteristic (ROC) analysis of lipid markers and the presence of aortic stenosis for patients aged $\leq$45; Table S2: Receiver operating characteristic (ROC) analysis of lipid markers and the presence of aortic stenosis for patients aged >45.

Author Contributions: Conceptualization, M.K., A.M., M.F., A.K. (Agnieszka Kuchta) and A.K. (Aleksandra Krzesińska); methodology, M.K., A.M., M.F., A.K. (Aleksandra Krzesińska) and A.K. (Agnieszka Kuchta); software, M.K. and A.K. (Agnieszka Kuchta); validation, M.F., A.M. and A.K. (Agnieszka Kuchta); formal analysis, M.K. and A.K. (Aleksandra Krzesińska); investigation, M.K., A.M., A.K. (Aleksandra Krzesińska) and A.K. (Agnieszka Kuchta); resources, M.K., A.M., A.K. (Aleksandra Krzesińska) and A.K. (Agnieszka Kuchta); data curation M.K., A.M.; writing—original draft preparation, M.K.; writing—review and editing, A.M., A.K. (Agnieszka Kuchta), M.F., M.G. and M.J.; visualization, M.K.; supervision, A.M., M.F., A.K. (Agnieszka Kuchta), M.J. and M.G.; project administration, A.M., M.K., A.K. (Agnieszka Kuchta) and M.F. All authors have read and agreed to the published version of the manuscript.

Funding: This research received no external funding.

Institutional Review Board Statement: The study was conducted in accordance with the Declaration of Helsinki, and approved by the Local Bioethics Committee at the Medical University of Gdansk (protocol no. NKBBN/487-517/2019).

Informed Consent Statement: Informed consent was obtained from all subjects involved in the study.

Data Availability Statement: The original contributions presented in this study are included in the article/Supplementary Material. Further inquiries can be directed to the corresponding author.

Conflicts of Interest: The authors declare no conflict of interest.

References

1. Braverman, A.; Guven, H.; Beardslee, M.; Makan, M.; Kates, A.; Moon, M. The Bicuspid Aortic Valve. *Curr. Probl. Cardiol.* **2005**, *30*, 470–522. [CrossRef] [PubMed]
2. Shah, S.Y.; Higgins, A.; Desai, M.Y. Bicuspid aortic valve: Basics and beyond. *Cleve Clin. J. Med.* **2018**, *85*, 779–784. [CrossRef] [PubMed]
3. Michelena, H.I.; Desjardins, V.A.; Avierinos, J.F.; Russo, A.; Nkomo, V.T.; Sundt, T.M.; Pellikka, P.A.; Tajik, A.J.; Enriquez-Sarano, M. Natural history of asymptomatic patients with normally functioning or minimally dysfunctional bicuspid aortic valve in the community. *Circulation* **2008**, *117*, 2776–2784. [CrossRef]
4. Siu, S.C.; Silversides, C.K. Bicuspid Aortic Valve Disease. *J. Am. Coll. Cardiol.* **2010**, *55*, 2789–2800. [CrossRef] [PubMed]
5. Lindman, B.R.; Clavel, M.A.; Mathieu, P.; Iung, B.; Lancellotti, P.; Otto, C.M.; Pibarot, P. Calcific aortic stenosis. *Nat. Rev. Dis. Prim.* **2016**, *2*, 16006. [CrossRef]
6. Beppu, S.; Suzuki, S.; Matsuda, H.; Ohmori, F.; Nagata, S.; Miyatake, K. Rapidity of progression of aortic stenosis in patients with congenital bicuspid aortic valves. *Am. J. Cardiol.* **1993**, *71*, 322–327. [CrossRef] [PubMed]
7. Yuan, M.; Yuan, S.-M. The anatomopathology of bicuspid aortic valve. *Folia Morphol.* **2011**, *70*, 217–227.
8. Mai, Z.; Guan, L.; Mu, Y. Association between bicuspid aortic valve phenotype and patterns of valvular dysfunction: A meta-analysis. *Clin. Cardiol.* **2021**, *44*, 1683. [CrossRef]
9. Tzemos, N.; Therrien, J.; Yip, J.; Thanassoulis, G.; Tremblay, S.; Jamorski, M.T.; Webb, G.D.; Siu, S.C. Outcomes in Adults With Bicuspid Aortic Valves. *JAMA* **2008**, *300*, 1317–1325. [CrossRef] [PubMed]
10. Ivert, T.; Hammar, N.; Talbäck, M.; Malmström, H.; Leander, K.; Walldius, G. Elevated Apolipoprotein B/A-1 Ratio is Associated With an Increased Risk of Aortic Stenosis: Experience From the AMORIS Cohort. *Heart. Lung Circ.* **2021**, *30*, 1050–1057. [CrossRef] [PubMed]
11. Yan, A.T.; Koh, M.; Chan, K.K.; Guo, H.; Alter, D.A.; Austin, P.C.; Tu, J.V.; Wijeysundera, H.C.; Ko, D.T. Association Between Cardiovascular Risk Factors and Aortic Stenosis: The CANHEART Aortic Stenosis Study. *J. Am. Coll. Cardiol.* **2017**, *69*, 1523–1532. [CrossRef] [PubMed]
12. Glavinovic, T.; Thanassoulis, G.; de Graaf, J.; Couture, P.; Hegele, R.A.; Sniderman, A.D. Physiological Bases for the Superiority of Apolipoprotein B Over Low-Density Lipoprotein Cholesterol and Non–High-Density Lipoprotein Cholesterol as a Marker of Cardiovascular Risk. *J. Am. Heart Assoc. Cardiovasc. Cerebrovasc. Dis.* **2022**, *11*, 25858. [CrossRef]
13. Nagao, M.; Nakajima, H.; Toh, R.; Hirata, K.I.; Ishida, T. Cardioprotective Effects of High-Density Lipoprotein Beyond its Anti-Atherogenic Action. *J. Atheroscler. Thromb.* **2018**, *25*, 985. [CrossRef] [PubMed]
14. Hofmanis, J.; Hofmane, D.; Svirskis, S.; Mackevics, V.; Tretjakovs, P.; Lejnieks, A.; Signorelli, S.S. HDL-C Role in Acquired Aortic Valve Stenosis Patients and Its Relationship with Oxidative Stress. *Medicina* **2019**, *55*, 416. [CrossRef]
15. Barter, P.J.; Nicholls, S.; Rye, K.A.; Anantharamaiah, G.M.; Navab, M.; Fogelman, A.M. Antiinflammatory properties of HDL. *Circ. Res.* **2004**, *95*, 764–772. [CrossRef] [PubMed]
16. Lommi, J.I.; Kovanen, P.T.; Jauhiainen, M.; Lee-Rueckert, M.; Kupari, M.; Helske, S. High-density lipoproteins (HDL) are present in stenotic aortic valves and may interfere with the mechanisms of valvular calcification. *Atherosclerosis* **2011**, *219*, 538–544. [CrossRef] [PubMed]
17. Tsompanidi, E.M.; Brinkmeier, M.S.; Fotiadou, E.H.; Giakoumi, S.M.; Kypreos, K.E. HDL biogenesis and functions: Role of HDL quality and quantity in atherosclerosis. *Atherosclerosis* **2010**, *208*, 3–9. [CrossRef] [PubMed]
18. Liu, C.; Dhindsa, D.; Almuwaqqat, Z.; Ko, Y.A.; Mehta, A.; Alkhoder, A.A.; Alras, Z.; Desai, S.R.; Patel, K.J.; Hooda, A.; et al. Association Between High-Density Lipoprotein Cholesterol Levels and Adverse Cardiovascular Outcomes in High-risk Populations. *JAMA Cardiol.* **2022**, *7*, 672–680. [CrossRef]
19. Sökmen, E.; Çelik, M.; Sivri, S.; Güçlü, K. Relationship between Paraoxonase-1 and Arylesterase Enzyme Activities and SYNTAX I and II Scores in Patients with ST-Elevation Myocardial Infarction. *J. Tehran Univ. Heart Cent.* **2019**, *14*, 156. [CrossRef]
20. Song, J.; Zheng, Q.; Ma, X.; Zhang, Q.; Xu, Z.; Zou, C.; Wang, Z. Expression levels of paraoxonase-1 in aortic valve tissue are associated with the progression of calcific aortic valve stenosis. *J. Thorac. Dis.* **2019**, *11*, 2890–2898. [CrossRef] [PubMed]
21. O'Brien, K.D.; Reichenbach, D.D.; Marcovina, S.M.; Kuusisto, J.; Alpers, C.E.; Otto, C.M. Apolipoproteins B, (a), and E accumulate in the morphologically early lesion of "degenerative" valvular aortic stenosis. *Arterioscler. Thromb. Vasc. Biol.* **1996**, *16*, 523–532. [CrossRef] [PubMed]
22. Gebhard, C.; Maafi, F.; Stähli, B.E.; Dang, J.; Nachar, W.; de Oliveira Moraes, A.B.; Kernaleguen, A.E.; Lavoie, V.; Mecteau, M.; Mihalache-Avram, T.; et al. Apolipoprotein A-I proteolysis in aortic valve stenosis: Role of cathepsin S. *Basic Res. Cardiol.* **2018**, *113*, 30. [CrossRef] [PubMed]
23. Kaneva, A.M.; Potolitsyna, N.N.; Bojko, E.R.; Odland, J. The Apolipoprotein B/Apolipoprotein A-I Ratio as a Potential Marker of Plasma Atherogenicity. *Dis. Markers* **2015**, *2015*, 591454. [CrossRef] [PubMed]

24. Zheng, K.H.; Arsenault, B.J.; Kaiser, Y.; Khaw, K.T.; Wareham, N.J.; Stroes, E.S.G.; Boekholdt, S.M. apoB/apoA-I Ratio and Lp(a) Associations With Aortic Valve Stenosis Incidence: Insights From the EPIC-Norfolk Prospective Population Study. *J. Am. Heart Assoc. Cardiovasc. Cerebrovasc. Dis.* **2019**, *8*, e013020. [CrossRef]
25. Duran Karaduman, B.; Ayhan, H.; Keleş, T.; Bozkurt, E. Association between monocyte to high-density lipoprotein cholesterol ratio and bicuspid aortic valve degeneration. *Turk. J. Med. Sci.* **2020**, *50*, 1307–1313. [CrossRef]
26. Endo, M.; Nabuchi, A.; Okuyama, H.; Muto, Y.; Hiranuma, S.; Miyazaki, T.; Hosokawa, J.; Enjoji, Y.; Shimura, Y.; Hashimoto, O. Differing relationship between hypercholesterolemia and a bicuspid aortic valve according to the presence of aortic valve stenosis or aortic valve regurgitation. *Gen. Thorac. Cardiovasc. Surg.* **2015**, *63*, 502–506. [CrossRef]
27. Magni, P. Bicuspid aortic valve, atherosclerosis and changes of lipid metabolism: Are there pathological molecular links? *J. Mol. Cell. Cardiol.* **2019**, *129*, 231–235. [CrossRef] [PubMed]
28. Aggarwal, A.; Srivastava, S.; Velmurugan, M. Newer perspectives of coronary artery disease in young. *World J. Cardiol.* **2016**, *8*, 728. [CrossRef]
29. Michos, E.D.; Choi, A.D. Coronary Artery Disease in Young Adults: A Hard Lesson But a Good Teacher. *J. Am. Coll. Cardiol.* **2019**, *74*, 1879–1882. [CrossRef] [PubMed]
30. Vahanian, A.; Beyersdorf, F.; Praz, F.; Milojevic, M.; Baldus, S.; Bauersachs, J.; Capodanno, D.; Conradi, L.; De Bonis, M.; De Paulis, R.; et al. 2021 ESC/EACTS Guidelines for the management of valvular heart diseaseDeveloped by the Task Force for the management of valvular heart disease of the European Society of Cardiology (ESC) and the European Association for Cardio-Thoracic Surgery (EACTS). *Eur. Heart J.* **2022**, *43*, 561–632. [CrossRef]
31. Friedewald, W.T.; Levy, R.I.; Fredrickson, D.S. Estimation of the Concentration of Low-Density Lipoprotein Cholesterol in Plasma, Without Use of the Preparative Ultracentrifuge. *Clin. Chem.* **1972**, *18*, 499–502. [CrossRef]
32. Fukuyama, N.; Homma, K.; Wakana, N.; Kudo, K.; Suyama, A.; Ohazama, H.; Tsuji, C.; Ishiwata, K.; Eguchi, Y.; Nakazawa, H.; et al. Validation of the Friedewald Equation for Evaluation of Plasma LDL-Cholesterol. *J. Clin. Biochem. Nutr.* **2007**, *43*, 1–5. [CrossRef] [PubMed]
33. Nakanishi, M.; Takanami, Y.; Maruyama, T.; Murata, M.; Motohashi, Y.; Nakano, S.; Uchida, K.; Maruyama, C.; Kyotani, S.; Tsushima, M. The ratio of serum paraoxonase/arylesterase activity using an improved assay for arylesterase activity to discriminate PON1(R192) from PON1(Q192). *J. Atheroscler. Thromb.* **2003**, *10*, 337–342. [CrossRef] [PubMed]
34. Fenoglio, J.J.; McAllister, H.A.; DeCastro, C.M.; Davia, J.E.; Cheitlin, M.D. Congenital bicuspid aortic valve after age 20. *Am. J. Cardiol.* **1977**, *39*, 164–169. [CrossRef]
35. Lewin, M.B.; Otto, C.M. The bicuspid aortic valve: Adverse outcomes from infancy to old age. *Circulation* **2005**, *111*, 832–834. [CrossRef] [PubMed]
36. Perrin, N.; Ibrahim, R.; Dürrleman, N.; Basmadjian, A.; Leroux, L.; Demers, P.; Modine, T.; Ali, W. Ben Bicuspid Aortic Valve Stenosis: From Pathophysiological Mechanism, Imaging Diagnosis, to Clinical Treatment Methods. *Front. Cardiovasc. Med.* **2022**, *8*, 798949. [CrossRef]
37. Lim, M.S.; Strange, G.; Playford, D.; Stewart, S.; Celermajer, D.S. Characteristics of Bicuspid Aortic Valve Disease and Stenosis: The National Echo Database of Australia. *J. Am. Heart Assoc. Cardiovasc. Cerebrovasc. Dis.* **2021**, *10*, e020785. [CrossRef]
38. Otto, C.M. Calcification of bicuspid aortic valves. *Heart* **2002**, *88*, 321–322. [CrossRef] [PubMed]
39. Faggiano, P.; Antonini-Canterin, F.; Baldessin, F.; Lorusso, R.; D'Aloia, A.; Dei Cas, L. Epidemiology and cardiovascular risk factors of aortic stenosis. *Cardiovasc. Ultrasound* **2006**, *4*, 27. [CrossRef] [PubMed]
40. Sticchi, E.; Giusti, B.; Cordisco, A.; Gori, A.M.; Sereni, A.; Sofi, F.; Mori, F.; Colonna, S.; Fugazzaro, M.P.; Pepe, G.; et al. Role of lipoprotein (a) and LPA KIV2 repeat polymorphism in bicuspid aortic valve stenosis and calcification: A proof of concept study. *Intern. Emerg. Med.* **2019**, *14*, 45–50. [CrossRef]
41. Alegret, J.M. Masana, L.; Martinez-micaelo, N.; Heras, M.; Beltrán-debón, R. LDL cholesterol and apolipoprotein B are associated with ascending aorta dilatation in bicuspid aortic valve patients. *QJM Int. J. Med.* **2015**, *108*, 795–801. [CrossRef] [PubMed]
42. Baigent, C.; Blackwell, L.; Emberson, J.; Holland, L.E.; Reith, C.; Bhala, N.; Peto, R.; Barnes, E.H.; Keech, A.; Simes, J.; et al. Efficacy and safety of more intensive lowering of LDL cholesterol: A meta-analysis of data from 170,000 participants in 26 randomised trials. *Lancet* **2010**, *376*, 1670–1681. [CrossRef]
43. Smith, J.G.; Luk, K.; Schulz, C.A.; Engert, J.C.; Do, R.; Hindy, G.; Rukh, G.; Dufresne, L.; Almgren, P.; Owens, D.S.; et al. Association of Low-Density Lipoprotein Cholesterol–Related Genetic Variants With Aortic Valve Calcium and Incident Aortic Stenosis. *JAMA* **2014**, *312*, 1764. [CrossRef] [PubMed]
44. Holmes, M.V.; Asselbergs, F.W.; Palmer, T.M.; Drenos, F.; Lanktree, M.B.; Nelson, C.P.; Dale, C.E.; Padmanabhan, S.; Finan, C.; Swerdlow, D.I.; et al. Mendelian randomization of blood lipids for coronary heart disease. *Eur. Heart J.* **2015**, *36*, 539–550. [CrossRef] [PubMed]
45. Nazarzadeh, M.; Pinho-Gomes, A.C.; Bidel, Z.; Dehghan, A.; Canoy, D.; Hassaine, A.; Ayala Solares, J.R.; Salimi-Khorshidi, G.; Smith, G.D.; Otto, C.M.; et al. Plasma lipids and risk of aortic valve stenosis: A Mendelian randomization study. *Eur. Heart J.* **2020**, *41*, 3913–3920. [CrossRef] [PubMed]

46. Stanciulescu, L.A.; Scafa-Udriste, A.; Dorobantu, M. Exploring the Association between Low-Density Lipoprotein Subfractions and Major Adverse Cardiovascular Outcomes—A Comprehensive Review. *Int. J. Mol. Sci.* **2023**, *24*, 6669. [CrossRef]
47. Galimberti, F.; Casula, M.; Olmastroni, E. Apolipoprotein B compared with low-density lipoprotein cholesterol in the atherosclerotic cardiovascular diseases risk assessment. *Pharmacol. Res.* **2023**, *195*, 106873. [CrossRef] [PubMed]
48. Behbodikhah, J.; Ahmed, S.; Elyasi, A.; Kasselman, L.J.; De Leon, J.; Glass, A.D.; Reiss, A.B. Apolipoprotein B and Cardiovascular Disease: Biomarker and Potential Therapeutic Target. *Metabolites* **2021**, *11*, 690. [CrossRef]
49. Walldius, G.; Jungner, I. Apolipoprotein A-I versus HDL cholesterol in the prediction of risk for myocardial infarction and stroke. *Curr. Opin. Cardiol.* **2007**, *22*, 359–367. [CrossRef] [PubMed]
50. Deng, F.; Li, D.; Lei, L.; Yang, Q.; Li, Q.; Wang, H.; Deng, J.; Zheng, Q.; Jiang, W. Association between apolipoprotein B/A1 ratio and coronary plaque vulnerability in patients with atherosclerotic cardiovascular disease: An intravascular optical coherence tomography study. *Cardiovasc. Diabetol.* **2021**, *20*, 188. [CrossRef] [PubMed]
51. Mach, F.; Baigent, C.; Catapano, A.L.; Koskina, K.C.; Casula, M.; Badimon, L.; Chapman, M.J.; De Backer, G.G.; Delgado, V.; Ference, B.A.; et al. 2019 ESC/EAS guidelines for the management of dyslipidaemias: Lipid modification to reduce cardiovascular risk. *Atherosclerosis* **2019**, *290*, 140–205. [CrossRef] [PubMed]
52. Küçük, H.O.; Küçük, U.; Demirtaş, C.; Özdemir, M. Role of serum high density lipoprotein levels and functions in calcific aortic valve stenosis progression. *Int. J. Clin. Exp. Med.* **2015**, *8*, 22543.
53. Endo, Y.; Fujita, M.; Ikewaki, K. HDL Functions—Current Status and Future Perspectives. *Biomolecules* **2023**, *13*, 105. [CrossRef] [PubMed]

antioxidants

MDPI

Article

PON-1 and PON-2 Polymorphisms and PON-1 Paraoxonase Activity in People Living with HIV-1

Cadiele Oliana Reichert [1], Débora Levy [1], Luciana Morganti Ferreira Maselli [1], Joel da Cunha [1], Sandra Fátima Menosi Gualandro [2] and Sérgio Paulo Bydlowski [1,2,3,*]

[1] Lipids, Oxidation, and Cell Biology Group, Laboratory of Immunology (LIM19), Heart Institute (InCor), Hospital das Clínicas HCFMUSP, Faculdade de Medicina, Universidade de Sao Paulo, Sao Paulo 05403-900, SP, Brazil; kadielli@hotmail.com or cadiele@usp.br (C.O.R.); d.levy@hc.fm.usp.br (D.L.); lu_morganti@yahoo.com.br (L.M.F.M.); joelbioq@gmail.com (J.d.C.)

[2] Department of Hematology, Hemotherapy, and Cell Therapy, Faculdade de Medicina FMUSP, Universidade de Sao Paulo, Sao Paulo 05419-000, SP, Brazil; sandrafmg@uol.com.br

[3] Instituto Nacional de Ciencia e Tecnologia em Medicina Regenerativa (INCT-Regenera), CNPq, Rio de Janeiro 21941-902, RJ, Brazil

* Correspondence: spbydlow@usp.br

Abstract: Antiretroviral therapy (ART) has significantly improved the life expectancy of people living with HIV-1 (PLWH). However, prolonged ART use is linked to metabolic alterations and oxidative stress. The paraoxonase (PON) enzymes, especially PON-1 and PON-2, are critical in maintaining antioxidant balance. Their activity can be influenced by polymorphisms such as Q192R and L55M in PON-1 and A148G and S311C in PON-2. This study examines the impact of these polymorphisms on paraoxonase activity, lipid metabolism, and infection markers in PLWH under various ART regimens. This is a case-control study with 525 participants, 175 healthy controls (HC) and 350 PLWH divided into subgroups: T0 (ART-naïve, $n = 48$), T1 (ART with reverse transcriptase inhibitors, $n = 159$), and T2 (ART with protease inhibitors, $n = 143$). Paraoxonase activity was higher in PLWH (123.0; IQR: 62.0–168.0) compared to HC (91.0; IQR: 48.0–136.0, $p < 0.001$) but similar between HC and T0 ($p = 0.594$). T1 (125.0; IQR: 65.5–166.0) and T2 (123.0; IQR: 61.0–182.0) showed higher activity than HC ($p = 0.002$ and 0.003). Among 61 complete genotypes, 13 were unique to PLWH and 6 to HC ($p < 0.001$). L55L was more frequent in HC (49.7% vs. 36.9% in PLWH), while M55M was higher in PLWH ($p = 0.004$). The S311C genotype was more frequent in HC (39.2%) than PLWH (24.9%) ($p = 0.003$). The L55L genotype conferred 59.9% protection against HIV-1 (OR: 0.401; 95% CI: 0.228–0.704), while the M allele increased susceptibility by ~69% (OR: 1.694; 95% CI: 1.173–2.446). The M55M genotype and/or M allele may be linked to HIV-1 susceptibility. Prolonged ART use elevates PON-1 activity in PLWH.

Keywords: ARV; HIV-1; lipids; paraoxonase; PON-1; PON-2

1. Introduction

The mechanisms associated with the oxidative balance in the human body act as a seesaw between oxidant and antioxidant factors [1]. This balance maintains physiological homeostasis through the action of antioxidant agents, which can neutralize and/or metabolize reactive species [2,3]. Some of the most effective mechanisms against the increase in both cellular and tissue oxidative stress (OS) are antioxidant enzymes, among which the paraoxonase (PON) family is of importance [4–6]. The PON enzymes are composed of three isoforms, paraoxonase-1 (PON-1, EC 3.1.1.2, 3.1.1.81, 3.1.8.1), paraoxonase-2 (PON-2,

EC 3.1.1.2, 3.1.1.81), and paraoxonase-3 (PON-3, EC 3.1.1.2, 3.1.1.81, 3.1.8.1), showing 52.4% sequence identity and 76.3% sequence similarity among the isoforms. The enzymes are located adjacent to human chromosome 7 (7q21-23) [7,8].

Although the three paraoxonase enzymes share a homologous protein structure, they are known to differ in their localization, function, and activity [9]. PON-1 is a calcium-dependent glycoprotein 43 kDa with 355 amino acid residues, synthesized in the liver [9]. In humans, the PON-1 enzyme is mainly associated with high-density lipoprotein 3 (HDL3) and in lower concentrations in very-low density lipoprotein (VLDL) and chylomicrons [10]. A small fraction of PON-1 can be found free in plasma [10]. PON-1 has esterase activity (arylesterase and lactonase), through the hydrolysis of aromatic ester compounds and aromatic and aliphatic lactones, and paraoxonase activity, through the hydrolysis of toxic oxonium metabolites [11–14].

The paraoxonase activity of the PON-1 enzyme can be regulated by environmental factors, different pathophysiological conditions, both genetic and epigenetic alterations, and the presence of single nucleotide polymorphisms (SNPs) in the regulatory region of the gene [15,16]. PON-1 exists in two isoforms, resulting from amino acid substitutions: glutamine (Gln) is replaced by arginine (Arg) at position 192, Q192R, and leucine (Leu) is substituted by methionine (Met) at position 55, L55M. These genetic polymorphisms have been linked to variations in PON-1 activity, either reduced or elevated, and the risk of developing certain diseases [17–20].

The PON-2 enzyme has approximately 40–43 kDa and is composed of 355 amino acids [18]. PON-2 is ubiquitously expressed intracellularly, particularly in the perinuclear region, endoplasmic reticulum, and mitochondria. The role of the PON-2 enzyme in the defense system against oxidative stress, and therefore apoptosis, is due to its high lactonase activity [21–23]. PON-2 has two SNPs that have clinical relevance. The A148G polymorphism, in which an alanine residue is exchanged for glycine at position 148 of the protein, and the S311C polymorphism, in which a serine is exchanged for a cysteine at position 311 [24]. Some studies associate the presence of both polymorphisms with the development of diseases related to increased oxidative stress, changes in lipid metabolism, type 2 diabetes, infection, and chronic inflammation with an antioxidative stress activity, but there is disagreement between the studies [25–28].

Human immunodeficiency virus type 1 (HIV-1) infection has been a subject of study since its discovery nearly four decades ago. Over the years there have been effective biotechnological advances in the diagnosis and introduction of antiretroviral therapy (ART), and people living with HIV (PLWH) have delayed the natural progression of the disease, wherein no disease symptoms appear and there is a decrease in co-infections and mortality and an increase in lifespan [29–31].

The World Health Organization (WHO) recommends a combination of different ARTs such as nucleotide and non-nucleotide reserve transcriptase inhibitors associated with each other or with protease inhibitors. The ART objective is to combat intense viral replication, which leads to a decrease in CD4 T lymphocytes (CD4-TLs). Such multi-drug combinations bring about significant improvements in the immune systems of PLWH. On the other hand, chronic use of antiretroviral therapy induces a prolonged pro-inflammatory state that is closely related to the development of chronic degenerative diseases caused, in part, by metabolic alteration, increased oxidative stress, and genomic instability [32–34].

The prolonged use of ART in PLWH has been associated with an increased incidence of comorbidities in this population. These alterations may also be associated with oxidative stress and genetic alterations resulting from the toxic effects of ART drug use and/or metabolism [35,36]. The presence of reactive species can negatively impact lipid metabolism, including lipoprotein dysfunction and lipid peroxidation [37,38]. This can exacerbate the dyslipidemia already linked to prolonged ART use, leading to changes such as increased triglyceride levels, reduced HDL cholesterol (HDL-C), and elevated low-density lipoprotein cholesterol (LDL-C). These metabolic changes heighten the risk of early atherosclerosis and cardiovascular diseases and lipodystrophy [39–41]. Given these characteristics, many studies have focused on improving the metabolic and antioxidant status of PLWH [42–44]. However, few studies have examined PON function in PLWH. In a study involving 624 PLWH, PON-1 paraoxonase activity was lower in ART-naïve individuals compared to those on ART and showed a positive correlation with the absolute number of CD4+ TL, suggesting a relationship with the immune system in PLWH [45].

The diverse functions of PON-1, including its antioxidant and anti-inflammatory roles, as well as its involvement in lipid metabolism, make this enzyme particularly attractive for studies focused on metabolic disorders and conditions related to oxidative stress, mainly because it is considered a cardioprotective enzyme [4,46–48]. Therefore, studying paraoxonase enzymes and their polymorphisms in PLWH is necessary. Understanding their role and activity in this population could provide valuable insights into the mechanisms underlying metabolic alterations, oxidative stress, and their associated comorbidities, particularly in the context of prolonged antiretroviral therapy.

Therefore, we designed this case-control study to evaluate whether the frequency of PON-1 (Q192R and L55M) and PON-2 (A148G and S311C) polymorphisms, as well as PON-1 paraoxonase activity, is different among PLWH when compared to healthy individuals. Furthermore, we conducted secondary analyses to verify whether PON-1 and PON-2 polymorphisms and paraoxonase activity are associated with lipid and infection markers in PLWH using different antiretroviral therapies.

2. Materials and Methods

2.1. Study Design

This is a case-control and multicentric study comprising 525 participants with ≥18 years of age (Figure 1). The participants were divided into two groups, 350 PLWH and 175 individuals considered clinically healthy (healthy control; HC). Study participants were matched by sex at a ratio of 2:1 (male:female).

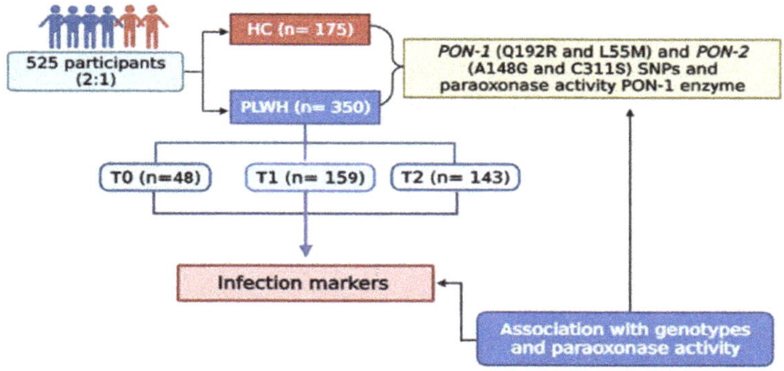

Figure 1. Flow-chart of this study.

2.2. Study Population Criteria

2.2.1. PLWH Group

The PLWH group was composed of individuals diagnosed with HIV type 1 (HIV-1) who were being monitored at the HIV-1 outpatient clinic at Casa da AIDS and the Hospital das Clínicas of the Faculty of Medicine of the University of São Paulo (HCFMUSP). All PLWH were positive for HIV type 1 (HIV-1) and each diagnosis was carried out in accordance with institutional standards recommended by the World Health Organization and Ministry of Health in Brazil [49].

PLWH were divided into three groups, T0, T1, and T2, according to their ART regimen. This classification aimed to assess whether different ART regimens influenced the paraoxonase activity of PON-1. Additionally, it is well established that ART regimens can impact lipid metabolism. The T0 group comprised 48 ART-naïve PLWH who had never undergone ART. These individuals were selected at the time of HIV-1 diagnosis. The T1 and T2 groups consisted of individuals who had been using ART for a minimum of six consecutive months.

The T1 group included 159 PLWH receiving ART based on non-nucleoside reverse transcriptase inhibitors (NNRTIs) in combination with nucleoside reverse transcriptase inhibitors (NRTIs). The treatment regimens included efavirenz (EFV) 600 mg once daily (qd) combined with azidovudine (AZT) 300 mg and lamivudine (3TC) 150 mg twice daily (bid); EFV 600 mg qd with estavudine (d4T) 40 mg and 3TC 150 mg bid; and EFV 600 mg (qd) with tenofovir (TDF) 300 mg and 3TC 150 mg (bid). Additional regimens included nevirapine (NVP) 200 mg bid combined with AZT 300 mg and 3TC 150 mg (bid); NVP 200 mg bid with d4T 40 mg and 3TC 150 mg bid; and NVP 200 mg bid with TDF 300 mg and 3TC 150 mg bid.

The T2 group consisted of 143 PLWH on ART regimens based on protease inhibitors (PIs) combined with NRTIs and/or NNRTIs. The treatment regimens also included lopinavir/ritonavir (LOP/r) 400 mg/100 mg bid combined with AZT 300 mg and 3TC 150 mg bid, as well as LOP/r 400 mg/100 mg bid with d4T 40 mg and 3TC 150 mg bid.

The selection criteria for PLWH were (I) no renal, cardiac, or hepatic function alterations and/or metabolic syndrome; (II) no co-infection, such as HPV, hepatitis B or C, or tuberculosis, in the last 6 months; (III) no use of anti-inflammatory drugs, hormones, or other medications except ART; and (IV) be positive only for HIV-1. These criteria were used to reduce the biases related to the paraoxonase activity of the PON-1 enzyme and both lipid and infection markers. The clinical and laboratory variables of infection markers were collected from medical records. For PLWH who were already under follow-up at the institution, blood samples were also collected on the day of HIV-1 infection monitoring to assess paraoxonase activity and lipid markers.

2.2.2. HC Group

The HC group consisted of 175 volunteer blood donors. Individuals in the HC group were evaluated according to the guidelines set by the World Health Organization and the National Health Surveillance Agency (ANVISA) for blood donation [50,51]. This group of individuals were regular blood donors, meaning they donated blood every six months. The selection criteria were to be between 18 and 69 years of age, be in good health, weigh at least 50 kg, not use medications or have received blood transfusions, and show no clinical or analytical evidence of renal insufficiency, liver disease, neurological disease, neoplasms, dyslipidemia, hematological disorders, or chronic infections or inflammation. Furthermore, they had to be negative for clinical and laboratory evidence of transmissible infectious diseases, including hepatitis B and C, AIDS or HIV-1/2, HTLV I and II viruses, and Chagas disease. The clinical evaluation was conducted by a hematologist during donor screening. Following this, the blood donation took place and all laboratory tests, including for infectious diseases, were performed. Participants who met all the criteria described above were included in this study.

2.3. Sample Preparation

The venous blood samples (15 mL) were collected after 8–12 h fasting using a vacuum system with and without EDTA. Blood without EDTA was immediately centrifuged at 420× *g* for 15 min and the serum was stored at −80 °C until use. The blood collected with EDTA was used for genomic DNA extraction from leukocytes by the salting out precipitation method [52].

2.4. PON-1 and PON-2 Genotypes

The PON-1 polymorphisms (Q192R and L55M) were analyzed using primers designed to introduce a recognition site for the Hinf I enzyme in one allele of each PCR product. This approach enabled the simultaneous identification of both polymorphisms in a single amplification, followed by restriction enzyme analysis [53]. The Q192 and R192 alleles were determined by the presence of a 111 bp undigested fragment, along with 77 and 34 bp digested fragments. For the L55M polymorphism, L and M alleles were distinguished by a 144 bp undigested fragment and 122 and 22 bp digested fragments. Genotyping of the A148G codon of PON-2 was performed as described by Hegele et al. [54], while the S311C polymorphism was determined according to the method outlined by Motti et al. [53].

2.5. PON-1 Activity, Biochemical Determination and Viral Load

Here, the paraoxonase activity of PON-1 was used a marker of oxidative stress. The paraoxonase activity of PON-1 was determined according to Sentí et al. [55] and Agachan et al. [56]. The enzymatic hydrolysis of paraoxon releases *p*-nitrophenol, whose rate of formation was evaluated spectrophotometrically with absorbance readings at 405 nm at 37 °C for 10 min. PON-1 enzyme paraoxonase activity was performed in all groups.

The concentrations of serum total cholesterol (TC) as well as their fractions (HDL, LDL, and VLDL), triglycerides (TG), complete blood count/leucogram, viral load, and CD4-TL and CD8-TL lymphocyte count were measured by standard methods in a Modular 48 Analytics P-800 (Roche and Hitachi, Basel, Switzerland) automated analyzer. These clinical variables were measured in PLWH.

The HIV-1 viral load was quantified using the Nucleic Acid Sequence-Based Amplification (NASBA) kit (Organon Teknika, Boxtel, The Netherlands). The detection limit for the viral load was 50 copies/mL of HIV-1 RNA. This test was performed in both groups, PLWH and HC.

To reduce biases related to the correlation between biochemical variables, infection markers, and paraoxonase activity, all samples were collected on the same day.

2.6. Statistical Data Analysis

The data analysis of this research was carried out in two stages. First, we performed the comparison of demographic characteristics (sex and age), paraoxonase activity, and distribution of polymorphisms between the groups HC and PLWH. Here, the analysis performed matched sex. Second, we evaluated the difference in lipid metabolism markers and infection markers, as well as the influence of polymorphisms under these variables between the PLWH groups: T0, T1, and T2. To verify the adherence of the numerical data to a Gaussian distribution, we used the Shapiro–Wilk test, the histogram plot, and the qq-plot (quantile–quantile).

Numerical data are presented as a measure of central tendency, median with 25 and 75 percentiles, or interquartile range (IQR). Categorical variables are presented as absolute count number and frequency (n-%). The Student's *t* test and the non-parametric Mann–Whitney u test were used to compare the quantitative variables between the groups. One-way or two-way analysis of variance with Tukey's post-test or Kruskal–Wallis test was used for comparison among groups. The genotype frequencies of the polymorphisms were calculated using the Hardy–Weinberg Equilibrium (HWE), Chi-squared test (χ^2), and Fisher's exact test. Pearson (r^2) or Spearman (ρ) correlation analysis was performed between the PON-1 activities and all other data.

Binary logistic regression analysis was used to investigate the relationship between the presence or absence of HIV-1 and the polymorphisms Q192R, L55M, A148G, and S311C. In other words, this approach assesses whether the presence of a polymorphism may be associated with the likelihood of having HIV-1. The HC and PWHL groups were defined as the dependent variable, while the polymorphisms of PON-1 and PON-2 enzymes were used as independent variables. The "wild-type" polymorphisms of each SNP were used as the reference. The forward conditional method was employed to identify significant SNPs in final multivariate analysis. The interpretation of the results was based on established mathematical parameters [57]. The results of the binary logistic regression are presented as odds ratios (ORs) with a 95% confidence interval (95% CI).

The linear regression was used to establish the relationship between lipid markers, PON-1 activity with viral load, CD4-LT, and CD8+-LT. Mathematical criteria were used to conduct the regression analysis. Briefly, (1) Linearity: the relationship between the dependent variable and each independent variable. All dependent variables (viral load, CD4-LT, and CD8+-LT) were log-transformed to reduce data dispersion and adhere to the Gaussian distribution. (2) Assessment of the independence of errors/residuals using the Durbin–Watson statistic. (3) Assessment of homoscedasticity, which should be constant, by plotting the residuals in relation to the predicted values. (4) Assessment of the Gaussian distribution of the residuals, as previously mentioned. (5) Assessment of multicollinearity using the Variance Inflation Factor (VIF) values and/or correlation matrices. VIF values above 10 were considered as the presence of multicollinearity. (6) Assessment of significant outliers using Cook's distance statistics. Only continuous dependent variables were used in the regression analysis.

$p \leq 0.05$ values were considered as significant. SPSS Statistics software (IBM SPSS version 30.0) was used for all analyses and the GraphPad Prism version 8.0 program was used to make the figures.

3. Results

3.1. Gender and Age of PLWH Subjects and Healthy Control Group

The population of this study consisted of 350 PLWH patients and 175 healthy individuals (Table 1). The percentage of men was higher than that of women in both groups. The mean age was higher in PLWH individuals when compared with healthy controls ($p < 0.001$).

Table 1. Gender and age of patients with HIV-1 and healthy controls.

Gender	Groups (n = 525)		
	HC (n = 175)	**PLWH (n = 350)**	**p Value (1)**
Female	43 (24.6%)	86 (24.6%)	1.000
Male	132 (75.4%)	264 (75. 4%)	1.000
Age (years)	37.4 ± 9.0	41.5 ± 10.9	<0.001

(1) Comparison between groups using Chi-squared test (χ^2) and Student's t test. Abbreviation: HC = healthy control; PLWH = people living with HIV-1; n = number of individuals; % = percentage.

Due to the age difference observed between the groups, we assessed whether there was a correlation between age and paraoxonase activity. No significant correlation was observed in the total population (ρ = 0.015; $p = 0.738$), nor in the HC (ρ = 0.015; $p = 0.738$), T0 (ρ = 0.016; $p = 0.912$), T1 (ρ = −0.104; $p = 0.192$), and T2 (ρ = −0.022; $p = 0.796$) groups.

3.2. PON-1 and PON-2 Polymorphisms

In this study, we verified whether the Q192R and L55M polymorphisms of the PON-1 gene and the A148G and S311C polymorphisms of the PON-2 gene were in Hardy–Weinberg equilibrium between the populations studied. We observed that the L55M PON-1 ($p = 0.004$) and S311C PON-2 ($p = 0.003$) polymorphisms were not in Hardy–Weinberg equilibrium (HWE). Regarding the L55M PON-1 polymorphism, we observed that there was a higher frequency of the homozygous L55L genotype in the HC group when compared to the PLWH group (49.7% and 36.9%, respectively) and, inversely, there was an increase in the frequency of the homozygous M55M in PLWH ($p = 0.004$). Interestingly, in the analysis of the genotype frequency of the S311C PON-2 genotype, we observed that the heterozygous S311C PON-2 polymorphism was more frequent in the HC group (39.2%) when compared to PLWH (24.9%) ($p = 0.003$). The other polymorphisms, C311C and S311S showed similar frequencies in both groups (Table 2).

Table 2. Distribution of genotypes and allelic frequency of *PON-1* Q192R and L55M polymorphisms and *PON-2* A148G and C311S polymorphisms in HC and PLWH.

Gene-Polymorphism		Group ($n = 525$)				
		HC ($n = 175$)		PLWH ($n = 350$)		p Value (1)
PON-1 Q192R	QQ	75	42.9%	152	43.6%	0.970
	QR	71	40.6%	142	40.7%	
	RR	29	16.6%	55	15.8%	
	Q allele	221	63.1%	446	63.9%	
	R allele	129	36.9%	252	36.1%	
PON-1 L55M	LL	87	49.7%	129	36.9%	0.004
	LM	68	38.9%	147	42.0%	
	MM	20	11.4%	74	21.1%	
	L allele	242	69.1%	405	57.9%	
	M allele	108	30.9%	295	42.1%	
PON-2 A148G	AA	99	56.9%	209	59.7%	0.811
	AG	63	36.2%	117	33.4%	
	GG	12	6.9%	24	6.9%	
	A allele	262	75.0%	535	76.4%	
	G allele	87	25.0%	165	23.6%	
PON-2 S311C	SS	76	44.4%	186	53.1%	0.003
	CS	67	39.2%	87	24.9%	
	CC	28	16.4%	77	22.0%	
	C allele	123	36.0%	241	34.4%	
	S allele	219	64.0%	459	65.6%	

Results are expressed as n (%); (1) Comparison between groups using Chi-squared test (χ^2) or Fisher's exact test. Abbreviation: HC = healthy control; PLWH = people living with HIV-1; n = number of individuals; % = percentage.

In both populations studied, 61 combinations of complete genotypes were found (Figure 2) ($p < 0.001$). The frequency of 100% homozygous genotypes was higher in the

PLWH group compared to the HC group. Of the eleven homozygous genotypes, eight were more frequent in the PLWH group: L55L-R192R-G148G-C311C (67.0%), L55L-Q192Q-A148A-S311S (73.0%), L55L-R192R-A148A-S311S (79.0%), M55M-Q192Q-A148A-S311S (86.0%), M55M-R192R-G148G-C311C (100.0%), L55L-Q192Q-G148G-C311C (60.0%), M55M-Q192Q-A148A-C311C (100.0%), and M55M-R192R-A148A-S311S (100.0%); and only three in the HC group: L55L-Q192Q-G148G-S311S (33.0%) L55L-R192R-A148A-C311C (75.0%), and L55L-Q192Q-A148A-C311C (100.0%).

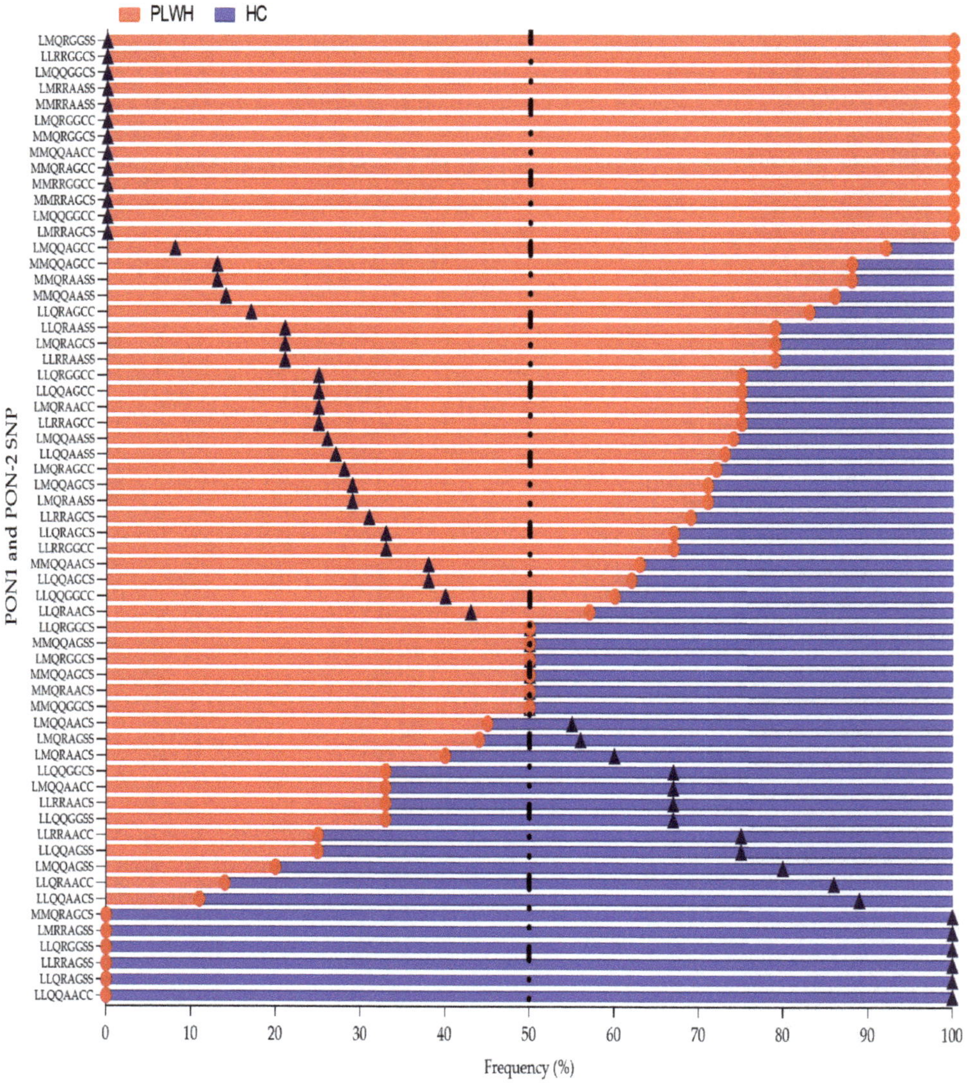

Figure 2. PON-1 and PON-2 genotypic frequencies. Distribution of PON-1 and PON-2 genotypic frequencies between PLWH (in red) and HC (in blue) groups. The red dots in the figure represent the genotypic frequencies for the PLWH group, while the blue triangles indicate the genotypic frequencies for the HC group. The position of the dot and triangle indicates the frequency of the genotype combination. The black dotted line marks the 50% frequency. The frequency between the groups was assessed by the Chi-squared test ($p < 0.001$)

In addition, the frequency of genotypes L55M-R192R-G148G-S311S, L55M-Q192Q-G148G-S311S, L55M-Q192Q-G148G-S311C, L55M-Q192R-A148A-C311C, L55M-Q192R-G148G-S311S, L55M-R192R-A148A-S311S, L55M-R192R-A148G-S311C, M55M-Q192Q-A148A-C311C, M55M-Q192R-A148G-C311C, M55M-Q192R-G418G-S311C, M55M-R192R-A148A-S311S, M55M-R192R-A148G-S311C, and M55M-R192R-G148G-C311C were 100% present only in the PLWH group.

On the other hand, the frequency of genotypes M55M-Q192R-A148G-C311S, L55M-R192R-A148G-S311S, L55L-R192R-A148G-S311S, L55L-Q192R-G148G-S311S, L55L-Q192R-A148G-S311S, and L55L-Q192Q-A148A-C311C were 100% present only in the HC group ($p < 0.001$). Through the analysis of these frequencies, it is possible to observe the higher frequency of the M allele in the PLWH population, in contrast with the higher frequency of the L allele in the HC population.

The PON-1 and PON-2 genes are part of the same genetic cluster and the strength of the relationships between PON-1 and PON-2 polymorphisms in HC and PLWH was evaluated (Figure 3). It was observed that the strength of the relationships between the genetic polymorphisms was different between the two populations studied. The relationship between the polymorphisms is associated with the frequency of the genotypes in the HC and PLWH groups. In the HC group, the polymorphisms Q192Q, Q192R, L55L, and L55M of the PON-1 gene and A148A, A148G, S311S, and C311S of the PON-2 gene present greater strength of integration with the other genotypes, while in the PLWH group these genotypes present lower interaction force.

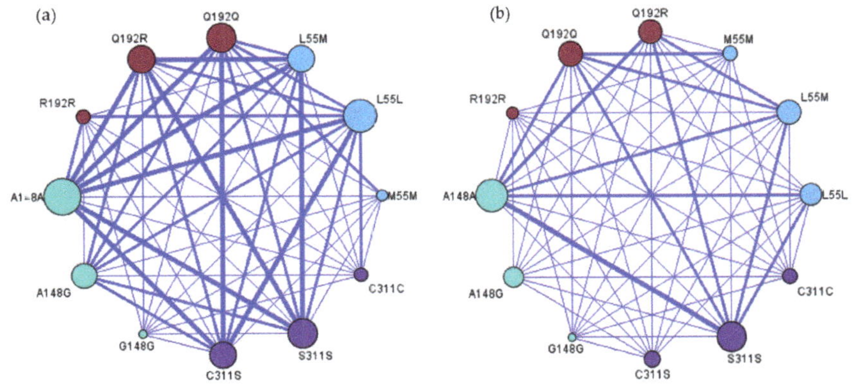

Figure 3. Relationship map of PON-1 and PON-2 polymorphisms in HC group (**a**) and PLWH group (**b**). The larger the circle, the greater the interaction with other polymorphisms. The blue lines represent interactions; the thicker the line, the stronger the interaction between genotypes.

Based on the results described, the odds ratio (OR) of the susceptibility to HIV-1 infection in relation to polymorphisms of the PON-1 and PON-2 genes was calculated using univariate binary logistic regression (Table 3). First, the OR calculation was performed using the dominant or greater genotype in relation to the others. Then, individuals were grouped according to the presence of a minor allele using univariate binary logistic regression. It was observed that the presence of the homozygous L55L polymorphism of PON-1 in relation to the homozygous M55M polymorphism was associated with a 59.9% reduction in the odds of HIV-1 susceptibility (OR: 0.401; 95% CI: 0.228–0.704). Additionally, the M (LM + MM) allele was associated with 69.4% increased odds of susceptibility to HIV-1 (OR: 1.694; 95% CI: 1.173–2.446). Interestingly, the presence of the heterozygous C311S polymorphism was also associated with an increased likelihood of susceptibility to HIV-1 (OR: 2.118; 95% CI: 1.238–3.624).

Table 3. Univariate binary logistic regression between the presence of polymorphisms PON-1 and PON-2 and susceptibility to HIV-1.

Polymorphism	β	SE	Wald	*p* Value	Exp(β)	Exp(β) CI 95%	
						Lower	Upper
Q192Q			0.032	0.984			
Q192R	0.013	0.203	0.004	0.948	1.013	0.681	0.507
R192R	0.048	0.269	0.032	0.857	1.050	0.620	1.777
Constant	−0.706	0.141	25.059	<0.001	0.493		
R allele	0.023	0.187	0.016	0.901	1.024	0.710	1.477
Constant	−0.730	0.308	50.622	0.018	0.482		
L55L			10.848	0.004			
L55M	−0.377	0.202	30.488	0.062	0.686	0.462	1.019
M55M	−0.914	0.288	10.104	0.001	0.401	0.228	0.704
Constant	−0.394	0.139	80.062	0.005	0.674		
M allele	0.527	0.187	7.902	0.005	1.694	1.173	2.446
Constant	−0.921	0.126	53.38	<0.001	0.398		
A148A			0.418	0.811			
A148G	0.128	0.198	0.418	0.518	1.137	0.771	1.677
G148G	0.054	0.374	0.021	0.885	1.056	0.507	2.197
Constant	−0.747	0.122	37.508	<0.001	0.474		
G allele	0.116	0.188	0.381	0.537	1.123	0.777	1.623
Constant	−0.747	0.122	37.508	<0.001	0.474		
C311C			11.332	0.003			
C311S	0.750	0.274	7.496	0.006	2.118	1.238	3.624
S311S	0.117	0.259	0.202	0.653	1.124	0.676	1.868
Constant	−1.012	0.221	21.013	<0.001	0.364		
S allele	0.365	0.244	2.244	0.134	1.440	0.894	2.322
Constant	−1.012	0.221	21.013	<0.001	0.364		

Binary logistic regression parameters and interpretation: The β (coefficient) indicates the direction and magnitude of the polymorphism's effect, with positive values increasing the chances of the event and negative values decreasing them. SE (standard error) reflects the precision of the coefficient. Wald assesses the relevance of the variable, with larger values indicating greater importance. *p*-value indicates statistical significance, being significant when less than 0.050. Exp(β) (odds ratio) shows how the chances of the event change with each unit of polymorphism change, with values > 1 increasing and <1 decreasing the chances. Exp(β) CI 95% shows the confidence interval for the OR, indicating the range of values with 95% certainty. The constant represents the probability of the event in the absence of independent variables; if negative, the chances are low, and if positive, high.

Subsequently, a multivariate analysis was conducted using only the significant SNPs, L55M and C311S. In the final model, the only SNPs that remained significant were the heterozygous C311S polymorphism (β = 0.860; OR: 2.195; 95% CI: 1.276–3.775) compared to C311C and the L55L polymorphism compared to M55M (β = −0.867; OR: 0.420; 95% CI: 0.228–0.704).

3.3. Paraoxonase Activity

The median paraoxonase activity of the PON-1 enzyme was higher in the PLWH group (123.0; IQR: 62.0–168.0) when compared to the HC group (91.0; IQR: 48.0–136.0)

($p < 0.001$) (Figure 4a). Interestingly, the comparison of the median of paraoxonase activity between the HC group and the T0 group (111.5; IQR: 54.0–161.0) was similar ($p = 0.594$). In addition, both the T1 (125.0; IQR: 65.5–166.0) and T2 (123.0; IQR: 61.0–182.0) groups showed higher paraoxonase activity when compared to the HC group ($p = 0.002$ and $p = 0.003$, respectively) (Figure 4b).

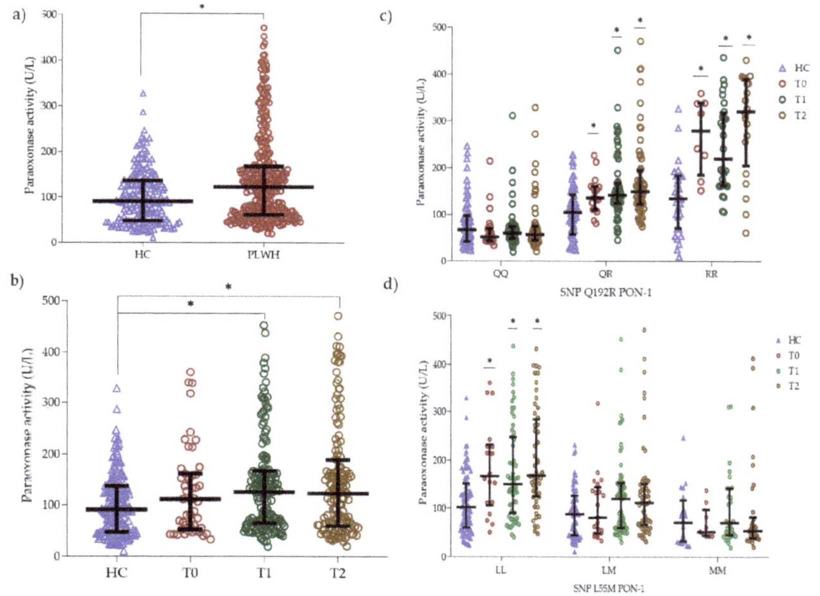

Figure 4. PON-1 activity. (**a**) Comparison of paraoxonase activity between the HC (in blue) and PLWH (in red) groups. (**b**) Comparison of paraoxonase activity between the HC (in blue), T0 (in red), T1 (in green), and T2 (in brown) groups. (**c**) Comparison of paraoxonase activity between the HC, T0, T1, and T2 groups by Q192R polymorphism. (**d**) Comparison of paraoxonase activity between the HC, T0, T1, and T2 groups by L55M polymorphism. The black bar represents the median and interquartile range. The HC group is represented by a triangle symbol. The PLWH group is represented by a circle. Each point represents an observation from the case series. The symbol (*) represents that the group is different from the others. The comparison between two groups was performed using the Mann–Whitney U test. The comparison between more than two groups was performed using the Kruskal–Wallis test.

Regarding the Q192R polymorphism, the presence of the homozygous Q192Q genotype showed no difference in paraoxonase activity between the groups evaluated ($p > 0.050$). However, different paraoxonase activity was observed between the groups considering the heterozygous Q192R polymorphism, as well as in the group itself when compared to the Q192Q polymorphism. The highest activity was related to the homozygous R192R polymorphism and the activity was higher in the T0, T1, and T2 groups when compared to the HC group. Thus, the polymorphisms influence paraoxonase activity ($p < 0.001$) as well as HIV-1 infection ($p < 0.001$). Moreover, there is an interaction between the polymorphism and HIV-1 infection, regardless of the ART treatment stage, that increases the PON-1 paraoxonase activity ($p < 0.001$) (Figure 4c).

The analysis of the paraoxonase activity associated with the L55M SNP of PON-1 showed that the highest activity of the enzyme is associated with the homozygous L55L genotype when compared to the other genotypes ($p < 0.001$), being similar between the heterozygous L55M and M55M genotypes, in all groups ($p > 0.050$). Furthermore, the highest paraoxonase activity observed was in the L55L genotype in the T2, T1, and T0 groups when compared to the HC group ($p < 0.001$) (Figure 4d).

3.4. Cholesterol, Lipoproteins, T Lymphocytes, and Viral Load

The effects of antiretroviral therapy on cholesterol, lipoproteins, CD4 and 8 T lymphocytes, and viral load were evaluated in the three groups of PLWH (Table 4). The lowest concentration of total cholesterol ($p = 0.050$), as well as triglycerides ($p < 0.001$) and VLDL ($p < 0.001$), was observed in the T0 group when compared to the other groups. The HDL concentration was higher in the T1 group when compared to the other groups ($p < 0.007$). The LDL concentration was similar between groups ($p = 0.106$).

Table 4. Cholesterol, lipoproteins, CD4 and CD8 T lymphocytes, and viral load in PLWH.

	PLWH (n = 350)									
	T0 (n = 48)			T1 (n = 159)			T2 (n = 143)			
	Median	P25	P75	Median	P25	P75	Median	P25	P75	p Value
CD4-TLs (mil/mm^3)	462.0	351.0	629.0	534.0	376.0	704.0	455.0	269.0	632.0	0.004
CD8-TLs (mil/mm^3)	1001.5	746.0	1289.0	796.0	604.0	1042.0	952.0	726.0	1295.0	<0.001
Viral load (Log)	4.4	3.7	5.0	3.9	3.1	4.6	4.5	3.8	5.1	0.048
Cholesterol (mg/dL)	173.0	150.0	192.0	187.0	160.0	214.0	172.0	151.0	210.0	0.050
HDL-C (mg/dL)	41.5	38.0	58.0	50.0	39.0	62.0	43.0	35.0	53.0	0.007
LDL-C (mg/dL)	94.5	67.0	119.0	105.0	81.0	131.0	98.0	70.0	121.0	0.106
VLDL-C (mg/dL)	24.5	18.0	36.0	25.0	18.0	40.0	34.0	23.0	44.0	<0.001
TG (mg/dL)	124.5	91.0	190.0	131.0	92.0	220.0	185.0	124.0	247.0	<0.001

Comparison among the groups using Kruskal–Wallis test. Abbreviations: PLWH = people living with HIV-1; n = number of individuals; TL: T lymphocyte; HDL-C: high-density lipoprotein cholesterol; LDL-C: low-density lipoprotein cholesterol; TG: triglycerides; VLDL-C: very low-density lipoprotein cholesterol. Data are presented as median and 25 percentile (P25) and 75 percentile (P75).

3.5. PON-1 and PON-2 Gene Polymorphisms and Paraoxonase Activity Association with Infection and Lipid Markers in PLWH

Based on previous data, we conducted secondary analyses to assess whether the presence of polymorphisms was associated with alterations in lipid metabolism markers and infection markers. All analyses are presented in the Supplementary Materials. Here we present the most relevant findings that can be used to generate hypotheses for future studies. Due to the low number of participants in each polymorphism subgroup we chose to group heterozygous individuals with smaller homozygotes. Therefore, analyses were conducted on a case-by-case basis in each antiretroviral therapy.

In the T0 group, a lower concentration of total cholesterol was observed in PLWH carriers of the R allele compared to the Q allele ($p = 0.046$) in SNP Q192R PON-1 gene. In addition, PLWH patients with R allele had a higher number of CD4-LT ($p = 0.077$), as well as a lower concentration of LDL-C ($p = 0.065$), although the statistical significance was borderline, Table S1.

In the T1 group, the highest number of CD4-TLs was observed in the patients carrying the G allele in PON-2 gene polymorphisms (A148G and G148G compared with A148A) ($p = 0.010$). As for the C311S SNP, a higher number of CD4-TLs was observed in homozygous C311C when compared to the other genotypes ($p = 0.018$). The polymorphisms in the other genes were not related with any changes in these patients (Table S2). In the T2 group, the only difference observed was in the Q192R polymorphism group of the PON-1 gene. Heterozygous (Q192R) and homozygous (R192R) had lower concentrations of LDL ($p = 0.008$) and total cholesterol ($p = 0.052$) when compared to homozygous Q192Q individuals, Table S3.

In the total PLWH group, it was observed that the highest number of CD4-LTs was associated with the R allele (59.1%) when compared with the Q allele (40.9%), while the lowest number of CD4-LTs was associated with the Q allele (51.6%) ($p = 0.048$). In the T0 group, the S311C genotype was associated with the presence of the S allele ($p = 0.031$). However, the presence of the S allele was associated with a decrease in CD4-LTs ($p = 0.008$) as well as the presence of viral load ($p = 0.050$). In the other groups, no association was observed between PON-1 and PON-2 gene polymorphisms and the decrease in CD4-LTs and detectable viral load (Table S4).

In this cohort, 96 (27.4%) PLWH had a CD4-LT count below 350 (cell/mm^3) and 112 (32.0%) PLWH had a detectable viral load both independent of the use of ART. However, we observed a difference between the groups (T0, T1, and T2) regarding the frequency of CD4-LTs ($p = 0.035$). The low CD4-LT count in the T0 group was 11 (23.9%), that in the T1 group was 35 (22.0%), and that in the T2 group was 50 (35.0%).

The detectable viral load was 33 (68.8%) from the T0 group, 28 (17.6%) from the T1 group, and 51 (35.7%) from the T2 group ($p < 0.001$). As for the paraoxonase activity of the PON-1 enzyme, no difference was observed between PLWH for the viral load ($p = 0.254$). On the other hand, paraoxonase activity was lower in PLWH with a low CD4-LT count when compared to PLWH with a high CD4-LT ($p = 0.010$).

To assess the influence of lipids on the number of CD4-LTs and CD8-LTs, univariate linear regression analyses were performed with each of the biochemical parameters studied (Table S5). In the T0 group, serum HDL concentration was associated with the amount of CD8-LTs, which was about 31% ($R^2 = 0.317$; $p = 0.008$). Similarly, in the T2 group, total cholesterol concentration was associated with an increase in CD4-LTs ($\beta = 0.008$; $R^2 = 0.115$; $p = 0.030$). In this study, it was not possible to perform multivariate regression analysis.

4. Discussion

In this study, we evaluated paraoxonase 1 and 2 polymorphisms, as well as PON-1 paraoxonase activity, in PLWH and healthy individuals. To determine whether polymorphisms in the PON-1 and PON-2 genes, along with paraoxonase activity, are associated with HIV-1 infection in PLWH, we conducted a sex-matched case-control study. This is the first study to assess these polymorphisms together in PLWH. Among the four single nucleotide polymorphisms analyzed, we found that the L55M PON-1 and C311S PON-2 polymorphisms deviated from a Hardy–Weinberg equilibrium between the PLWH and HC groups. The PON-1 and PON-2 genes are part of the same genetic cluster on human chromosome 7, and their respective polymorphisms—L55M, Q192R, A148G, and C311S—have been linked to the development of various metabolic disorders, particularly those related to lipid metabolism and cardiovascular diseases [27,58–60].

A predominance of genotypes associated with the L55M and M55M PON-1 polymorphisms was observed in the PLWH group, whereas the L55L PON-1 genotype was predominantly found in the HC group. Additionally, the M allele was more frequent in PLWH. In the odds ratio analysis, individuals homozygous for L55L exhibited an approximately 60% protective effect against HIV-1. This is the first time that the L55M PON-1 polymorphism has been associated with HIV-1 infection. Although this finding needs to be confirmed in further studies, the presence of the M variant (LM and/or MM), compared to the L allele (LL), has been linked to the development of several diseases [61], including increased susceptibility to non-alcoholic fatty liver disease [62], cancer [6,63], and other conditions [14,64–66].

Regarding the S311C polymorphism of PON-2, the homozygous C311C genotype was more prevalent in the PLWH group compared to the HC group. The PON-2 enzyme is located on the plasma membrane, and in vitro studies have shown that its lactonase activity and pro-apoptotic function contribute to defense against Gram-negative bacterial infections by regulating biofilm formation and the production of virulence factors [23]. Additionally, in vitro evidence suggests that the A148G and S311C polymorphisms may influence post-translational modifications, indicating a direct modulatory effect of these SNPs. Mutant C311C proteins exhibit a 30-fold reduction in esterase catalytic activity [67].

The Q192R and A148G polymorphisms exhibited similar frequencies between the groups. However, differences were observed in the distribution of complete genotypes and the interaction strengths of these genotypes within the evaluated groups. Association studies between PON-1 and PON-2 genetic cluster polymorphisms are scarce. We found 61 different combinations between the genotypes Q192R, L55M, A148G, and S311C, and these combinations were different between PLWH and HC, showing that the difference may be associated with HIV-1 infection. However, these results must be proven in future studies.

Although the physiological substrates of PON-1 remain unknown, in vitro studies have described three main classes of substrates for PON-1 that may be related to its enzymatic antioxidant activity in humans: the hydrolysis of lactones through lactonase activity, the hydrolysis of aryl esters through arylesterase activity, and the hydrolysis of organophosphates, primarily paraoxon, through paraoxonase activity [68]. The paraoxonase activity of the PON-1 enzyme is one of the most extensively studied in diseases associated with increased oxidative stress, inflammation, and lipid metabolism disorder [69–72].

Here, the paraoxonase activity was higher in PLWH when compared with healthy individuals. This result suggests that the increased paraoxonase activity of PON-1 in PLWH is a metabolic antioxidant response to the oxidative stress caused by HIV-1 infection and prolonged ART use. In fact, in PLWH with an undetectable viral load, prolonged ART use for approximately 10 years has been shown to result in a pronounced redox imbalance and triple ART therapies have been associated with increased oxidative stress. Furthermore, the use of protease inhibitors has been linked to a higher production of reactive oxygen metabolites [73].

PLWH using both NRTI- and PI-based ART presented increased paraoxonase activity, which is inconsistent with findings from previous studies on the lactonase, arilesterase, and paraoxonase activities of the PON-1 in this population [74–76]. These divergent results may be related to the mechanism of action of the PON-1 enzyme in detoxifying different xenobiotics, as well as to the use of distinct substrates to measure PON-1 activity [76–80]. Furthermore, the median paraoxonase activity was similar between the HC and ART-naïve group. These findings are particularly interesting as they highlight the influence of antiretroviral treatment on paraoxonase activity. It is likely that, at the onset of HIV-1 infection, paraoxonase activity related to oxidative stress remains unchanged, whereas prolonged antiretroviral therapy contributes to increased oxidative stress. As a compensatory mechanism, these combined factors may enhance PON-1 paraoxonase activity in an attempt to maintain oxidative homeostasis [77–80].

Conversely, a separate study revealed lower concentrations of paraoxonase PON-1, PON-3, and HDL in the PLWH cohort when compared to the control group. Furthermore, paraoxonase activity was significantly elevated in the control group relative to both the ART-naïve group and those receiving NNRTI-based ART, regardless of whether they had a detectable viral load or were treated with protease inhibitors [81]. Prolonged use of NNRTIs was too associated with a reduction in serum PON-3 concentrations [82]. All these findings, including those observed in our study, suggest that antiretroviral treatments may induce oxidative stress through the downregulation of the paraoxonase family. The increase in paraoxonase activity observed here may provide important insights into the development of comorbidities in PLWH.

The PON-1 enzyme exhibits anti-inflammatory and antioxidant functions, which are believed, in part, to be linked to its relationship with HDL, as well as to be due to its affinity for various substrates [83,84]. PON-1 circulates in the human body bound to HDL. HDL contains other enzymes in its structure, such as Apo-A1. It is suggested that both HDL and Apo-A1 are associated with PON-1 activities and that reduced enzyme activity is associated with the development of diseases or a pro-disease status [85]. Due to these characteristics related to metabolism, paraoxonase activity is known to be cardioprotective, primarily with anti-atherogenic functions. However, it is important to note that this function is not exclusive to PON-1, as it is shared with HDL [86,87].

The subjects in the T0 group had low concentrations of serum total cholesterol, VLDL-C, and triglycerides when compared to T1 and T2 groups. These results demonstrate that at the onset of HIV-1 infection, there are no evident changes in lipid metabolism. In this study, the ART in the T1 group was a combination of efavirenz, zidovudine, lamivudine, stavudine, tenofovir, and nevirapine. In an in vitro model of liver cells, Marinho and colleagues [88] reported that both nevirapine and its metabolite 12-hydroxy-nevirapine increased paraoxonase activity. These results were confirmed in a human study, where nevirapine and its metabolite were associated with increased HDL-C and paraoxonase activity [89]. In a study with rats that received the protease inhibitors ritonavir, atazanavir, and saquinavir for four weeks, paraoxonase activity was decreased, suggesting that these medications may lead to an exhaustion of PON-1 paraoxonase activity [90]. Furthermore, the prolonged use of protease inhibitors, particularly lopinavir/ritonavir, is associated with the development of dyslipidemia, characterized by increase in both LDL-C and cardiovascular risk [91,92].

Here, no difference in LDL-C concentration was observed between the T0, T1, and T2 groups. However, triglyceride and VLDL-C concentrations were higher in the T2 group, which used protease inhibitors. Although paraoxonase activity was increased in both the NNRTI-based and protease inhibitor groups compared to healthy controls, our study did not demonstrate any strong correlation between paraoxonase activity, infection, and lipid markers in any of the groups analyzed. Thus, based on all the observed results related to paraoxonase activity in the different groups of PLWH evaluated, we can observe that, while there is no increase in oxidative stress in the T0 group, the paraoxonase activity under PON-1 is similar to that of healthy controls. On the other hand, the increase in paraoxonase activity in the groups with different ARTs can be considered an indication of oxidative stress in this population.

Indeed, environmental and molecular–genetic factors alter the enzyme's function regarding the hydrolysis of substrates, which favors an increase in oxidative stress [14,15,66]. In addition, the highest paraoxonase activity was associated with the Q192R and R192R genotypes. In PLWH, the enzyme activity in these genotypes was approximately 1.5 times higher than in healthy individuals. Interestingly, the highest CD4-TL cell count was observed in individuals with the R allele. On the other hand, the lowest enzyme activity was found in genotypes Q192Q, L55M, and M55M. Both genotypes are known to be slow metabolizers, especially in individuals carrying the M and Q alleles [93]. Through these results, it is possible to observe the joint influence of antiretroviral treatment and the presence of L55M and Q192R polymorphisms on the paraoxonase activity of PON-1.

Our results of association between paraoxonase activity and imbalance in the presence of polymorphisms in the populations studied can be used to infer that HIV-1-infected individuals are likely to have an imbalance in their antioxidant status associated with the gene cluster of the paraoxonase family. In addition, these characteristics may contribute to viral infection, in part, by maintaining an environment conducive to the development of the virus disease progression [94–98]. The mean age of the PLWH group was higher compared to the HC group. However, no correlation was observed here between participant age and PON-1 paraoxonase activity. The relationship between age and PON-1 paraoxonase activity remains controversial [99,100]. However, it is possible that paraoxonase activity decreases with aging [101].

Systemic alterations in lipid metabolism, such as reduced HDL cholesterol levels and changes in triglycerides, were observed, indicating that the impact of HIV-1 and ART extends beyond viral control, encompassing potential metabolic and cardiovascular risks. These findings emphasize the need for personalized therapeutic strategies for PLWH, considering both genetic and metabolic factors associated with prolonged ART use. Additionally, monitoring paraoxonase activity and lipid profiles based on polymorphisms may be useful for preventing related complications in PLWH. Prolonged ART use in PLWH can lead to lipodystrophy, bone mass loss, diarrhea, lean tissue depletion, increased lipids, insulin resistance, diabetes, atherosclerosis, and cardiovascular diseases, all of which contribute to an elevated risk of mortality [102–104].

This study has some limitations. First, sample size biases may have affected the genotypic frequencies observed. Additionally, the Hardy–Weinberg imbalance for the L55M and S311C polymorphisms could be due to a lack of genetic representativeness in the populations studied. The cross-sectional design also limits the ability to establish causal relationships between the PON-1 and PON-2 gene polymorphisms, ART, lipid profile alterations, and paraoxonase activity. While we controlled for sex in our case-control design, other factors such as environmental exposure, lifestyle, demographics, ethnicity, and epigenetics, which can influence oxidative stress and lipid changes, were not considered.

Future studies should adopt a longitudinal approach to better understand the causal links between genetic polymorphisms, ART, and metabolic changes, with a focus on sample diversification. Additionally, it is important to explore the molecular and pathophysiological mechanisms underlying HIV-1 infection and the role of PON-1 and PON-2 polymorphisms, along with their enzyme activities, to reduce oxidative stress in PLWH. This could involve introducing potential antioxidant compounds that could enhance PON-1 function.

In conclusion, our data show that the frequency of the M55M genotype and/or the M allele is higher in PLWH. Specifically, the M allele may be linked to the susceptibility to HIV-1, while the L55L genotype may offer partial protection against infection. In addition, paraoxonase activity in PLWH was higher in groups using ART, suggesting that prolonged use of ART may positively influence the antioxidant activity of this enzyme in response to increased oxidative stress caused by both infection and treatment and that polymorphisms such as L55M and Q192R in the PON-1 gene are associated with variations in enzyme activity.

Supplementary Materials: The following supporting information can be downloaded at: https://www.mdpi.com/article/10.3390/antiox14020209/s1, Table S1: Comparison of biochemical variables between the SNPs in the T0 group (n = 48); Table S2: Comparison of biochemical variables between the SNPs in the T1 group (n = 159); Table S3: Comparison of biochemical variables between the SNPs in the T2 group (n = 143); Table S4: Association between SNPs of PON-1 e PON-2 genes with CD4-LT number 19 and viral load in PLWH; Table S5: Association between biochemical variables with viral load, CD4-TLs, and 24 CD8-TLs in the PLWH group.

Author Contributions: Conceptualization, D.L., C.O.R., J.d.C., L.M.F.M., S.F.M.G. and S.P.B.; methodology, D.L., C.O.R. and S.P.B.; writing—original draft preparation, C.O.R. and S.P.B.; writing—review and editing, C.O.R. and S.P.B.; supervision, S.P.B. All authors have read and agreed to the published version of the manuscript.

Funding: This research received no external funding.

Institutional Review Board Statement: This study was approved by the Ethics Committee of the Institution (HCFMUSP) (research protocol n° 0539, 26 August 2004). All study participants provided informed consent and the complete anonymity of all data used in this research was guaranteed.

Informed Consent Statement: Informed consent was obtained from all subjects involved in this study.

Data Availability Statement: The data generated in this research can be made available upon consultation with the main researcher, S.P.B. The data will be made available anonymously. Data on genotyping and PON-1 enzyme activity will be available. Data from medical records of study participants cannot be made available.

Acknowledgments: We are thankful to Conselho Nacional de Desenvolvimento Científico e Tecnológico (CNPq), Brazil and Coordenação de Aperfeiçoamento de Pessoal de Nível Superior (CAPES), Brazil.

Conflicts of Interest: The authors have no conflicting interests.

References

1. Mazuryk, O.; Gurgul, I.; Oszajca, M.; Polaczek, J.; Kieca, K.; Bieszczad-Żak, E.; Martyka, T.; Stochel, G. Nitric Oxide Signaling and Sensing in Age-Related Diseases. *Antioxidants* **2024**, *13*, 1213. [CrossRef] [PubMed]
2. Bartolini, D.; Giustarini, D.; Pietrella, D.; Rossi, R.; Galli, F. Glutathione S-Transferase P Influences the Nrf2-Dependent Response of Cellular Thiols to Seleno-Compounds. *Cell Biol. Toxicol.* **2020**, *36*, 379–386. [CrossRef] [PubMed]
3. Liguori, I.; Russo, G.; Curcio, F.; Bulli, G.; Aran, L.; Della-Morte, D.; Gargiulo, G.; Testa, G.; Cacciatore, F.; Bonaduce, D.; et al. Oxidative Stress, Aging, and Diseases. *Clin. Interv. Aging* **2018**, *13*, 757–772. [CrossRef] [PubMed]
4. Camps, J.; Castañé, H.; Rodríguez-Tomàs, E.; Baiges-Gaya, G.; Hernández-Aguilera, A.; Arenas, M.; Iftimie, S.; Joven, J. On the Role of Paraoxonase-1 and Chemokine Ligand 2 (C-c Motif) in Metabolic Alterations Linked to Inflammation and Disease. A 2021 Update. *Biomolecules* **2021**, *11*, 971. [CrossRef]
5. Arab, Z.N.; Khayatan, D.; Razavi, S.M.; Zare, K.; Kheradkhah, E.; Momtaz, S.; Ferretti, G.; Bacchetti, T.; Sathyapalan, T.; Emami, S.A.; et al. Phytochemicals as Modulators of Paraoxonase-1 in Health and Diseases. *Antioxidants* **2022**, *11*, 1273. [CrossRef]
6. Medina-Díaz, I.M.; Ponce-Ruíz, N.; Rojas-García, A.E.; Zambrano-Zargoza, J.F.; Bernal-Hernández, Y.Y.; González-Arias, C.A.; Barrón-Vivanco, B.S.; Herrera-Moreno, J.F. The Relationship between Cancer and Paraoxonase 1. *Antioxidants* **2022**, *11*, 697. [CrossRef]
7. Mackness, M.I.; Durrington, P.N.; Mackness, B. How High-Density Lipoprotein Protects against the Effects of Lipid Peroxidation. *Curr. Opin. Lipidol.* **2000**, *11*, 383–388. [CrossRef]
8. Parween, F.; Gupta, R.D. Insights into the Role of Paraoxonase 2 in Human Pathophysiology. *J. Biosci.* **2022**, *47*, 4. [CrossRef]
9. Taler-Verčič, A.; Goličnik, M.; Bavec, A. The Structure and Function of Paraoxonase-1 and Its Comparison to Paraoxonase-2 and -3. *Molecules* **2020**, *25*, 5980. [CrossRef]
10. Mackness, B.; Durrington, P.N.; Mackness, M.I. Human Serum Paraoxonase. *Gen. Pharmacol. Vasc. Syst.* **1998**, *31*, 329–336. [CrossRef]
11. Bayrak, A.; Bayrak, T.; Demirpençe, E.; Kilinç, K. Differential Hydrolysis of Homocysteine Thiolactone by Purified Human Serum 192Q and 192R PON1 Isoenzymes. *J. Chromatogr. B Anal. Technol. Biomed. Life Sci.* **2011**, *879*, 49–55. [CrossRef] [PubMed]
12. Gençer, N.; Arslan, O. Purification Human PON1Q192 and PON1R192 Isoenzymes by Hydrophobic Interaction Chromatography and Investigation of the Inhibition by Metals. *J. Chromatogr. B Anal. Technol. Biomed. Life Sci.* **2009**, *877*, 134–140. [CrossRef] [PubMed]
13. Goličnik, M.; Bavec, A. Evaluation of the Paraoxonase-1 Kinetic Parameters of the Lactonase Activity by Nonlinear Fit of Progress Curves. *J. Enzym. Inhib. Med. Chem.* **2020**, *35*, 261–264. [CrossRef] [PubMed]
14. Levy, D.; Reichert, C.O.; Bydlowski, S.P. Paraoxonases Activities and Polymorphisms in Elderly and Old-Age Diseases: An Overview. *Antioxidants* **2019**, *8*, 118. [CrossRef] [PubMed]
15. Mahrooz, A.; Mackness, M. Courrent Pinion: Epigenetics of Paraoxonases. *Curr. Opin. Lipidol.* **2020**, *31*, 200–205. [CrossRef]
16. Mahrooz, A.; Mackness, M.; Bagheri, A.; Ghaffari-Cherati, M.; Masoumi, P. The Epigenetic Regulation of Paraoxonase 1 (PON1) as an Important Enzyme in HDL Function: The Missing Link between Environmental and Genetic Regulation. *Clin. Biochem.* **2019**, *73*, 1–10. [CrossRef]
17. La Du, B.N. The Human Serum Paraoxonase/Arylesterase Polymorphism. *Am. J. Hum. Genet.* **1988**, *43*, 227–229.
18. Yigittürk, O.; Turgay, F.; Kızıldağ, S.; Özsoylu, D.; Balcı, G.A. Do PON1–Q192R and PON1–L55M Polymorphisms Modify the Effects of Hypoxic Training on Paraoxonase and Arylesterase Activity? *J. Sport. Health Sci.* **2021**, *12*, 266–274. [CrossRef]

19. Shenhar-Tsarfaty, S.; Waiskopf, N.; Ofek, K.; Shopin, L.; Usher, S.; Berliner, S.; Shapira, I.; Bornstein, N.M.; Ritov, Y.; Soreq, H.; et al. Atherosclerosis and Arteriosclerosis Parameters in Stroke Patients Associate with Paraoxonase Polymorphism and Esterase Activities. *Eur. J. Neurol.* **2013**, *20*, 891–898. [CrossRef]
20. Ashiq, S.; Ashiq, K. The Role of Paraoxonase 1 (PON1) Gene Polymorphisms in Coronary Artery Disease: A Systematic Review and Meta-Analysis. *Biochem. Genet.* **2021**, *59*, 919–939. [CrossRef]
21. Ravi, R.; Subramaniam Rajesh, B. Paraoxonase 2 Protects Against the CML Mediated Mitochondrial Dysfunction Through Modulating JNK Pathway in Human Retinal Cells. *Biochim. Biophys. Acta Gen. Subj.* **2022**, *1866*, 130043. [CrossRef] [PubMed]
22. Sulaiman, D.; Li, J.; Devarajan, A.; Cunningham, C.M.; Li, M.; Fishbein, G.A.; Fogelman, A.M.; Eghbali, M.; Reddy, S.T. Paraoxonase 2 Protects against Acute Myocardial Ischemia-Reperfusion Injury by Modulating Mitochondrial Function and Oxidative Stress via the PI3K/Akt/GSK-3β RISK Pathway. *J. Mol. Cell Cardiol.* **2019**, *129*, 154–164. [CrossRef] [PubMed]
23. Schwarzer, C.; Fu, Z.; Morita, T.; Whitt, A.G.; Neely, A.M.; Li, C.; Machen, T.E. Paraoxonase 2 Serves a Proapopotic Function in Mouse and Human Cells in Response to the Pseudomonas Aeruginosa Quorum-Sensing Molecule N-(3-Oxododecanoyl)-Homoserine Lactone. *J. Biol. Chem.* **2015**, *290*, 7247–7258. [CrossRef] [PubMed]
24. Mochizuki, H.; Scherer, S.W.; Xi, T.; Nickle, D.C.; Majer, M.; Huizenga, J.J.; Tsui, L.-C.; Prochazka, M. Human *PON2* Gene at 7q21.3: Cloning, Multiple MRNA Forms, and Missense Polymorphisms in the Coding Sequence1. *Gene* **1998**, *213*, 149–157. [CrossRef]
25. Li, B.H.; Zhang, L.L.; Yin, Y.W.; Pi, Y.; Yang, Q.W.; Gao, C.Y.; Fang, C.Q.; Wang, J.Z.; Li, J.C. Association Between Paraoxonase 2 Ser311Cys Polymorphism and Ischemic Stroke Risk: A Meta-Analysis Involving 5008 Subjects. *Mol. Biol. Rep.* **2012**, *39*, 5623–5630. [CrossRef]
26. Andalib, S.; Vaseghi, G.; Motavallian, A.; Sadeghi, H.M.; Eshraghi, A.; Amini, M.; Majlesi, A.-R. Association of Polymorphism of *Ser311cys Paraoxonase-2* Gene with Type 2 Diabetes Mellitus in Iran. *Int. J. Prev. Med.* **2013**, *4*, 517–522.
27. Paszek, E.; Godlewski, J.; Wołkow, P.; Żmudka, K.; Słowik, A.; Legutko, J.; Kleczyński, P. Paraoxonase 2 C311S Single Nucleotide Polymorphism Is Associated with Type C Lesions in Coronary Atherosclerosis. *Clin. Biochem.* **2022**, *105–106*, 64–69. [CrossRef]
28. Xie, C.; Jin, R.; Zhao, Y.; Lin, L.; Li, L.; Chen, J.; Zhang, Y. *Paraoxonase 2* Gene Polymorphisms and Prenatal Phthalates' Exposure in Chinese Newborns. *Environ. Res.* **2015**, *140*, 354–359. [CrossRef]
29. Chen, Q.; Liu, J.; Fu, X.; Yang, F.; Liu, Q.; Li, J.; Tan, Z.; Li, J.; Lin, K.; Yan, Y.; et al. Effect of Late Testing and Antiretroviral Treatment on Mortality Among People Living with HIV in the Era of Treat-All in Guangdong Province, China, 1992–2018: A Cohort Study. *Front Public Health* **2022**, *10*, 851117. [CrossRef]
30. Baisley, K.; Orne-Gliemann, J.; Larmarange, J.; Plazy, M.; Collier, D.; Dreyer, J.; Mngomezulu, T.; Herbst, K.; Hanekom, W.; Dabis, F.; et al. Treat-All Strategy and Long-Term Survival Among People Living with HIV in South Africa: Results After 6 Years of Observation in the ANRS 12249 Treatment as Prevention Trial. *HIV Med.* **2022**, *23*, 922–928. [CrossRef]
31. Naito, T.; Mori, H.; Fujibayashi, K.; Fukushima, S.; Yuda, M.; Fukui, N.; Tsukamoto, S.; Suzuki, M.; Goto-Hirano, K.; Kuwatsuru, R. Analysis of Antiretroviral Therapy Switch Rate and Switching Pattern for People Living with HIV from a National Database in Japan. *Sci. Rep.* **2022**, *12*, 1732. [CrossRef] [PubMed]
32. Spooner, R.K.; Taylor, B.K.; Moshfegh, C.M.; Ahmad, I.M.; Dyball, K.N.; Emanuel, K.; Schlichte, S.L.; Schantell, M.; May, P.E.; O'Neill, J.; et al. Neuroinflammatory Profiles Regulated by the Redox Environment Predicted Cognitive Dysfunction in People Living with HIV: A Cross-Sectional Study. *EBioMedicine* **2021**, *70*, 103487. [CrossRef] [PubMed]
33. Gutiérrez-García, G.; García-Herrera, A.; Cardesa, T.; Martínez, A.; Villamor, N.; Ghita, G.; Martínez-Trillos, A.; Colomo, L.; Setoain, X.; Rodríguez, S.; et al. Comparison of Four Prognostic Scores in Peripheral T-Cell Lymphoma. *Ann. Oncol.* **2011**, *22*, 397–404. [CrossRef]
34. Schwenger, K.J.P.; Arendt, B.M.; Smieja, M.; Ma, D.W.L.; Smaill, F.; Allard, J.P. Relationships between Atherosclerosis and Plasma Antioxidant Micronutrients or Red Blood Cell Polyunsaturated Fatty Acids in People Living with HIV. *Nutrients* **2019**, *11*, 1292. [CrossRef] [PubMed]
35. Shyamveer; Khan, A.A.; Singh, H.O. Effect of Genetic Variations in Drug Transporters, Metabolizing Enzyme and Regulatory Genes on the Development of HIV-Associated Lipodystrophy. *J. Gene Med.* **2023**, *25*, e3493. [CrossRef] [PubMed]
36. Zhang, J.; Sehl, M.E.; Shih, R.; Breen, E.C.; Li, F.; Lu, A.T.; Bream, J.H.; Duggal, P.; Martinson, J.; Wolinsky, S.M.; et al. Effects of Highly Active Antiretroviral Therapy Initiation on Epigenomic DNA Methylation in Persons Living with HIV. *Front. Bioinform.* **2024**, *4*, 1357889. [CrossRef]
37. Hamed, M.A.; Aremu, G.O.; Akhigbe, R.E. Concomitant Administration of HAART Aggravates Anti-Koch-Induced Oxidative Hepatorenal Damage via Dysregulation of Glutathione and Elevation of Uric Acid Production. *Biomed. Pharmacother.* **2021**, *137*, 111309. [CrossRef]
38. Mebrat, Y.; Amogne, W.; Mekasha, A.; Gleason, R.L.; Seifu, D. Lipid Peroxidation and Altered Antioxidant Profiles with Pediatric HIV Infection and Antiretroviral Therapy in Addis Ababa, Ethiopia. *J. Trop. Pediatr.* **2017**, *63*, 196–202. [CrossRef]
39. Brunet, L.; Mallon, P.; Fusco, J.S.; Wohlfeiler, M.B.; Prajapati, G.; Beyer, A.; Fusco, G.P. Switch from Tenofovir Disoproxil Fumarate to Tenofovir Alafenamide in People Living with HIV: Lipid Changes and Statin Underutilization. *Clin. Drug Investig.* **2021**, *41*, 955–965. [CrossRef]

40. Camps-Vilaró, A.; Pérez-Fernández, S.; Subirana, I.; Teira, R.; Estrada, V.; Domingo, P.; Dégano, I.R.; Marrugat, J. Standardized Comparison of Cardiovascular Risk Factors Prevalence in Spanish Women and Men Living with Hiv and in the General Population. *J. Pers. Med.* **2021**, *11*, 1085. [CrossRef]
41. McComsey, G.A.; Emond, B.; Shah, A.; Bookhart, B.K.; Rossi, C.; Milbers, K.; Lafeuille, M.-H.; Donga, P. Association Between Weight Gain and the Incidence of Cardiometabolic Conditions Among People Living with HIV-1 at High Risk of Weight Gain Initiated on Antiretroviral Therapy. *Infect. Dis. Ther.* **2022**, *11*, 1883–1899. [CrossRef] [PubMed]
42. Cusato, J.; Mulasso, A.; Ferrara, M.; Manca, A.; Antonucci, M.; Accardo, G.; Palermiti, A.; Bianco, G.; Chiara, F.; Mula, J.; et al. Studying the Changes in Physical Functioning and Oxidative Stress-Related Molecules in People Living with HIV after Switching from Triple to Dual Therapy. *Antioxidants* **2024**, *13*, 518. [CrossRef]
43. Wobeser, W.L.; McBane, J.E.; Balfour, L.; Conway, B.; Gill, M.J.; Huff, H.; Kilby, D.L.P.; Fergusson, D.A.; Mallick, R.; Mills, E.J.; et al. A Randomized Control Trial of High-Dose Micronutrient-Antioxidant Supplementation in Healthy Persons with Untreated HIV Infection. *PLoS ONE* **2022**, *17*, e0270590. [CrossRef] [PubMed]
44. Visser, M.E.; Durao, S.; Sinclair, D.; Irlam, J.H.; Siegfried, N. Micronutrient Supplementation in Adults with HIV Infection. *Cochrane Database Syst. Rev.* **2017**, *2017*, CD003650. [CrossRef]
45. Maselli, L.M.F.; da Cunha, J.; Gutierrez, E.B.; Maranhão, R.C.; Spada, C.; Bydlowski, S.P. Human Paraoxonase-1 Activity Is Related to the Number of CD4+ T-Cells and Is Restored by Antiretroviral Therapy in HIV-1-Infected Individuals. *Dis. Markers* **2014**, *2014*, 480201. [CrossRef]
46. Dornas, W.; Silva, M. Modulation of the Antioxidant Enzyme Paraoxonase-1 for Protection against Cardiovascular Diseases. *Nutr. Metab. Cardiovasc. Dis.* **2024**, *34*, 2611–2622. [CrossRef]
47. Kaya, M.O.; Sinan, S.; Güler, Ö.Ö.; Arslan, O. Is There a Relation Between Genetic Susceptibility with Cancer? A Study About Paraoxanase (PON1) Enzyme Activity in Breast Cancer Cases. *J. Enzym. Inhib. Med. Chem.* **2016**, *31*, 1349–1355. [CrossRef]
48. Rodríguez-Tomàs, E.; Murcia, M.; Arenas, M.; Arguís, M.; Gil, M.; Amigó, N.; Correig, X.; Torres, L.; Sabater, S.; Baiges-Gayà, G.; et al. Serum Paraoxonase-1-Related Variables and Lipoprotein Profile in Patients with Lung or Head and Neck Cancer: Effect of Radiotherapy. *Antioxidants* **2019**, *8*, 213. [CrossRef]
49. Ministry of Health Technical Manual for Diagnosis of HIV Infection in Adults and Children. Brasilia, Brazil; 2018. Available online: https://www.gov.br/aids/pt-br/central-de-conteudo/publicacoes/2018/manual_tecnico_hiv_27_11_2018_web.pdf (accessed on 7 February 2025).
50. World Health Organization. *Blood Donor Selection: Guidelines on Assessing Donor Suitability for Blood Donation*; World Health Organization: Geneva, Switzerland, 2013; ISBN 9789241548519.
51. Ministry of Health Implementation and Routine of Nucleic Acid Tests (NAT) in Hemotherapy Services: Operational Manual; Brasilia, Brazil. 2013; ISBN 978-85-334-2086-1. Available online: https://bvsms.saude.gov.br/bvs/publicacoes/implantacao_rotina_acidos_nucleicos_manual.pdf (accessed on 7 February 2025).
52. Miller, S.A.; Dykes, D.D.; Polesky, H.F. A Simple Salting out Procedure for Extracting DNA from Human Nucleated Cells. *Nucleic Acids Res.* **1988**, *16*, 1215. [CrossRef]
53. Motti, C.; Dessì, M.; Gnasso, A.; Irace, C.; Indigeno, P.; Angelucci, C.B.; Bernardini, S.; Fucci, G.; Federici, G.; Cortese, C. A Multiplex PCR-Based DNA Assay for the Detection of Paraoxonase Gene Cluster Polymorphisms. *Atherosclerosis* **2001**, *158*, 35–40. [CrossRef]
54. Hegele, R.A.; Connelly, P.W.; Scherer, S.W.; Hanley, A.J.G.; Harris, S.B.; Tsui, L.C.; Zinman, B. *Paraoxonase-2* Gene (PON2) G148 Variant Associated with Elevated Fasting Plasma Glucose in Noninsulin-Dependent Diabetes Mellitus. *J. Clin. Endocrinol. Metab.* **1997**, *82*, 3373–3377. [CrossRef] [PubMed]
55. Sentí, M.; Tomás, M.; Anglada, R.; Elosua, R.; Marrugat, J.; Covas, M.I.; Fitó, M. Interrelationship of Smoking, Paraoxonase Activity, and Leisure Time Physical Activity: A Population-Based Study. *Eur. J. Intern. Med.* **2003**, *14*, 178–184. [CrossRef]
56. Agachan, B.; Yilmaz, H.; Karaali, Z.; Isbir, T. Paraoxonase 55 and 192 Polymorphism and Its Relationship to Serum Paraoxonase Activity and Serum Lipids in Turkish Patients with Non-Insulin Dependent Diabetes Mellitus. *Cell Biochem. Funct.* **2004**, *22*, 163–168. [CrossRef] [PubMed]
57. Peng, C.Y.J.; Lee, K.L.; Ingersoll, G.M. An Introduction to Logistic Regression Analysis and Reporting. *J. Educ. Res.* **2002**, *96*, 3–14. [CrossRef]
58. Ayan, D.; Gül, M.A.; Karabay, U.; Bulut, S.M. Bioinformatic Investigation of Genetic Changes in Paraoxonase Genes in Breast Cancer and Breast Cancer Subtypes. *Eur. J. Breast Health* **2024**, *20*, 178–184. [CrossRef] [PubMed]
59. Sanghera, D.K.; Aston, C.E.; Saha, N.; Kamboh, M.I. DNA Polymorphisms in Two Paraoxonase Genes (*PON1* and *PON2*) Are Associated with the Risk of Coronary Heart Disease. *Am. J. Hum. Genet.* **1998**, *62*, 36–44. [CrossRef]
60. Chen, C.C.; Chen, C.C.; Tu, J.D.; Wu, Y.L.; Leu, S.J. Associations between Genetic Polymorphisms of Paraoxonase Genes and Coronary Artery Disease in a Taiwanese Population. *Clin. Biochem.* **2013**, *46*, 1664–1667. [CrossRef]

61. Doneva-Basheva, K.I.; Gospodinov, K.; Tacheva, T.; Dimov, D.; Vlaykova, T.I. Role of Single Nucleotide Polymorphism L55M in the *Paraoxonase 1* Gene as a Risk and Prognostic Factor in Acute Coronary Syndrome. *Curr. Issues Mol. Biol.* **2022**, *44*, 5915–5932. [CrossRef]
62. Milaciu, M.V.; Vesa, Ș.C.; Bocșan, I.C.; Ciumărnean, L.; Sâmpelean, D.; Negrean, V.; Pop, R.M.; Matei, D.M.; Pașca, S.; Răchișan, A.L.; et al. Paraoxonase-1 Serum Concentration and PON1 Gene Polymorphisms: Relationship with Non-Alcoholic Fatty Liver Disease. *J. Clin. Med.* **2019**, *8*, 2200. [CrossRef]
63. Eraldemir, F.C.; Üren, N.; Kum, T.; Erbay, B.; Sahin, D.; Ergül, E.; Acar, E.; Özsoy, D.; Çekmen, M.; Klr, H.; et al. Association of Serum Paraoxonase 1 Activities, Polymorphisms and Oxidative Stress in Breast Cancer Patients with Type 2 Diabetes Mellitus. *J. Med. Biochem.* **2019**, *38*, 368–375. [CrossRef]
64. Bizoń, A.; Ołdakowska, M.; Milnerowicz, H. Changes in Lipid Profile Parameters and PON1 Status Associated with L55M PON1 Polymorphism, Overweight and Exposure to Tobacco Smoke. *Inhal. Toxicol.* **2018**, *30*, 463–471. [CrossRef]
65. Salari, N.; Rasoulpoor, S.; Hosseinian-Far, A.; Razazian, N.; Mansouri, K.; Mohammadi, M.; Vaisi-Raygani, A.; Jalali, R.; Shabani, S.; Shabani Sherwin, S. Association Between Serum Paraoxonase 1 Activity and Its Polymorphisms with Multiple Sclerosis: A Systematic Review. *Neurol. Sci.* **2020**, *42*, 491–500. [CrossRef] [PubMed]
66. Reichert, C.O.; Levy, D.; Bydlowski, S.P. Paraoxonase Role in Human Neurodegenerative Diseases. *Antioxidants* **2021**, *10*, 11. [CrossRef] [PubMed]
67. Carusone, T.M.; Cardiero, G.; Cerreta, M.; Mandrich, L.; Moran, O.; Porzio, E.; Catara, G.; Lacerra, G.; Manco, G. WTAP and BIRC3 Are Involved in the Posttranscriptional Mechanisms That Impact on the Expression and Activity of the Human Lactonase PON2. *Cell Death Dis.* **2020**, *11*, 324. [CrossRef]
68. Mohammed, C.J.; Lamichhane, S.; Connolly, J.A.; Soehnlen, S.M.; Khalaf, F.K.; Malhotra, D.; Haller, S.T.; Isailovic, D.; Kennedy, D.J. A PON for All Seasons: Comparing Paraoxonase Enzyme Substrates, Activity and Action Including the Role of PON3 in Health and Disease. *Antioxidants* **2022**, *11*, 590. [CrossRef]
69. Erre, G.L.; Bassu, S.; Giordo, R.; Mangoni, A.A.; Carru, C.; Pintus, G.; Zinellu, A. Association Between Paraoxonase/Arylesterase Activity of Serum PON-1 Enzyme and Rheumatoid Arthritis: A Systematic Review and Meta-Analysis. *Antioxidants* **2022**, *11*, 2317. [CrossRef]
70. Charles-Schoeman, C.; Hyde, C.; Guan, S.; Parikh, N.; Wang, J.; Shahbazian, A.; Stockert, L.; Andrews, J. Relationship Between Paraoxonase-1 Genotype and Activity, and Major Adverse Cardiovascular Events and Malignancies in Patients with Rheumatoid Arthritis Receiving Tofacitinib. *J. Rheumatol.* **2023**, *50*, 1573–1580. [CrossRef]
71. Leocádio, P.C.L.; Goulart, A.C.; Santos, I.S.; Lotufo, P.A.; Bensenor, I.M.; Alvarez-Leite, J.I. Lower Paraoxonase 1 Paraoxonase Activity Is Associated with a Worse Prognosis in Patients with Non-ST-Segment Elevation Myocardial Infarction in Long-Term Follow-Up. *Coron. Artery Dis.* **2022**, *33*, 515–522. [CrossRef]
72. Mirdamadi, H.Z.; Sztanek, F.; Derdak, Z.; Seres, I.; Harangi, M.; Paragh, G. The Human Paraoxonase-1 Phenotype Modifies the Effect of Statins on Paraoxonase Activity and Lipid Parameters. *Br. J. Clin. Pharmacol.* **2008**, *66*, 366–374. [CrossRef]
73. Lombardi, F.; Belmonti, S.; Sanfilippo, A.; Borghetti, A.; Iannone, V.; Salvo, P.F.; Fabbiani, M.; Visconti, E.; Di Giambenedetto, S. Factors Associated with Oxidative Stress in Virologically Suppressed People Living with HIV on Long-Term Antiretroviral Therapy. *AIDS Res. Ther.* **2024**, *21*, 100. [CrossRef]
74. Dias, C.; Marinho, A.; Morello, J.; Almeida, G.; Caixas, U.; Soto, K.; Monteiro, E.; Pereira, S. Monitoring of the Lactonase Activity of Paraoxonase-1 Enzyme in HIV-1-infection. *J. Int. AIDS Soc.* **2014**, *17*, 19682. [CrossRef] [PubMed]
75. Bobin-Dubigeon, C.; Biron, C.; Volteau, C.; Piroth, L.; Biron, A.; Perré, P.; Leport, C.; Prazuck, T.; Sébille-Rivain, V.; Raffi, F.; et al. Short Communication: Paraoxonase 1 (PON1) in French HIV-Infected Patients under Antiretroviral Therapy: Relationship with the Metabolic Syndrome and Inflammation. *AIDS Res. Hum. Retroviruses* **2013**, *29*, 1571–1574. [CrossRef] [PubMed]
76. Parra, S.; Marsillach, J.; Aragonès, G.; Rull, A.; Beltrán-Debón, R.; Alonso-Villaverde, C.; Joven, J.; Camps, J. Methodological Constraints in Interpreting Serum Paraoxonase-1 Activity Measurements: An Example from a Study in HIV-Infected Patients. *Lipids Health Dis.* **2010**, *9*, 32. [CrossRef] [PubMed]
77. Ishizuka, T.; Fujimori, I.; Nishida, A.; Sakurai, H.; Yoshigae, Y.; Nakahara, K.; Kurihara, A.; Ikeda, T.; Izumi, T. Paraoxonase 1 as a Major Bioactivating Hydrolase for Olmesartan Medoxomil in Human Blood Circulation: Molecular Identification and Contribution to Plasma Metabolism. *Drug Metab. Dispos.* **2012**, *40*, 374–380. [CrossRef]
78. Zayed, A.A.; Ahmed, A.I.; Khattab, A.M.T.; Mekdad, A.A.H.; AbdelAal, A.G. Paraoxonase 1 and Cytochrome P450 Polymorphisms in Susceptibility to Acute Organophosphorus Poisoning in Egyptians. *Neurotoxicology* **2015**, *51*, 20–26. [CrossRef]
79. Tsatsakis, A.M.; Androutsopoulos, V.P.; Zafiropoulos, A.; Babatsikou, F.; Alegakis, T.; Dialyna, I.; Tzatzarakis, M.; Koutis, C. Associations of Xenobiotic-Metabolizing Enzyme Genotypes PON1Q192R, PON1L55M and CYP1A1*2A MspI with Pathological Symptoms of a Rural Population in South Greece. *Xenobiotica* **2011**, *41*, 914–925. [CrossRef]
80. Milnerowicz, H.; Kowalska, K.; Socha, E. Paraoxonase Activity as a Marker of Exposure to Xenobiotics in Tobacco Smoke. *Int. J. Toxicol.* **2015**, *34*, 224–232. [CrossRef]

81. Siegel, M.O.; Borkowska, A.G.; Dubrovsky, L.; Roth, M.; Welti, R.; Roberts, A.D.; Parenti, D.M.; Simon, G.L.; Sviridov, D.; Simmens, S.; et al. HIV Infection Induces Structural and Functional Changes in High Density Lipoproteins. *Atherosclerosis* **2015**, *243*, 19–29. [CrossRef]
82. Aragonès, G.; García-Heredia, A.; Guardiola, M.; Rull, A.; Beltrán-Debón, R.; Marsillach, J.; Alonso-Villaverde, C.; Mackness, B.; Mackness, M.; Pedro-Botet, J.; et al. Serum Paraoxonase-3 Concentration in HIV-Infected Patients. Evidence for a Protective Role against Oxidation. *J. Lipid Res.* **2012**, *53*, 168–174. [CrossRef]
83. Jakubowski, H. The Molecular Bases of Anti-Oxidative and Anti-Inflammatory Properties of Paraoxonase 1. *Antioxidants* **2024**, *13*, 1292. [CrossRef]
84. Lewoń-Mrozek, D.; Kurzynoga, J.; Jędrzejewski, P.; Kędzierska, K.; Partyka, A.; Kuriata-Kordek, M.; Ściskalska, M. Molecular Structure of Paraoxonase-1 and Its Modifications in Relation to Enzyme Activity and Biological Functions—A Comprehensive Review. *Int. J. Mol. Sci.* **2024**, *25*, 13129. [CrossRef]
85. Jakubowski, H. Proteomic Exploration of Paraoxonase 1 Function in Health and Disease. *Int. J. Mol. Sci.* **2023**, *24*, 7764. [CrossRef] [PubMed]
86. Kempegowda, S.N.; Sugur, K.; Thimmulappa, R.K. Dysfunctional HDL Diagnostic Metrics for Cardiovascular Disease Risk Stratification: Are We Ready to Implement in Clinics? *J. Cardiovasc. Transl. Res.* **2024**, 1–16. [CrossRef] [PubMed]
87. Celik, H.; Tuysuz, M.Z.; Aktas, Y.; Eren, M.A.; Demirbag, R. Assessment of Paraoxonase 1 and Arylesterase Activities and Lipid Profile in Bodybuilders: A Comparative Study of Physical Activity and Anthropometry on Atherosclerosis. *Medicina* **2024**, *60*, 1717. [CrossRef]
88. Marinho, A.T.; Dias, C.G.; Pinheiro, P.F.; Lemos, A.R.; Antunes, A.M.M.; Marques, M.M.; Monteiro, E.C.; Miranda, J.P.; Pereira, S.A. Nevirapine Modulation of Paraoxonase-1 in the Liver: An in Vitro Three-Model Approach. *Eur. J. Pharm. Sci.* **2016**, *82*, 147–153. [CrossRef]
89. Marinho, A.T.; Batuca, J.R.; Miranda, J.P.; Caixas, U.; Dias, C.G.; Branco, T.; Soto, K.; Pinheiro, P.; Bourbon, M.; Marques, M.M.; et al. The 2-Hydroxy-Nevirapine Metabolite as a Candidate for Boosting Apolipoprotein A1 and for Modulating Anti-HDL Antibodies. *Pharmacol. Res.* **2021**, *165*, 105446. [CrossRef]
90. Pastryk, J.E.; Rusek, M.; Bełtowski, J. Effects of Antiretroviral Treatment on Paraoxonase 1 (PON1) Activity in Rats. *Chem. Biol. Interact.* **2016**, *259*, 407–412. [CrossRef]
91. Limsreng, S.; Marcy, O.; Ly, S.; Ouk, V.; Chanroeurn, H.; Thavary, S.; Boroath, B.; Canestri, A.; Viretto, G.; Delfraissy, J.F.; et al. Dyslipidemias and Elevated Cardiovascular Risk on Lopinavir-Based Antiretroviral Therapy in Cambodia. *PLoS ONE* **2016**, *11*, e0160306. [CrossRef]
92. Dai, L.; Liu, A.; Zhang, H.; Wu, H.; Zhang, T.; Su, B.; Shao, Y.; Li, J.; Ye, J.; Scott, S.R.; et al. Impact of Lopinavir/Ritonavir and Efavirenz-Based Antiretroviral Therapy on the Lipid Profile of Chinese HIV/AIDS Treatment-Naïve Patients in Beijing: A Retrospective Study. *Curr. HIV Res.* **2019**, *17*, 324–334. [CrossRef]
93. Reichert, C.O.; de Macedo, C.G.; Levy, D.; Sini, B.C.; Monteiro, A.M.; Gidlund, M.; Maselli, L.M.F.; Gualandro, S.F.M.; Bydlowski, S.P. Paraoxonases (PON) 1, 2, and 3 Polymorphisms and PON-1 Activities in Patients with Sickle Cell Disease. *Antioxidants* **2019**, *8*, 252. [CrossRef]
94. Guillin, O.M.; Vindry, C.; Ohlmann, T.; Chavatte, L. Interplay Between Selenium, Selenoproteins and HIV-1 Replication in Human CD4 T-Lymphocytes. *Int. J. Mol. Sci.* **2022**, *23*, 1394. [CrossRef] [PubMed]
95. Thangaraj, A.; Chivero, E.T.; Tripathi, A.; Singh, S.; Niu, F.; Guo, M.L.; Pillai, P.; Periyasamy, P.; Buch, S. HIV TAT-Mediated Microglial Senescence: Role of SIRT3-Dependent Mitochondrial Oxidative Stress. *Redox Biol.* **2021**, *40*, 101843. [CrossRef] [PubMed]
96. Zeng, X.F.; Li, Q.; Li, J.; Wong, N.; Li, Z.; Huang, J.; Yang, G.; Sham, P.C.; Li, S.B.; Lu, G. HIV-1 Tat and Methamphetamine Co-Induced Oxidative Cellular Injury Is Mitigated by N-Acetylcysteine Amide (NACA) Through Rectifying MTOR Signaling. *Toxicol. Lett.* **2018**, *299*, 159–171. [CrossRef] [PubMed]
97. Burini, R.C.; Borges-Santos, M.D.; Moreto, F.; Yu, Y.M. Comparative Effects of Acute-Methionine Loading on the Plasma Sulfur-Amino Acids in NAC-Supplemented HIV+ Patients and Healthy Controls. *Amino Acids* **2018**, *50*, 569–576. [CrossRef]
98. Camps, J.; Iftimie, S.; Arenas, M.; Castañé, H.; Jiménez-Franco, A.; Castro, A.; Joven, J. Paraoxonase-1: How a Xenobiotic Detoxifying Enzyme Has Become an Actor in the Pathophysiology of Infectious Diseases and Cancer. *Chem. Biol. Interact.* **2023**, *380*, 110553. [CrossRef]
99. Meisinger, C.; Freuer, D.; Bub, A.; Linseisen, J. Association Between Inflammatory Markers and Serum Paraoxonase and Arylesterase Activities in the General Population: A Cross-Sectional Study. *Lipids Health Dis.* **2021**, *20*, 81. [CrossRef]
100. Orlando, P.; Silvestri, S.; Galeazzi, R.; Antonicelli, R.; Marcheggiani, F.; Cirilli, I.; Bacchetti, T.; Tiano, L. Effect of Ubiquinol Supplementation on Biochemical and Oxidative Stress Indexes After Intense Exercise in Young Athletes. *Redox Rep.* **2018**, *23*, 136–145. [CrossRef]

101. Parker, D.; Sloane, R.; Pieper, C.F.; Hall, K.S.; Kraus, V.B.; Kraus, W.E.; Huebner, J.L.; Ilkayeva, O.R.; Bain, J.R.; Newby, L.K.; et al. Age-Related Adverse Inflammatory and Metabolic Changes Begin Early in Adulthood. *J. Gerontol. Ser. A Biol. Sci. Med. Sci.* **2019**, *74*, 283–289. [CrossRef]
102. Basta, D.; Latinovic, O.S.; Silvestri, G. Potential Advantages of a Well-Balanced Nutrition Regimen for People Living with Human Immunodeficiency Virus Type-1. *J. AIDS HIV Treat.* **2024**, *6*, 11–27. [CrossRef]
103. Ciccacci, F.; Lucaroni, F.; Latagliata, R.; Morciano, L.; Mondlane, E.; Balama, M.; Tembo, D.; Gondwe, J.; Orlando, S.; Palombi, L.; et al. Hematologic Alterations and Early Mortality in a Cohort of HIV Positive African Patients. *PLoS ONE* **2020**, *15*, e0242068. [CrossRef]
104. Cummins, N.W. Metabolic Complications of Chronic HIV Infection: A Narrative Review. *Pathogens* **2022**, *11*, 197. [CrossRef]

antioxidants

MDPI

Review

Protective Role of High-Density Lipoprotein in Multiple Sclerosis

Agnieszka Damiza-Detmer *, Małgorzata Pawełczyk and Andrzej Głąbiński

Department of Neurology and Stroke, Medical University of Lodz, ul. Zeromskiego 113, 90-549 Lodz, Poland; andrzej.glabinski@umed.lodz.pl (A.G.)
* Correspondence: damiza@vp.pl

Abstract: Multiple sclerosis (MS) is a chronic, progressive demyelinating disease with a most likely autoimmune background and a neurodegenerative component. Besides the demyelinating process caused by autoreactive antibodies, an increased permeability in the blood–brain barrier (BBB) also plays a key role. Recently, there has been growing interest in assessing lipid profile alterations in patients with MS. As a result of myelin destruction, there is an increase in the level of cholesterol released from cells, which in turn causes disruptions in lipid metabolism homeostasis both in the central nervous system (CNS) and peripheral tissues. Currently, there is a growing body of evidence suggesting a protective role of HDL in MS through its effect on the BBB by decreasing its permeability. This follows from the impact of HDL on the endothelium and its anti-inflammatory effect, mostly by interacting with adhesion molecules like vascular cell adhesion molecule 1 (VCAM-1), intercellular adhesion molecule 1 (ICAM-1), and E-selectin. HDL, through its action via sphingosine-1-phosphate, exerts an inhibitory effect on leukocyte migration, and its antioxidant properties contribute to the improvement of the BBB function. In this review, we want to summarize these studies and focus on HDL as a mediator of the anti-inflammatory response in MS.

Keywords: multiple sclerosis; HDL; antioxidant; anti-inflammatory; BBB; lipid alteration; apolipoprotein

1. Introduction

HDL, along with LDL, is the main lipoprotein responsible for transporting cholesterol in the blood. Its primary function is to transport cholesterol from peripheral tissues to the liver. HDLs, similar to other lipoproteins—LDL, VLDL, IDL, are primarily made up of apolipoproteins (apo), non-structural proteins, and lipids. Their surface consists of a monolayer that includes amphipathic phospholipids, sphingolipids, and unesterified cholesterol, which encloses a core containing triglycerides and cholesteryl esters. HDLs differ in terms of size, density, and their specific lipid and protein makeup. The main apolipoprotein of HDL is apoA1 [1–3].

HDLs are known for their protective, antiatherogenic properties, particularly their ability to promote cholesterol removal from vascular cells and aid in its elimination. Beyond cholesterol efflux, they also have anti-inflammatory antioxidant effects and can stimulate nitric oxide (NO) production in the endothelium. Recent research has emphasized HDL functionality, revealing that its role in cardiovascular health may be more predictive than simply measuring HDL-C levels in the blood [2,4,5].

MS is a disorder that is of unwavering interest to researchers. Despite many years of study, the pathophysiology remains unclear. Yet, most investigators are convinced about the autoimmune nature of MS, with an emphasis on its neurodegenerative component. It is still unknown if the trigger for the cascade leading to the demyelinating process occurs within or outside the CNS [6]. Clinically, we can distinguish four subtypes of MS. In total, 80% of patients suffer from relapsing-remitting MS (RRMS). Patients have acute relapses followed by periods of remission. Unfortunately, for over 40% of patients, these remissions are partial, leading to disability over time. Untreated RRMS, or RRMS treated with insufficient response, can transform into secondary progressive MS (SPMS)—this occurs in 50–60% of RRMS cases. Primary-progressive MS (PPMS) is characterized by constant neurological worsening without acute relapses, and it affects about 10–15% of MS patients. The rarest subtype is progressive-relapsing MS (PRMS), where patients experience progressive worsening of the neurological state along with acute relapses [7].

Despite advances in understanding MS and treatments to reduce relapses, stopping and reversing disease progression remains a challenge. Current clinical approaches need to shift towards biologically based definitions of MS progression. Progression is driven by various mechanisms—non-resolving inflammation, neurodegeneration, oxidative stress, mitochondrial dysfunction, and failed compensatory responses like remyelination. These processes differ among patients and over time, highlighting the need for personalized tracking methods. New tools are needed to correlate clinical, radiological, and biological data, shifting from traditional MS classifications to a biomarker-driven, individualized treatment model. Transitioning to this new framework will require collaboration across research, healthcare, and regulatory systems [8].

In the autoimmune background of MS, autoreactive lymphocytes play a key role, particularly T CD4+ and CD8+ cells, especially CD4+ Th cells [9]. Th1 and especially Th17 seem to be the most important factors leading to the damage of endothelial cells (ECs) forming the BBB. B lymphocytes, which, similarly to T lymphocytes, are activated in the periphery or in the CNS, pass through the damaged BBB, and, as plasma cells, secrete autoantibodies. Myelin oligodendrocyte glycoprotein (MOG), myelin basic protein (MBP), myelin-associated glycoprotein (MAG), or myelin proteolipid protein (PLP) are postulated as antigens for these cells. Newer research indicates that the target for these produced antibodies may be lipid elements that build cell membranes, with the most likely antigen being cholesterol [10–12].

A crucial pathomechanism for MS is BBB damage, which leads to increased permeability and is associated with disease severity [13]. It is still unclear whether the initiating event of autoimmunity leading to BBB impairment occurs within the CNS or in peripheral tissues. It is also unknown whether the dysfunction of the endothelium that forms the BBB is primary, due to a pathological response to oxidative stress, or secondary, in response to previously circulating autoreactive lymphocytes [6,7]. Recent studies have shown that a damaged BBB exhibits excessive expression of P-, E-, and L-selectins, as well as VCAM and ICAM on ECs, initiated by exaggerated production of proinflammatory chemokines [14,15].

2. Methods

This narrative review draws upon a selection of research studies investigating the antioxidant and anti-inflammatory roles of HDLs in MS, particularly in relation to BBB dysfunction. Relevant original research, editorials, and review articles published up to August 2024 were sourced from the PubMed database. The search utilized keywords such as "HDLs", "high-density lipoprotein", "apoA-I", "apoA1", "multiple sclerosis", "blood-brain barrier", "endothelial dysfunction", "antioxidative", and "anti-inflammatory" to identify pertinent studies for inclusion in this review.

3. Lipid Profile Alteration and Their Association with MS

The CNS is the most lipid-rich organ. Approximately 50–60% of its dry weight is constituted by lipids, and 20–25% of that is cholesterol. Up to 80% of brain cholesterol is used in building myelin sheaths. In addition to cholesterol, myelin also contains other lipids, such as phospholipids and glycosphingolipids [16,17]. Cholesterol is synthesized de novo in the brain, mostly by astrocytes in the mature CNS and by oligodendrocytes and neurons in the postnatal period. Due to the fact that the BBB is impermeable to cholesterol, its metabolism—from synthesis to transport and storage—is almost completely independent of metabolism in the periphery [16,18]. Similarly to peripheral tissues, cholesterol in the brain is transported by lipoproteins. Due to the impermeability of the BBB to these molecules, the profile of lipoproteins in the CSF and serum is different. CSF is abundant in apolipoprotein E (apoE), apolipoprotein A1 (apoA1), and apolipoprotein J (apoJ), while apolipoprotein B (apoB) is absent. Analysis of the density and lipid composition of lipoproteins in CSF reveals that they most closely resemble HDL found in the periphery, hence their name HDL-like. However, HDL-like particles are larger than their peripheral counterparts [19,20]. Proteins from the ATP-binding cassette transporter (ABC) family—ABCA1, ABCG1, and ABCA7—are required during the formation of lipoproteins. These transporters are located in the neuronal cell membrane [19]. They are the main proteins involved in the transmembrane transport of cholesterol from the cell. They are responsible for the incorporation of phospholipids into apoE, resulting in the formation of a lipoprotein disk—nascent HDL, which subsequently incorporates free cholesterol produced in the cell. This cholesterol undergoes esterification by enzymes, most likely cholesterol ester transfer protein (CETP) and lecithin cholesterol acyltransferase (LCAT), resulting in the formation of mature HDL-like lipoproteins. The transport of cholesterol across the cell membrane using ABC transporters is energy-consuming, requiring the use of ATP [21–23]. Neurons, microglia, and arachnoid cells use these mature lipoproteins via low-density lipoprotein receptors (LDLR), mostly LDLR-related protein 1 (LRP1). Transport through these receptors is strongly associated with apoE [17]. In order to maintain cholesterol homeostasis, in addition to its synthesis and metabolism, the process of its removal from cells must take place. Cholesterol is metabolized to oxysterols or undergoes esterification. This process takes place thanks to oxidizing enzymes—sterol hydroxylases. Most of these enzymes belong to the cytochrome P450 complex. The main route of elimination of excess cholesterol is hydroxylation by the enzyme CYP46A1, resulting in the metabolite 24S-hydroxycholesterol (24S-OHC). Due to its hydrophilic nature, 24S-OHC is able to cross the BBB and is found in serum. Peripherally located 24S-OHC undergoes esterification, binding with fatty acids to form LDL or HDL [18,24,25]. Oxysterols, apart from their function as cholesterol transporters, are also regulators of their metabolism, among other roles, by acting as ligands for liver X receptors (LXRs). LXRs activate the transcription of genes, promoting cholesterol efflux from the cell, which causes a decrease in its intracellular level [18,26,27]. Increased levels of oxysterols, especially 24S-OH, are found in the serum of MS patients [28–30]. Because they freely migrate across the BBB, they have an activating effect on LXRs [28]. These receptors affect inflammatory responses via T lymphocytes. They reduce their influx into the CNS, inhibit the differentiation in naive CD4+ T lymphocytes into Th17-producing cells, and inhibit Il-9-producing CD8+ T lymphocytes [31]. In addition, LXR activation has an anti-inflammatory effect, which is achieved by inhibiting proinflammatory genes responsible for the production of TNFα, IL-1β, IL6, and nitric oxide synthase [32]. The remyelination process is also associated with the activation of LXRs. This is evidenced by studies on mice, in which blocking LXRs inhibits the repair processes within myelin while their activation stimulates the maturation of oligodendrocytes and both myelin production and remyelination. This mechanism involves reverse cholesterol transport using ABCA1 and apoE [33]. Studies also suggest LXRs' role in reducing oxidative stress by stimulating antioxidant genes: glucose-6-phosphate dehydrogenase (G6PDH), isocitrate dehydrogenase 1 (IDH1), and 6-phosphogluconate dehydrogenase (6-PGDH) in damaged myelin sheaths in peripheral nerves [34]. Many studies provide evidence that MS is associated with serum lipid profile alteration. The most common findings in these patients are increased levels of TC, LDL, TG, and HDL [35–38]. However, it is not known whether the dyslipidemia described in the studies is the result of myelin damage associated with the development of the disease or if it is pathophysiologically unrelated to the processes underlying MS and is merely a comorbidity.

Many studies provide evidence that MS is associated with serum lipid profile alteration. The most common findings in these patients are increased levels of TC, LDL, TG, and HDL [24,35,39,40]. A recent study assessed the prevalence of normolipidemia and various types of dyslipidemia in a group of healthy individuals, those with RRMS, and those with progressive MS (PMS, which included patients with PPMS and SPMS). While it did not show differences in the occurrence of different types of dyslipidemia between the groups, it was observed that individuals with PMS and higher HDL levels demonstrated lower levels of disability [41]. There are also studies discussing the impact of diet on the course of MS. One study shows that patients following a diet high in saturated fats present greater disability and experience a more severe course of the disease [42]. Meanwhile, a more recent study—a randomized clinical trial—points to the Swank diet (low in saturated fats) and the Wahls diet (modified Paleolithic elimination) as diets that reduce chronic fatigue and improve quality of life [43]. However, it is not known whether the dyslipidemia described in the studies is the result of myelin damage associated with the development of the disease or if it is pathophysiologically unrelated to the processes underlying MS and is merely a comorbidity.

Various studies indicate a positive correlation between elevated levels of TC and the Expanded Disability Status Scale (EDSS), TC and disease duration, increased levels of LDL and EDSS, and LDL with disease duration. Moreover, levels of TC and LDL are significantly higher in PPMS and SPMS than in RRMS [44–47]. The relationship between high TC levels and a higher EDSS score may result from the impact of excess cholesterol on remyelination. Some studies suggest that the toxic effect of excess cholesterol in the CNS has an inhibitory effect on remyelination by limiting microglia's ability to clear myelin debris [33]. Other studies have shown an association between increased levels of LDL and contrast-enhancing lesions (CEL), the number of lesions, or the appearance of new lesions in T2 MRI sequences [38,48,49]. Increased levels of TC and its metabolites—24S-OHC and 27S-OHC—are also found to positively correlate with CEL. Furthermore, they are negatively correlated with brain volume in MS patients [45,50].

Other studies have shown an association between increased levels of LDL and CELs, the number of lesions, or the appearance of new lesions in T2 MRI sequences [40,51,52]. Increased levels of TC and its metabolites—24S-OHC and 27S-OHC—are also found to positively correlate with CELs. Furthermore, they are negatively correlated with brain volume in MS patients [30,47].

The lipid metabolism disorder described above results from disturbances in cholesterol homeostasis in the brain. The destruction of myelin—the process that underlies MS—leads to an overload of the CNS with released cholesterol. This necessitates enhanced activity of the processes responsible for its removal in order to reduce the risk of its toxic effects [36]. The activity of CYP46A1 hydroxylase is increased, which metabolizes excess cholesterol to 24S-OHC, allowing it to freely penetrate the BBB. In serum, 24S-OHC is mainly transported in the form of LDL (70–80%) and HDL (20–30%) and then eliminated in the liver as bile acids [37]. Through the damaged BBB, cholesterol originating from the demyelination process penetrates into the bloodstream, which may indirectly result in increasing levels of serum LDL and TC.

Activation of LXR receptors takes place both in the CNS and in the periphery, mainly in the liver. Ligands for these receptors (including 24S-OHC) elicit an increase in the transcription of genes for ABCA1, ABCG1, and apoE, which are responsible for reverse cholesterol transport. This indirectly leads to a further increase in LDL, HDL, and VLDL levels in the serum. The increase in apoE levels is a response to the increased need for cholesterol efflux from the cell. Activation of LXRs also induces the promotion of transcription of the SREBP1c gene, leading to an increase in the synthesis of fatty acids. Another extremely important function of LXR is its immunomodulatory role. These receptors, located on T lymphocytes and macrophages, inhibit the influx of these cells into the CNS under conditions of stimulation. Activation of LXR also leads to a decrease in the transcription of genes responsible for the production of TNFα, IL-6, and IL-1β and also promotes transcription of anti-inflammatory factors such as IL-10 and TGFβ [31,32,38].

The increase in LDL levels resulting from the mechanisms described above is also harmful in itself. Under normal conditions, even increased LDL does not affect the processes occurring in the CNS due to the preserved integrity of the BBB. However, in the course of MS, when there is damage to the BBB and a significant increase in its permeability, even particles as large as LDL can migrate through it freely. In the vessel walls, oxidation occurs, leading to the formation of ox-LDL, which has a very strong atherogenic and proinflammatory effect. Its proinflammatory effect results from the presence of a changed epitope of apoB, the main apolipoprotein of LDL [53,54]. The pathologically changed epitope becomes recognizable by macrophages, which "engulf" ox-LDL, leading to the formation of foam cells, whose role in demyelination has been suggested [50,55]. In this process, chemotaxis of monocytes occurs, promoting the production of proinflammatory cytokines such as TNFα, IL-6, and IL-8 [48]. As a consequence of these modifications, HDL shifted from being an anti-inflammatory particle to a proinflammatory one, as evidenced by its altered capacity to either prevent or promote LDL oxidation by arterial wall cells or to either inhibit or enhance LDL-induced monocyte chemotactic activity [49]. All this exaggerates the inflammatory and demyelinating processes in the CNS. This is reflected in previously conducted studies showing a positive relationship between the concentration of LDL, ox-LDL, and the level of EDSS, the duration of the disease, or the number of demyelinating plaques in the CNS [53,56].

4. HDL's Role in MS Pathophysiology

HDL is one of five classes of lipoproteins. This classification is based on molecular size, density, and the content of individual lipids and apolipoproteins. Both LDL and HDL are cholesterol-rich lipoproteins. The main apolipoprotein of HDL is apoA1 [3]. ApoA1 plays a crucial role in lipid metabolism. It facilitates the removal of fats from cells, including macrophages overloaded with oxidized LDL, by transporting them to other locations, such as the liver, for excretion. ApoA1 acts as a cofactor for LCAT, which forms plasma cholesteryl esters and may have an anticoagulant effect by stabilizing prostacyclin [57].

Research assessing HDL levels in patients with MS produces heterogeneous results. Most of the studies exhibit increased levels of HDL in MS. The adjustment of HDL varies among the different MS subtypes. The research conducted by Giubilei et al. assessed HDL levels in patients with clinically isolated syndrome (CIS). CIS is defined as the first episode of characteristic neurological symptoms that do not yet fulfill MS diagnostic criteria. In this study, patients with initially higher HDL levels also exhibited lower initial EDSS scores and a reduced number of CELs [51].

In the stable course of RRMS without recent relapses, HDL levels in serum are found to be significantly higher compared to healthy controls. Interestingly, the studies did not establish a significant correlation between EDSS scores, disease duration, and HDL levels [39,58,59].

Further, studies conducted by Meyers et al. and Gardner et al. showed reduced levels of HDL and apoA1—the main apolipoprotein for brain HDL, in the group of patients with MS. The results obtained by these researchers may be due to the fact that their RRMS patients were older and had more advanced diseases compared to the previous studies or had already been diagnosed with PPMS or SPMS [60,61].

In the study assessing the differences in lipid profiles in patients with RRMS and SPMS, it was shown that HDL levels are significantly lower in patients with SPMS, suggesting a potential association of this lipoprotein with disease progression and severity [46].

Differences observed in HDL levels, whether elevated or decreased, as seen in the aforementioned studies, may also depend on the assessment of specific HDL subfractions—such as small and large HDL particles—as well as the evaluation of oxidized HDL (ox-HDL).

Analyzing studies that evaluate HDL levels in relation to the pathophysiology of MS, it is hypothesized that elevated HDL levels are associated with better prognosis, slower disease progression, and improved BBB function. Initial support for this hypothesis comes from observed differences between the subtypes of multiple sclerosis.

Prospective studies evaluating patients with RRMS over a 5-year period have demonstrated that individuals with lower baseline HDL levels exhibit a significantly higher risk of developing SPMS [47]. Additionally, correlations have been observed between HDL levels and brain imaging findings on MRI. It has been demonstrated that during the course of the observations, patients with relative increases in HDL levels exhibited reduced gray matter atrophy [47,62]. Some available data indicate that higher levels of HDL and apoA1 are associated with improved cerebral perfusion in patients with MS [58].

Many studies also indicate a relationship between HDL and BBB integrity. An indirect marker of this correlation is the association between higher HDL levels and a reduced number of CELs, smaller lesion volumes, and a prospectively lower incidence of new plaque formation [39,40,58,63]. Fellows et al. designed a study to investigate the direct relationship between HDL and BBB integrity. They compared serum HDL levels with markers of BBB damage found in CSF. They discovered that higher levels of HDL and apoA1 are associated with lower total protein levels in CSF, lower albumin and IgG levels in CSF, and reduced concentrations of CD80+ and CD19+ cells [64]. These findings suggest that HDL is essential for maintaining proper BBB permeability. Similarly, the protective effects of HDL have been confirmed in Alzheimer's disease, and studies have also demonstrated a relationship between higher HDL levels and reduced BBB permeability [65].

5. Mechanisms of HDL Action in MS

The exact mechanism underlying the role of HDL in the pathophysiology of MS is not fully understood. However, based on the studies mentioned, the most likely explanation is its beneficial effect on the BBB through its influence on the vascular endothelium. HDL exerts its effects on the endothelium through its anti-inflammatory, antioxidant, antithrombotic, antiapoptotic, and nitric oxide synthesis properties [2,3].

5.1. Anti-Inflammatory Effect of HDL

The anti-inflammatory properties exhibited by HDL result from various mediated processes. One of these processes is the protective effect of HDL on the vascular endothelium through its interaction with endothelial adhesion molecules such as VCAM-1, intercellular adhesion molecule-1 (ICAM-1), and E-selectin [66]. These molecules are involved in the processes of leukocyte rolling along the endothelium, their activation, adhesion, and subsequent transendothelial migration to the target site. In addition to facilitating leukocyte migration to sites of inflammation, the endothelium also participates in the production of cytokines and growth factors. These include IL-1, IL-6, IL-18, TNF, and monocyte chemotactic protein 1 (MCP-1) [15,67–69]. The overexpression of these molecules and the consequent damage to the BBB are well-documented in MS [70]. The protective effect of HDL on the vascular endothelium that constitutes the BBB is attributed to the fact that this apoA1-containing lipoprotein exerts an inhibitory effect on cytokine-induced EC activation, preventing the expression of adhesion molecules. Some in vitro studies suggest that the inhibitory effect of HDL on the expression of VCAM-1, ICAM-1, and E-selectin is associated with TNF-α. In these studies, endothelial cells were activated by the addition of TNF-α and then incubated with HDL. Depending on the specific experimental setup, the expression levels of various adhesion molecules were subsequently assessed. The levels of VCAM-1 and E-selectin were significantly reduced in the presence of HDL [71,72].

Another mechanism by which HDL attenuates the endothelial activation response involves its modulation of E-selectin via nuclear factor kappa-light-chain-enhancer of activated B cells (NF-κB) and S1P [73,74]. HDL influences NF-κB by reducing S1P levels through the inhibition of the enzyme sphingosine kinase. Reduction in NF-κB levels leads to decreased expression of E-selectin [75,76]. While E-selectin contributes to leukocyte rolling, research indicates that its primary function is to facilitate the transition of leukocytes from rolling to firm adhesion to the endothelium. Experimental models lacking E- and P-selectin genes exhibit a complete absence of leukocyte migration across the BBB, an absence of leukocyte rolling, and increased leukocyte production [77]. Therefore, by reducing the expression of adhesion molecules, HDL reinforces the BBB, diminishes leukocyte migration into the CNS, and thereby reduces demyelination (Figure 1).

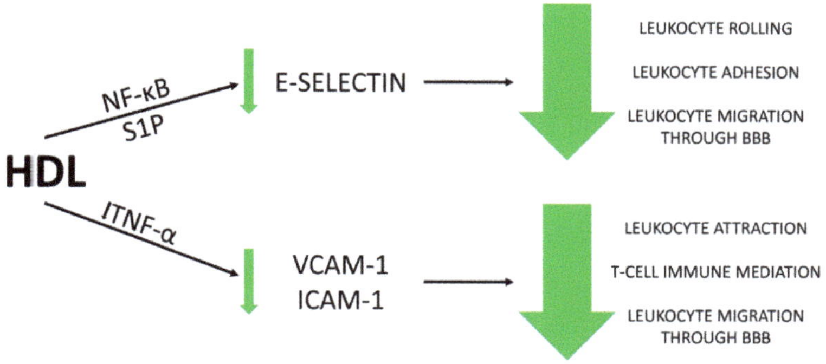

Figure 1. HDL reduces S1P levels by inhibiting sphingosine kinase, which in turn lowers NF-κB activity. This reduction in NF-κB activity leads to decreased expression of E-selectin, a molecule involved in leukocyte rolling, adhesion, and migration through the BBB. The downregulation of E-selectin by HDL results in a decrease in leukocyte rolling, adhesion, and migration through the BBB. HDL inhibits the effects of TNF-α, which is responsible for the upregulation of VCAM-1 and ICAM-1. By reducing the expression of VCAM-1 and ICAM-1, HDL diminishes leukocyte attraction and T-cell immune mediation, thereby reducing leukocyte migration through the BBB. BBB- blood–brain barrier, S1P—sphingosine-1-phosphate, NF-κB—nuclear factor kappa-light-chain-enhancer of activated B cells, HDL—high-density lipoprotein, TNF-α—tumor necrosis factor-alpha, VCAM-1—vascular cell adhesion molecule-1, ICAM-1—intercellular adhesion molecule-1.

5.2. S1P Interactions with HDL

Changes in sphingolipid metabolism also play a significant role in the pathophysiology of MS. These changes involve not only the levels of sphingolipids themselves but also the signaling pathways mediated by them. Disruptions in sphingolipid metabolism are implicated in various neurodegenerative and inflammatory CNS diseases [78]. Sphingolipids participate in modulating the immune response, including through the induction of apoptosis in autoreactive T lymphocytes [79]. Sphingosine-1-phosphate (S1P) is a representative sphingolipid with a well-documented impact on immune response and neurodegeneration in MS [80]. S1P is involved in neuronal apoptosis and exhibits proinflammatory activity [80]. Increased expression of S1P receptors—primarily S1PR1, S1PR2, S1PR3, and S1PR5—has been observed in astrocytes and oligodendrocytes in MS patients [79,81].

S1P is also modulated by HDL. Approximately 50–65% of serum S1P is bound to apolipoprotein M (apoM) and transported by HDL in the HDL-apoM-S1P complex. S1P receptors are responsible for various functions related to immune responses. Among them, S1PR1 is responsible for regulating the migration of leukocytes from secondary lymphoid organs to the bloodstream and lymph nodes [72,82–84]. One of the drugs used in the treatment of MS, fingolimod, is an agonist of S1P receptors. By binding to these receptors on autoreactive T and B lymphocytes, it prevents their migration into the CNS and retains them within lymphoid organs. In a study evaluating HDL levels in patients undergoing fingolimod therapy, it was demonstrated that HDL levels increased during treatment, which was associated with a deceleration of disease progression and a reduction in the frequency of relapses [85]. The results of this study suggest that the beneficial effect of HDL on the course and severity of MS is attributable to its interaction with S1P (Figure 2).

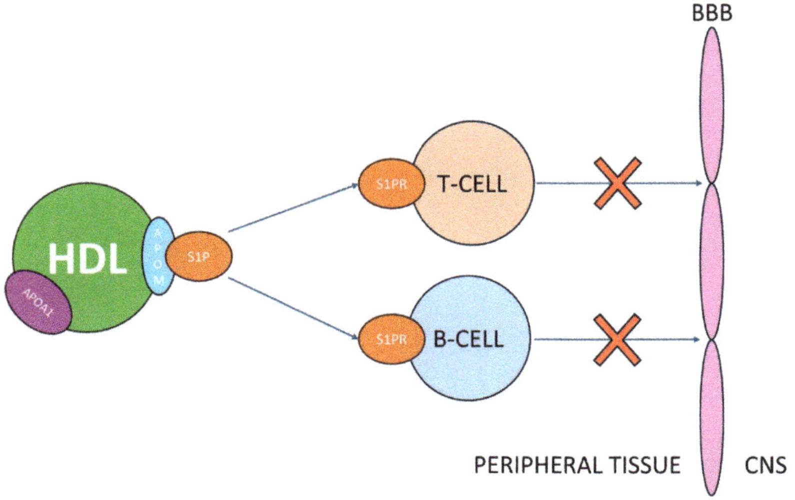

Figure 2. S1PRs (1–5) are abundantly expressed on immune cells, particularly on T and B lymphocytes. The primary function of these receptors is to regulate the movement of these cells between lymphoid organs, including lymph nodes, and peripheral tissues, such as the CNS. S1P molecules bound to HDL via apoM act as agonists for these receptors by binding them. Consequently, HDL indirectly influences immune response modulation and prevents activated T and B lymphocytes from migrating from lymphoid organs to the CNS, thereby inhibiting demyelination processes. HDL—high-density protein, CNS—central nervous system, BBB—blood–brain barrier, apoM- apolipoprotein M, S1PR—sphingosine-1-phosphate receptor, S1P—sphingosine-1-phosphate.

5.3. Antioxidant Effect of HDL

The role of oxidative stress in the development of MS is highly emphasized. The studies that were conducted support evidence of increased levels of oxidation and decreased activity of antioxidants in MS patients [86]. As mentioned before, in MS, we deal with the demyelination of neurons, axonal injury, and neurodegenerative components. These impairments could be associated with oxidative stress due to the high sensitivity of glial cells and neurons to its negative effects, such as DNA damage, mitochondrial dysfunction, or defective enzyme activities [86,87]. In patients with MS, elevated markers indicative of nitrosative stress are also observed, primarily including increased levels of nitrotyrosine [88,89].

The antioxidant properties exhibited by HDL are also linked to their beneficial impact on the course of MS. These properties are attributed to HDL-associated enzymes, such as paraoxonase-1 (PON1) and glutathione selenoperoxidase (GSPx), whose dysfunction has been reported in the development of MS [90,91]. PON1 activity is found to be decreased in patients with MS compared to healthy individuals [92,93]. Moreover, patients with SPMS indicate lower PON1 activity compared to other subtypes [94]. The primary function of PON1 is to prevent the oxidation of LDL to ox-LDL, a process that occurs through the hydrolysis of the lactone ring in homocysteine thiolactone (HTL) molecules. Ox-LDL is known for its proinflammatory properties [95]. As previously mentioned, ox-LDL levels are elevated in patients with MS and are associated with higher EDSS scores and markers of endothelial dysfunction [53]. Those patients have also reduced levels of serum HDL. The relationship between HDL levels and ox-LDL has also been well-known for a long time, particularly in relation to atherosclerosis. Higher HDL levels reduce LDL oxidation, thereby exerting a protective effect on the vascular walls (Figure 3) [5].

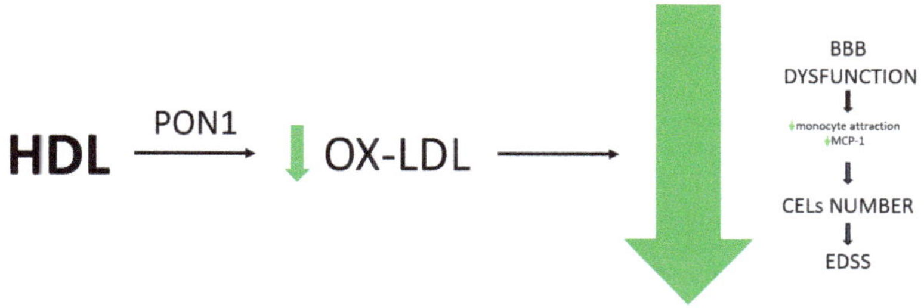

Figure 3. PON1 is an enzyme anchored in HDL. The activity of PON1 comprises the lactonase, homocysteine-thiolactonase (HTase), and arylesterase (AREase) activities. Through the hydrolysis of reactive compounds—PON1 is anticipating oxidation of LDL. The reduction in LDL oxidation to harmful proinflammatory ox-LDL in the course of MS leads to a decrease in the number of CELs. This is due to the fact that ox-LDL no longer exacerbates BBB endothelial dysfunction via increasing monocyte attraction or MCP-1 activation. As a result, there is a slowdown in the progression of disability, as measured by tools such as the EDSS.HDL—high-density lipoprotein, LDL—low-density lipoprotein, PON1—paraoxonase-1, BBB—blood–brain barrier, CELs—contrast-enhancing lesions, MCP-1—monocyte chemoattractant protein-1, EDSS—Expanded Disability Status Scale.

Patients with MS who have higher HDL levels demonstrate better brain perfusion parameters [58]. This association may be attributed to the relationship between HDL and apoA1 with NO synthesis. Some studies suggest that HDL interacts with scavenger receptor-BI on brain vascular cells, stimulating endothelial NO synthase (eNOS) [96,97]. This enzyme is responsible for the synthesis of NO, which has vasodilatory properties. It has been shown that anti-ApoA1 antibodies can block eNOS-dependent vascular relaxation [97]. Another mechanism by which HDL exerts its vasodilatory effects on the vessel wall likely involves the mimicry of HDL-bound S1P3, which activates the Akt-mediated pathway leading to eNOS activation [98].

5.4. Ox-HDL in MS

The mechanisms outlined above highlight the potentially critical role of HDL in the pathogenesis of MS. However, several studies suggest that serum HDL levels may be diminished in patients with MS, particularly in those with more severe disease phenotypes such as PPMS, SPMS, or chronic RRMS [46,60,61]. This reduction may be linked to structural abnormalities in HDL, its oxidation to the proinflammatory ox-HDL, or potential dysfunctions in LXRs, which are pivotal in regulating cholesterol homeostasis within the CNS [99]. Ox-HDL In a study conducted by Jorissen et al., it was demonstrated that patients with RRMS with reduced HDL levels exhibit nitration and oxidation of tyrosine and tryptophan, along with a +126 amu modification on tyrosine residues in HDL3-derived apoA1 [99]. In these patients, the presence of ox-HDL was also observed, which correlates positively with higher EDSS scores [93]. The formation of this harmful molecule in MS patients is attributed to prolonged oxidative stress, nitrosative stress, and the dysregulated activity of heme oxygenase 1 (HO-1). HO-1 exerts a protective role against reactive oxygen species (ROS) and oxidative stress, and its upregulation mitigates the harmful impact of oxidized HDL. Several studies have reported increased activity of this enzyme in patients with MS [100–104].

6. Conclusions

1. HDL's Role in MS Pathophysiology: HDL plays a potentially critical role in MS by influencing BBB integrity and vascular endothelium through its anti-inflammatory, antioxidant, and nitric oxide synthesis properties.
2. Mechanisms of HDL Action: HDL protects the endothelial cells forming the BBB by interacting with adhesion molecules like VCAM-1, ICAM-1, and E-selectin, thereby

reducing leukocyte migration and BBB permeability. HDL also modulates endothelial activation through NF-κB and sphingosine-1-phosphate (S1P) pathways, enhancing its protective effect.

3. Impact of HDL on S1P and Nitric Oxide: HDL modulates S1P, a crucial molecule in MS pathogenesis, by binding it to apolipoprotein M (apoM). This interaction impacts leukocyte migration and is linked to therapeutic effects observed with fingolimod, an agonist drug that targets S1P receptors.
4. Antioxidant Properties: HDL's antioxidant properties, linked to enzymes such as PON1 and GSPx, contribute to its protective role. Increased ox-HDL levels are associated with MS, potentially worsening disease outcomes. Due to the reduced PON1 activity, elevated ox-LDL levels are associated with increased disease severity, higher EDSS scores, and endothelial dysfunction

Author Contributions: Conceptualization A.D.-D., writing—original draft preparation A.D.-D.; figures preparation—A.D.-D., writing—review and editing M.P.; supervision, final revision A.G. All authors have read and agreed to the published version of the manuscript.

Funding: This research received no external funding.

Conflicts of Interest: The authors declare no conflicts of interest.

References

1. Denimal, D. Antioxidant and Anti-Inflammatory Functions of High-Density Lipoprotein in Type 1 and Type 2 Diabetes. *Antioxidants* **2023**, *13*, 57. [CrossRef] [PubMed]
2. Shao, B.; Heinecke, J.W. HDL, lipid peroxidation, and atherosclerosis. *J. Lipid Res.* **2009**, *50*, 599–601. [CrossRef] [PubMed]
3. Deng, S.; Xu, Y.; Zheng, L. HDL Structure. In *HDL Metabolism and Diseases*; Advances in Experimental Medicine and Biology; Springer: Singapore, 2022; Volume 1377, pp. 1–11. [CrossRef]
4. Denimal, D. Rethinking 'good cholesterol' for cardiovascular risk stratification. *QJM Int. J. Med.* **2024**, *117*, 243–245. [CrossRef] [PubMed]
5. Mertens, A.; Holvoet, P. Oxidized LDL and HDL: Antagonists in atherothrombosis. *FASEB J.* **2001**, *15*, 2073–2084. [CrossRef]
6. Compston, A.; Coles, A. Multiple sclerosis. *Lancet* **2008**, *372*, 1502–1517. [CrossRef]
7. Thompson, A.J.; Baranzini, S.E.; Geurts, J.; Hemmer, B.; Ciccarelli, O. Multiple sclerosis. *Lancet* **2018**, *391*, 1622–1636. [CrossRef]
8. Kuhlmann, T.; Moccia, M.; Coetzee, T.; Cohen, J.A.; Correale, J.; Graves, J.; Marrie, R.A.; Montalban, X.; Yong, V.W.; Thompson, A.J.; et al. Multiple sclerosis progression: Time for a new mechanism-driven framework. *Lancet Neurol.* **2023**, *22*, 78–88. [CrossRef]
9. Bar-Or, A.; Darlington, P.J. The immunology of multiple sclerosis. In *Multiple Sclerosis Therapeutics*, 4th ed.; Cambridge University Press: Cambridge, UK, 2011. [CrossRef]
10. Krumbholz, M.; Derfuss, T.; Hohlfeld, R.; Meinl, E. B cells and antibodies in multiple sclerosis pathogenesis and therapy. *Nat. Rev. Neurol.* **2012**, *8*, 613–623. [CrossRef]
11. Greenfield, A.L.; Hauser, S.L. B-cell Therapy for Multiple Sclerosis: Entering an era. *Ann. Neurol.* **2018**, *83*, 13–26. [CrossRef]
12. Jurewicz, A.; Domowicz, M.; Galazka, G.; Raine, C.S.; Selmaj, K. Multiple sclerosis: Presence of serum antibodies to lipids and predominance of cholesterol recognition. *J. Neurosci. Res.* **2017**, *95*, 1984–1992. [CrossRef]
13. Leech, S.; Kirk, J.; Plumb, J.; McQuaid, S. Persistent endothelial abnormalities and blood–brain barrier leak in primary and secondary progressive multiple sclerosis. *Neuropathol. Appl. Neurobiol.* **2007**, *33*, 86–98. [CrossRef] [PubMed]
14. Liebner, S.; Dijkhuizen, R.M.; Reiss, Y.; Plate, K.H.; Agalliu, D.; Constantin, G. Functional morphology of the blood–brain barrier in health and disease. *Acta Neuropathol.* **2018**, *135*, 311–336. [CrossRef] [PubMed]
15. Vestweber, D. How leukocytes cross the vascular endothelium. *Nat. Rev. Immunol.* **2015**, *15*, 692–704. [CrossRef] [PubMed]
16. Stadelmann, C.; Timmler, S.; Barrantes-Freer, A.; Simons, M. Myelin in the Central Nervous System: Structure, Function, and Pathology. *Physiol. Rev.* **2019**, *99*, 1381–1431. [CrossRef]
17. Loving, B.A.; Bruce, K.D. Lipid and Lipoprotein Metabolism in Microglia. *Front. Physiol.* **2020**, *11*, 393. [CrossRef]
18. Ho, W.Y.; Hartmann, H.; Ling, S. Central nervous system cholesterol metabolism in health and disease. *IUBMB Life* **2022**, *74*, 826–841. [CrossRef]
19. Raulin, A.-C.; Martens, Y.A.; Bu, G. Lipoproteins in the Central Nervous System: From Biology to Pathobiology. *Annu. Rev. Biochem.* **2022**, *91*, 731–759. [CrossRef]
20. Koch, S.; Donarski, N.; Goetze, K.; Kreckel, M.; Stuerenburg, H.-J.; Buhmann, C.; Beisiegel, U. Characterization of four lipoprotein classes in human cerebrospinal fluid. *J. Lipid Res.* **2001**, *42*, 1143–1151. [CrossRef]
21. Wahrle, S.E.; Jiang, H.; Parsadanian, M.; Legleiter, J.; Han, X.; Fryer, J.D.; Kowalewski, T.; Holtzman, D.M. ABCA1 Is Required for Normal Central Nervous System ApoE Levels and for Lipidation of Astrocyte-secreted apoE. *J. Biol. Chem.* **2004**, *279*, 40987–40993. [CrossRef]

22. Kim, W.S.; Guillemin, G.J.; Glaros, E.N.; Lim, C.K.; Garner, B. Quantitation of ATP-binding cassette subfamily-A transporter gene expression in primary human brain cells. *NeuroReport* **2006**, *17*, 891–896. [CrossRef]
23. Kim, W.S.; Rahmanto, A.S.; Kamili, A.; Rye, K.-A.; Guillemin, G.J.; Gelissen, I.C.; Jessup, W.; Hill, A.F.; Garner, B. Role of ABCG1 and ABCA1 in Regulation of Neuronal Cholesterol Efflux to Apolipoprotein E Discs and Suppression of Amyloid-β Peptide Generation. *J. Biol. Chem.* **2007**, *282*, 2851–2861. [CrossRef] [PubMed]
24. Podbielska, M.; O'keeffe, J.; Pokryszko-Dragan, A. New Insights into Multiple Sclerosis Mechanisms: Lipids on the Track to Control Inflammation and Neurodegeneration. *Int. J. Mol. Sci.* **2021**, *22*, 7319. [CrossRef] [PubMed]
25. Saher, G.; Stumpf, S.K. Cholesterol in myelin biogenesis and hypomyelinating disorders. *Biochim. Biophys. Acta (BBA)—Mol. Cell Biol. Lipids* **2015**, *1851*, 1083–1094. [CrossRef]
26. Luo, J.; Yang, H.; Song, B.-L. Mechanisms and regulation of cholesterol homeostasis. *Nat. Rev. Mol. Cell Biol.* **2020**, *21*, 225–245. [CrossRef] [PubMed]
27. Zhang, J.; Liu, Q. Cholesterol metabolism and homeostasis in the brain. *Protein Cell* **2015**, *6*, 254–264. [CrossRef] [PubMed]
28. Vejux, A.; Ghzaiel, I.; Nury, T.; Schneider, V.; Charrière, K.; Sghaier, R.; Zarrouk, A.; Leoni, V.; Moreau, T.; Lizard, G. Oxysterols and multiple sclerosis: Physiopathology, evolutive biomarkers and therapeutic strategy. *J. Steroid Biochem. Mol. Biol.* **2021**, *210*, 105870. [CrossRef] [PubMed]
29. Leoni, V.; Masterman, T.; Diczfalusy, U.; De Luca, G.; Hillert, J.; Björkhem, I. Changes in human plasma levels of the brain specific oxysterol 24S-hydroxycholesterol during progression of multiple sclerosis. *Neurosci. Lett.* **2002**, *331*, 163–166. [CrossRef]
30. van de Kraats, C.; Killestein, J.; Popescu, V.; Rijkers, E.; Vrenken, H.; Lütjohann, D.; Barkhof, F.; Polman, C.; Teunissen, C. Oxysterols and cholesterol precursors correlate to magnetic resonance imaging measures of neurodegeneration in multiple sclerosis. *Mult. Scler. J.* **2014**, *20*, 412–417. [CrossRef]
31. Ma, X.; Bi, E.; Huang, C.; Lu, Y.; Xue, G.; Guo, X.; Wang, A.; Yang, M.; Qian, J.; Dong, C.; et al. Cholesterol negatively regulates IL-9–producing CD8+ T cell differentiation and antitumor activity. *J. Exp. Med.* **2018**, *215*, 1555–1569. [CrossRef]
32. Pineda-Torra, I.; Siddique, S.; Waddington, K.E.; Farrell, R.; Jury, E.C. Disrupted Lipid Metabolism in Multiple Sclerosis: A Role for Liver X Receptors? *Front. Endocrinol.* **2021**, *12*, 639757. [CrossRef]
33. Cantuti-Castelvetri, L.; Fitzner, D.; Bosch-Queralt, M.; Weil, M.-T.; Su, M.; Sen, P.; Ruhwedel, T.; Mitkovski, M.; Trendelenburg, G.; Lütjohann, D.; et al. Defective cholesterol clearance limits remyelination in the aged central nervous system. *Science* **2018**, *359*, 684–688. [CrossRef] [PubMed]
34. Hichor, M.; Sundaram, V.K.; Eid, S.A.; Abdel-Rassoul, R.; Petit, P.X.; Borderie, D.; Bastin, J.; Eid, A.A.; Manuel, M.; Grenier, J.; et al. Liver X Receptor exerts a protective effect against the oxidative stress in the peripheral nerve. *Sci. Rep.* **2018**, *8*, 2524. [CrossRef] [PubMed]
35. Uher, T.; Fellows, K.; Horakova, D.; Zivadinov, R.; Vaneckova, M.; Sobisek, L.; Tyblova, M.; Seidl, Z.; Krasensky, J.; Bergsland, N.; et al. Serum lipid profile changes predict neurodegeneration in interferon-β1a-treated multiple sclerosis patients. *J. Lipid Res.* **2017**, *58*, 403–411. [CrossRef] [PubMed]
36. Zhornitsky, S.; McKay, K.A.; Metz, L.M.; Teunissen, C.E.; Rangachari, M. Cholesterol and markers of cholesterol turnover in multiple sclerosis: Relationship with disease outcomes. *Mult. Scler. Relat. Disord.* **2015**, *5*, 53–65. [CrossRef] [PubMed]
37. Nunes, V.S.; da Silva, E.J.; Ferreira, G.d.S.; de Assis, S.I.S.; Cazita, P.M.; Nakandakare, E.R.; Zago, V.H.d.S.; de Faria, E.C.; Quintão, E.C.R. The Plasma Distribution of Non-cholesterol Sterol Precursors and Products of Cholesterol Synthesis and Phytosterols Depend on HDL Concentration. *Front. Nutr.* **2022**, *9*, 723555. [CrossRef]
38. Yang, T.-M.; Miao, M.; Yu, W.-Q.; Wang, X.; Xia, F.-J.; Li, Y.-J.; Guo, S.-D. Targeting macrophages in atherosclerosis using nanocarriers loaded with liver X receptor agonists: A narrow review. *Front. Mol. Biosci.* **2023**, *10*, 1147699. [CrossRef]
39. Weinstock-Guttman, B.; Zivadinov, R.; Mahfooz, N.; Carl, E.; Drake, A.; Schneider, J.; Teter, B.; Hussein, S.; Mehta, B.; Weiskopf, M.; et al. Serum lipid profiles are associated with disability and MRI outcomes in multiple sclerosis. *J. Neuroinflamm.* **2011**, *8*, 127. [CrossRef]
40. Weinstock-Guttman, B.; Zivadinov, R.; Horakova, D.; Havrdova, E.; Qu, J.; Shyh, G.; Lakota, E.; O'Connor, K.; Badgett, D.; Tamaño-Blanco, M.; et al. Lipid profiles are associated with lesion formation over 24 months in interferon-β treated patients following the first demyelinating event. *J. Neurol. Neurosurg. Psychiatry* **2013**, *84*, 1186–1191. [CrossRef]
41. Wicks, T.R.; Nehzat, N.; Wolska, A.; Shalaurova, I.; Browne, R.W.; Weinstock-Guttman, B.; Jakimovski, D.; Zivadinov, R.; Remaley, A.T.; Otvos, J.; et al. Dyslipidemias in multiple sclerosis. *Mult. Scler. Relat. Disord.* **2024**, *91*, 105841. [CrossRef]
42. Swank, R.L.; Grimsgaard, A. Multiple sclerosis: The lipid relationship. *Am. J. Clin. Nutr.* **1988**, *48*, 1387–1393. [CrossRef]
43. Wahls, T.L.; Titcomb, T.J.; Bisht, B.; Eyck, P.T.; Rubenstein, L.M.; Carr, L.J.; Darling, W.G.; Hoth, K.F.; Kamholz, J.; Snetselaar, L.G. Impact of the Swank and Wahls elimination dietary interventions on fatigue and quality of life in relapsing-remitting multiple sclerosis: The WAVES randomized parallel-arm clinical trial. *Mult. Scler. J.—Exp. Transl. Clin.* **2021**, *7*, 20552173211035400. [CrossRef] [PubMed]
44. Ortí, J.E.d.l.R.; Armero, J.L.P.; Cuerda-Ballester, M.; Sanchis-Sanchis, C.E.; Navarro-Illana, E.; Lajara-Romance, J.M.; Benlloch, M.; Ceron, J.J.; Tvarijonaviciute, A.; Proaño, B. Lipid Profile in Multiple Sclerosis: Functional Capacity and Therapeutic Potential of Its Regulation after Intervention with Epigallocatechin Gallate and Coconut Oil. *Foods* **2023**, *12*, 3730. [CrossRef] [PubMed]
45. Mandoj, C.; Renna, R.; Plantone, D.; Sperduti, I.; Cigliana, G.; Conti, L.; Koudriavtseva, T. Anti-annexin antibodies, cholesterol levels and disability in multiple sclerosis. *Neurosci. Lett.* **2015**, *606*, 156–160. [CrossRef] [PubMed]

46. Ďurfinová, M.; Procházková, L'.; Petrleničová, D.; Bystrická, Z.; Orešanská, K.; Kuračka, L'.; Líška, B. Cholesterol level correlate with disability score in patients with relapsing-remitting form of multiple sclerosis. *Neurosci. Lett.* **2018**, *687*, 304–307. [CrossRef]
47. Murali, N.; Browne, R.W.; Fellows Maxwell, K.; Bodziak, M.L.; Jakimovski, D.; Hagemeier, J.; Bergsland, N.; Weinstock-Guttman, B.; Zivadinov, R.; Ramanathan, M. Cholesterol and neurodegeneration: Longitudinal changes in serum cholesterol biomarkers are associated with new lesions and gray matter atrophy in multiple sclerosis over 5 years of follow-up. *Eur. J. Neurol.* **2020**, *27*, 188-e4. [CrossRef]
48. Rhoads, J.P.; Major, A.S. How Oxidized Low-Density Lipoprotein Activates Inflammatory Responses. *Crit. Rev. Immunol.* **2018**, *38*, 333–342. [CrossRef]
49. Navab, M.; Berliner, J.A.; Subbanagounder, G.; Hama, S.; Lusis, A.J.; Castellani, L.W.; Reddy, S.; Shih, D.; Shi, W.; Watson, A.D.; et al. HDL and the Inflammatory Response Induced by LDL-Derived Oxidized Phospholipids. *Arterioscler. Thromb. Vasc. Biol.* **2001**, *21*, 481–488. [CrossRef]
50. Newcombe, J.; Li, H.; Cuzner, M.L. Low density lipoprotein uptake by macrophages in multiple sclerosis plaques: Implications for pathogenesis. *Neuropathol. Appl. Neurobiol.* **1994**, *20*, 152–162. [CrossRef]
51. Giubilei, F.; Antonini, G.; Di Legge, S.; Sormani, M.P.; Pantano, P.; Antonini, R.; Sepe-Monti, M.; Caramia, F.; Pozzilli, C. Blood cholesterol and MRI activity in first clinical episode suggestive of multiple sclerosis. *Acta Neurol. Scand.* **2002**, *106*, 109–112. [CrossRef]
52. Yuan, S.; Xiong, Y.; Larsson, S.C. An atlas on risk factors for multiple sclerosis: A Mendelian randomization study. *J. Neurol.* **2021**, *268*, 114–124. [CrossRef]
53. Palavra, F.; Marado, D.; Mascarenhas-Melo, F.; Sereno, J.; Teixeira-Lemos, E.; Nunes, C.C.; Gonçalves, G.; Teixeira, F.; Reis, F. New Markers of Early Cardiovascular Risk in Multiple Sclerosis Patients: Oxidized-LDL Correlates with Clinical Staging. *Dis. Markers* **2013**, *34*, 341–348. [CrossRef] [PubMed]
54. Salomonsson, L. Oxidised LDL decreases VEGFR-1 expression in human monocyte-derived macrophages. *Atherosclerosis* **2003**, *169*, 259–267. [CrossRef] [PubMed]
55. Keller, J.N.; Hanni, K.B.; Gabbita, S.; Friebe, V.; Mattson, M.P.; Kindy, M.S. Oxidized lipoproteins increase reactive oxygen species formation in microglia and astrocyte cell lines. *Brain Res.* **1999**, *830*, 10–15. [CrossRef] [PubMed]
56. Haider, L.; Fischer, M.T.; Frischer, J.M.; Bauer, J.; Höftberger, R.; Botond, G.; Esterbauer, H.; Binder, C.J.; Witztum, J.L.; Lassmann, H. Oxidative damage in multiple sclerosis lesions. *Brain* **2011**, *134*, 1914–1924. [CrossRef] [PubMed]
57. Van der Vorst, E.P.C. High-Density Lipoproteins and Apolipoprotein A1. In *Vertebrate and Invertebrate Respiratory Proteins, Lipoproteins and Other Body Fluid Proteins*; Springer: Cham, Switzerland, 2020; pp. 399–420. [CrossRef]
58. Jakimovski, D.; Zivadinov, R.; Dwyer, M.G.; Bergsland, N.; Ramasamy, D.P.; Browne, R.W.; Weinstock-Guttman, B.; Ramanathan, M. High density lipoprotein cholesterol and apolipoprotein A-I are associated with greater cerebral perfusion in multiple sclerosis. *J. Neurol. Sci.* **2020**, *418*, 117120. [CrossRef]
59. Tettey, P.; Simpson, S.; Taylor, B.; Blizzard, L.; Ponsonby, A.-L.; Dwyer, T.; Kostner, K.; van der Mei, I. An adverse lipid profile is associated with disability and progression in disability, in people with MS. *Mult. Scler. J.* **2014**, *20*, 1737–1744. [CrossRef]
60. Meyers, L.; Groover, C.J.; Douglas, J.; Lee, S.; Brand, D.; Levin, M.C.; Gardner, L.A. A role for Apolipoprotein A-I in the pathogenesis of multiple sclerosis. *J. Neuroimmunol.* **2014**, *277*, 176–185. [CrossRef]
61. Gardner, L.A.; Levin, M.C. Importance of Apolipoprotein A-I in Multiple Sclerosis. *Front. Pharmacol.* **2015**, *6*, 278. [CrossRef]
62. McComb, M.; Parambi, R.; Browne, R.W.; Bodziak, M.L.; Jakimovski, D.; Bergsland, N.; Maceski, A.; Weinstock-Guttman, B.; Kuhle, J.; Zivadinov, R.; et al. Apolipoproteins AI and E are associated with neuroaxonal injury to gray matter in multiple sclerosis. *Mult. Scler. Relat. Disord.* **2020**, *45*, 102389. [CrossRef]
63. Browne, R.W.; Weinstock-Guttman, B.; Horakova, D.; Zivadinov, R.; Bodziak, M.L.; Tamaño-Blanco, M.; Badgett, D.; Tyblova, M.; Vaneckova, M.; Seidl, Z.; et al. Apolipoproteins are associated with new MRI lesions and deep grey matter atrophy in clinically isolated syndromes. *J. Neurol. Neurosurg. Psychiatry* **2014**, *85*, 859–864. [CrossRef]
64. Fellows, K.; Uher, T.; Browne, R.W.; Weinstock-Guttman, B.; Horakova, D.; Posova, H.; Vaneckova, M.; Seidl, Z.; Krasensky, J.; Tyblova, M.; et al. Protective associations of HDL with blood-brain barrier injury in multiple sclerosis patients. *J. Lipid Res.* **2015**, *56*, 2010–2018. [CrossRef] [PubMed]
65. Bowman, G.L.; Kaye, J.A.; Quinn, J.F. Dyslipidemia and Blood-Brain Barrier Integrity in Alzheimer's Disease. *Curr. Gerontol. Geriatr. Res.* **2012**, *2012*, 184042. [CrossRef] [PubMed]
66. Barter, P.J.; Nicholls, S.; Rye, K.-A.; Anantharamaiah, G.; Navab, M.; Fogelman, A.M. Antiinflammatory Properties of HDL. *Circ. Res.* **2004**, *95*, 764–772. [CrossRef] [PubMed]
67. Zhang, J. Biomarkers of endothelial activation and dysfunction in cardiovascular diseases. *Rev. Cardiovasc. Med.* **2022**, *23*, 73. [CrossRef]
68. Calabresia, L.; Franceschinia, G.; Sirtori, C.R.; De Palma, A.; Saresellac, M.; Ferrantec, P.; Taramellib, D. Inhibition of VCAM-1 Expression in Endothelial Cells by Reconstituted High Density Lipoproteins. *Biochem. Biophys. Res. Commun.* **1997**, *238*, 61–65. [CrossRef]
69. Siddiqui, K.; George, T.P.; Mujammami, M.; Isnani, A.; Alfadda, A.A. The association of cell adhesion molecules and selectins (VCAM-1, ICAM-1, E-selectin, L-selectin, and P-selectin) with microvascular complications in patients with type 2 diabetes: A follow-up study. *Front. Endocrinol.* **2023**, *14*, 1072288. [CrossRef]

70. Gauberti, M.; Fournier, A.P.; Docagne, F.; Vivien, D.; de Lizarrondo, S.M. Molecular Magnetic Resonance Imaging of Endothelial Activation in the Central Nervous System. *Theranostics* **2018**, *8*, 1195–1212. [CrossRef]
71. Cockerill, G.W.; Saklatvala, J.; Ridley, S.H.; Yarwood, H.; Miller, N.E.; Oral, B.; Nithyanathan, S.; Taylor, G.; Haskard, D.O. High-Density Lipoproteins Differentially Modulate Cytokine-Induced Expression of E-Selectin and Cyclooxygenase-2. *Arterioscler. Thromb. Vasc. Biol.* **1999**, *19*, 910–917. [CrossRef]
72. Baker, P.W.; Rye, K.-A.; Gamble, J.R.; Vadas, M.A.; Barter, P.J. Ability of reconstituted high density lipoproteins to inhibit cytokine-induced expression of vascular cell adhesion molecule-1 in human umbilical vein endothelial cells. *J. Lipid Res.* **1999**, *40*, 345–353. [CrossRef]
73. Gilmore, T.D. Introduction to NF-κB: Players, pathways, perspectives. *Oncogene* **2006**, *25*, 6680–6684. [CrossRef]
74. Christoffersen, C.; Obinata, H.; Kumaraswamy, S.B.; Galvani, S.; Ahnström, J.; Sevvana, M.; Egerer-Sieber, C.; Muller, Y.A.; Hla, T.; Nielsen, L.B.; et al. Endothelium-protective sphingosine-1-phosphate provided by HDL-associated apolipoprotein M. *Proc. Natl. Acad. Sci. USA* **2011**, *108*, 9613–9618. [CrossRef] [PubMed]
75. Xia, P.; Vadas, M.A.; Rye, K.-A.; Barter, P.J.; Gamble, J.R. High Density Lipoproteins (HDL) Interrupt the Sphingosine Kinase Signaling Pathway. *J. Biol. Chem.* **1999**, *274*, 33143–33147. [CrossRef] [PubMed]
76. Park, S.-H.; Park, J.H.Y.; Kang, J.-S.; Kang, Y.-H. Involvement of transcription factors in plasma HDL protection against TNF-α-induced vascular cell adhesion molecule-1 expression. *Int. J. Biochem. Cell Biol.* **2003**, *35*, 168–182. [CrossRef] [PubMed]
77. Frenette, P.S.; Wagner, D.D. Insights into Selectin Function from Knockout Mice. *Thromb. Haemost.* **1997**, *78*, 060–064. [CrossRef]
78. van Kruining, D.; Luo, Q.; van Echten-Deckert, G.; Mielke, M.M.; Bowman, A.; Ellis, S.; Oliveira, T.G.; Martinez-Martinez, P. Sphingolipids as prognostic biomarkers of neurodegeneration, neuroinflammation, and psychiatric diseases and their emerging role in lipidomic investigation methods. *Adv. Drug Deliv. Rev.* **2020**, *159*, 232–244. [CrossRef]
79. Podbielska, M.; Ariga, T.; Pokryszko-Dragan, A. Sphingolipid Players in Multiple Sclerosis: Their Influence on the Initiation and Course of the Disease. *Int. J. Mol. Sci.* **2022**, *23*, 5330. [CrossRef]
80. Obinata, H.; Hla, T. Sphingosine 1-phosphate and inflammation. *Int. Immunol.* **2019**, *31*, 617–625. [CrossRef]
81. Roy, R.; Alotaibi, A.A.; Freedman, M.S. Sphingosine 1-Phosphate Receptor Modulators for Multiple Sclerosis. *CNS Drugs* **2021**, *35*, 385–402. [CrossRef]
82. Jozefczuk, E.; Guzik, T.; Siedlinski, M. Significance of sphingosine-1-phosphate in cardiovascular physiology and pathology. *Pharmacol. Res.* **2020**, *156*, 104793. [CrossRef]
83. Parra, S.; Castro, A.; Masana, L. The pleiotropic role of HDL in autoimmune diseases. *Clin. Investig. Arterioscler.* **2015**, *27*, 97–106. [CrossRef]
84. Levkau, B. HDL-S1P: Cardiovascular functions, disease-associated alterations, and therapeutic applications. *Front. Pharmacol.* **2015**, *6*, 243. [CrossRef] [PubMed]
85. Kan, S.B.; Staun-Ram, E.; Golan, D.; Miller, A. HDL-cholesterol elevation associated with fingolimod and dimethyl fumarate therapies in multiple sclerosis. *Mult. Scler. J. Exp. Transl. Clin.* **2019**, *5*, 205521731988272. [CrossRef]
86. Jiménez-Jiménez, F.J.; Alonso-Navarro, H.; Salgado-Cámara, P.; García-Martín, E.; Agúndez, J.A.G. Oxidative Stress Markers in Multiple Sclerosis. *Int. J. Mol. Sci.* **2024**, *25*, 6289. [CrossRef] [PubMed]
87. Pegoretti, V.; Swanson, K.A.; Bethea, J.R.; Probert, L.; Eisel, U.L.M.; Fischer, R. Inflammation and Oxidative Stress in Multiple Sclerosis: Consequences for Therapy Development. *Oxidative Med. Cell. Longev.* **2020**, *2020*, 7191080. [CrossRef] [PubMed]
88. Van Horssen, J.; Schreibelt, G.; Drexhage, J.; Hazes, T.; Dijkstra, C.; van der Valk, P.; de Vries, H. Severe oxidative damage in multiple sclerosis lesions coincides with enhanced antioxidant enzyme expression. *Free Radic. Biol. Med.* **2008**, *45*, 1729–1737. [CrossRef] [PubMed]
89. Penkowa, M.; Espejo, C.; Ortega-Aznar, A.; Hidalgo, J.; Montalban, X.; Cáceres, E.M.M. Metallothionein expression in the central nervous system of multiple sclerosis patients. *Cell. Mol. Life Sci.* **2003**, *60*, 1258–1266. [CrossRef]
90. Essenburg, C.; Browne, R.W.; Ghazal, D.; Tamaño-Blanco, M.; Jakimovski, D.; Weinstock-Guttman, B.; Zivadinov, R.; Ramanathan, M. Antioxidant defense enzymes in multiple sclerosis: A 5-year follow-up study. *Eur. J. Neurol.* **2023**, *30*, 2338–2347. [CrossRef]
91. Bizoń, A.; Chojdak-Łukasiewicz, J.; Kołtuniuk, A.; Budrewicz, S.; Pokryszko-Dragan, A.; Piwowar, A. Evaluation of Selected Oxidant/Antioxidant Parameters in Patients with Relapsing-Remitting Multiple Sclerosis Undergoing Disease-Modifying Therapies. *Antioxidants* **2022**, *11*, 2416. [CrossRef]
92. Kirbas, A.; Kirbas, S.; Anlar, O.; Efe, H.; Yilmaz, A. Serum paraoxonase and arylesterase activity and oxidative status in patients with multiple sclerosis. *J. Clin. Neurosci.* **2013**, *20*, 1106–1109. [CrossRef]
93. Ferretti, G.; Bacchetti, T.; Principi, F.; Di Ludovico, F.; Viti, B.; Angeleri, V.A.; Danni, M.; Provinciali, L. Increased levels of lipid hydroperoxides in plasma of patients with multiple sclerosis: A relationship with paraoxonase activity. *Mult. Scler. J.* **2005**, *11*, 677–682. [CrossRef]
94. Jamroz-Wisniewska, A.; Beltowski, J.; Stelmasiak, Z.; Bartosik-Psujek, H. Paraoxonase 1 activity in different types of multiple sclerosis. *Mult. Scler. J.* **2009**, *15*, 399–402. [CrossRef] [PubMed]
95. Bacchetti, T.; Ferretti, G.; Carbone, F.; Ministrini, S.; Montecucco, F.; Jamialahmadi, T.; Sahebkar, A. Dysfunctional High-density Lipoprotein: The Role of Myeloperoxidase and Paraoxonase-1. *Curr. Med. Chem.* **2021**, *28*, 2842–2850. [CrossRef] [PubMed]
96. Mineo, C.; Yuhanna, I.S.; Quon, M.J.; Shaul, P.W. High Density Lipoprotein-induced Endothelial Nitric-oxide Synthase Activation Is Mediated by Akt and MAP Kinases. *J. Biol. Chem.* **2003**, *278*, 9142–9149. [CrossRef] [PubMed]

97. Yuhanna, I.S.; Zhu, Y.; Cox, B.E.; Hahner, L.D.; Osborne-Lawrence, S.; Lu, P.; Marcel, Y.L.; Anderson, R.G.; Mendelsohn, M.E.; Hobbs, H.H.; et al. High-density lipoprotein binding to scavenger receptor-BI activates endothelial nitric oxide synthase. *Nat. Med.* **2001**, *7*, 853–857. [CrossRef]
98. Nofer, J.-R.; van der Giet, M.; Tölle, M.; Wolinska, I.; Lipinski, K.v.W.; Baba, H.A.; Tietge, U.J.; Gödecke, A.; Ishii, I.; Kleuser, B.; et al. HDL induces NO-dependent vasorelaxation via the lysophospholipid receptor S1P3. *J. Clin. Investig.* **2004**, *113*, 569–581. [CrossRef]
99. Jorissen, W.; Wouters, E.; Bogie, J.F.; Vanmierlo, T.; Noben, J.-P.; Sviridov, D.; Hellings, N.; Somers, V.; Valcke, R.; Vanwijmeersch, B.; et al. Relapsing-remitting multiple sclerosis patients display an altered lipoprotein profile with dysfunctional HDL. *Sci. Rep.* **2017**, *7*, srep43410. [CrossRef]
100. Mehindate, K.; Sahlas, D.J.; Frankel, D.; Mawal, Y.; Liberman, A.; Corcos, J.; Dion, S.; Schipper, H.M. Proinflammatory cytokines promote glial heme oxygenase-1 expression and mitochondrial iron deposition: Implications for multiple sclerosis. *J. Neurochem.* **2001**, *77*, 1386–1395. [CrossRef]
101. Jhelum, P.; Zandee, S.; Ryan, F.; Zarruk, J.G.; Michalke, B.; Venkataramani, V.; Curran, L.; Klement, W.; Prat, A.; David, S. Ferroptosis induces detrimental effects in chronic EAE and its implications for progressive MS. *Acta Neuropathol. Commun.* **2023**, *11*, 1–22. [CrossRef]
102. Pennisi, G.; Cornelius, C.; Cavallaro, M.; Salinaro, A.T.; Cambria, M.; Pennisi, M.; Bella, R.; Milone, P.; Ventimiglia, B.; Migliore, M.; et al. Redox regulation of cellular stress response in multiple sclerosis. *Biochem. Pharmacol.* **2011**, *82*, 1490–1499. [CrossRef]
103. Stahnke, T.; Richter-Landsberg, C.; Stadelmann, C.; Netzler, A.; Brück, W. Differential upregulation of heme oxygenase-1 (HSP32) in glial cells after oxidative stress and in demyelinating disorders. *J. Mol. Neurosci.* **2007**, *32*, 25–37. [CrossRef]
104. Ferretti, G.; Bacchetti, T. Peroxidation of lipoproteins in multiple sclerosis. *J. Neurol. Sci.* **2011**, *311*, 92–97. [CrossRef] [PubMed]

antioxidants

Article

Oxidative Status and Lipid Metabolism Analytes in Dogs with Mast Cell Tumors: A Preliminary Study

Argyrios Ginoudis [1], Dimitra Pardali [1], Mathios E. Mylonakis [2], Androniki Tamvakis [3], Asta Tvarijonaviciute [4], Evgenia Lymperaki [5], Jose Joaquin Ceron [4] and Zoe Polizopoulou [1,*]

1 Diagnostic Laboratory, School of Veterinary Medicine, Faculty of Health Sciences, Aristotle University of Thessaloniki, 546 27 Thessaloniki, Greece; agkinou@vet.auth.gr (A.G.); dpardali@vet.auth.gr (D.P.)
2 Companion Animal Clinic, School of Veterinary Medicine, Faculty of Health Sciences, Aristotle University of Thessaloniki, 546 27 Thessaloniki, Greece; mmylonak@vet.auth.gr
3 Laboratory of Ecology and System Dynamics, Department of Marine Sciences, University of the Aegean, 811 00 Mytilene, Greece; atamvaki@mar.aegean.gr
4 Interdisciplinary Laboratory of Clinical Analysis, Interlab-UMU, Regional Campus of International Excellence Campus Mare Nostrum, University of Murcia, 30100 Murcia, Spain; asta@um.es (A.T.); jjceron@um.es (J.J.C.)
5 Department of Biomedical Sciences, International Hellenic University, 570 22 Sindos, Greece; evlimper@ihu.gr
* Correspondence: poliz@vet.auth.gr

Abstract: Mast cell tumors (MCTs) are common skin neoplasms in dogs. Prognostic indicators include histologic grade, clinical stage, high Ki-67 index, elevated argyrophilic nucleolus organizer regions (AgNOR) index, *c-kit* mutations, and recurrence after surgery. Blood serum redox status has been shown to correlate with prognostic factors in canine lymphoma and mammary tumors. This study aimed to assess the correlation between established prognostic factors and serum redox status and lipid metabolism analytes in dogs with MCTs. Dogs with cutaneous ($n = 33$) or subcutaneous ($n = 6$) MCTs, without comorbidities, were studied. Staging was evaluated based on cytology of regional lymph nodes and ultrasound-guided liver and spleen aspiration cytology. Histologic grading and immunohistochemical staining for Ki-67 and KIT patterns were performed on excised tumor specimens. Dogs were categorized by Patnaik grading (1–3), Kiupel grading (low/high), metastatic status, Ki-67 positive nuclei per cm^2 (>23 or ≤23), and KIT pattern (I, II–III). Paraoxonase-1, Butyrylcholinesterase, Cupric Reducing Antioxidant Capacity (CUPRAC), Diacron Reactive Oxygen Metabolites (d-ROMs), and oxy-adsorbent levels were measured before any therapeutic intervention. ANOVA and independent t-tests were used to detect differences in the mean values among groups. Paraoxonase-1 activity was significantly lower in Patnaik grade 3 ($p = 0.003$) and Kiupel high-grade ($p = 0.022$) MCTs. No significant differences were found in CUPRAC, d-ROMs, or oxy-adsorbent levels across different prognostic groups. This study found a significant correlation between histologic grading and Paraoxonase-1 activity, suggesting a potential role of Paraoxonase-1 as a prognostic biomarker in canine MCTs.

Keywords: canine; mast cell tumors; Paraoxonase-1 (PON-1); metabolomics; redox status; biomarkers

1. Introduction

Mast cell tumors (MCTs) are the most common malignant skin neoplasm in dogs with an incidence rate of 16–21% [1]. The biological behavior of canine MCTs varies considerably, ranging from benign tumors amenable to curative surgery, to extremely aggressive tumors, with a survival time of less than four months, regardless of the treatment approach [2]. Subcutaneous MCTs tend to have a more favorable prognosis compared to cutaneous MCTs in dogs [3,4].

Historically, the most important prognostic markers in dogs with MCT included histologic grading (based mostly on a 2-tier system) and the clinical stage of the neoplasm [2,5].

In addition to this, molecular markers, including c-kit expression pattern, *c-kit* mutations and proliferation indices such as the Ki-67 index, which correlates with the growth fraction of the tumor, and the argyrophilic nucleolus organizer regions (AgNORs) index, which correlates with the proliferation rate of the neoplastic cells, are of particular prognostic importance [6–11].

Redox status is defined as the dynamic balance between oxidants and antioxidants to maintain cell and tissue function [12]. Disruption of this balance triggers oxidative stress, which has been linked to the pathogenesis of many diseases such as cancer, cardiovascular disease, and diabetes mellitus in humans [13]. The total oxidative status of blood can be assessed by direct measurement of Reactive Oxygen Species (ROS), with methods assessing the oxidation of ROS-sensitive molecules [14–16] or by determining the concentration of molecules derived from oxidation of biomolecules, including proteins, lipids, and nucleic acids using various assays [17]. Oxidative stress can be estimated indirectly by measuring enzymes that induce the body's antioxidant response (Thioredoxin, Peroxiredoxins), high concentrations of which are indicative of oxidative stress [18]. Finally, oxidative stress is assessed by determining the concentration of antioxidants such as ascorbic acid, glutathione, paraoxonase 1 (PON-1) and vitamin E compounds (α-, γ-tocopherol) [19–21]. Determination of total antioxidants can be performed by estimating the oxidant reducing capacity contained in commercially available reagents [22].

PON-1 in particular is an important enzyme involved in lipid metabolism and has gained attention as biomarker of oxidative stress and disease. Primarily associated with high-density lipoproteins (HDL), PON-1 plays a key role in protecting lipids from oxidative damage by hydrolyzing lipid peroxides, thus maintaining the antioxidant capacity of HDL and preventing atherosclerosis [23,24]. Its activity is decreased in various pathological conditions, including cancer, where oxidative stress plays a pivotal role in disease progression [25]. Butyrylcholinesterase (BChE), although primarily recognized for its role in hydrolyzing choline-based esters, is increasingly implicated in lipid metabolism and inflammation. Elevated or reduced BChE levels have been associated with metabolic disorders, chronic inflammation, and cancer, making it a potential biomarker for disease states [26–28].

Several studies have reported on the measurement of blood redox status in human cancers. For instance, oxidative stress measured by 8-hydroxydeoxyguanosine (8-OHdG) has been linked to cancer risk, while elevated Malondialdehyde (MDA) and reduced vitamin E levels are associated with poor breast cancer prognosis [29,30]. Similarly, higher 8-OHdG concentrations have been linked to worse outcomes in ovarian carcinoma [31].

In canine medicine, blood redox status has been used to monitor treatment outcomes for leishmaniosis. A study showed significant increases in antioxidant markers [Cupric Reducing Antioxidant Capacity (CUPRAC), serum thiol, PON-1] after 30 and 180 days of treatment [32]. Redox status has also been evaluated in canine inflammatory bowel disease (IBD), where oxidative markers were higher and antioxidant markers lower in affected dogs, suggesting oxidative stress plays a role in IBD pathogenesis [33]. However, no correlation between these markers and treatment success was assessed.

In a study that assessed oxidative damage in dogs with multicentric lymphoma or with cutaneous MCT, serum levels of O^{2-}, and NO appeared reduced in diseased compared to clinically healthy dogs, with the antioxidant response showing no statistically significant difference [34]. In another study including dogs with MCT, the oxidative status of the diseased dogs was assessed by measuring d-ROMs, which were found to be increased compared to a healthy dog population, while antioxidant capacity (assessed by the BAP method) was found to be reduced in the diseased animals, providing a basis for further study [35]. In the above studies, the potential prognostic significance of oxidative stress was not addressed, particularly in relation to well-established prognostic markers such as the clinical stage and histologic grade of the disease.

The objectives of this study were to assess the blood redox status and lipid metabolism markers in dogs with MCTs and to investigate their possible correlation with the clinical stage, the histologic grade, and the immunohistochemical assessment of the disease.

2. Materials and Methods

2.1. Study Population

Adult dogs with confirmed cutaneous or subcutaneous MCTs based on cytologic examination were included in the study. The patients were required to have not undergone surgical or chemotherapy treatment for the MCTs prior to inclusion in the study, and to have no comorbidities that might affect the redox status of the dogs.

2.2 History, Physical Examination, and Clinical Staging

In all cases, a detailed history was obtained, followed by a physical examination with particular attention being paid to the presence of any cutaneous and subcutaneous masses, or any manifestations implying comorbidity. The anatomic location of the mass(es) was mapped and its size was measured with a thickness gauge. All masses and palpable lymph nodes were fine needle aspirated. Diagnostic imaging included abdominal ultrasound followed by fine needle aspiration of the liver and spleen according to the methodology for staging [36,37]. All aspirates were Giemsa-stained and examined for the presence of mast cells. Metastasis was diagnosed by the presence of atypical mast cells and/or clusters of normal-looking mast cells in the lymph nodes, the liver, and the spleen.

2.3. Clinicopathologic Testing

All the dogs included in the study underwent a complete blood count (CBC) (ADVIA 2120 Hematology System, Siemens Healthcare Diagnostics, Tarrytown, NY, USA) and serum biochemistry panel (Vitalab Flexor E Chemistry Analyzer, Vital Scientific N.V., Dieren, The Netherlands) to exclude any underlying conditions that could influence the biomarkers being studied. These tests ensured that no severe comorbidities were present, allowing for a more accurate assessment of the relationship between the biomarkers and mast cell tumors (MCTs) without interference from other health issues.

2.4. Histologic and Immunohistochemical Examination

After surgical excision of the primary neoplasms and/or any lymph nodes with cytologic evidence of metastasis, the excised tissues were sent for histologic examination in order to confirm the diagnosis, definitively characterize the MCT as cutaneous or subcutaneous, and grade the cutaneous MCTs based on the Patnaik and Kiupel classification systems (VET MED LABOR GMBH—Division of IDEXX Laboratories, Leipzig, Germany). All tumors were also stained in the same commercial laboratory with antibodies for the Ki-67 marker and the number of positive cells per 1 cm^2 grid-area with the highest proliferation activity were recorded. In addition, the KIT expression pattern was described as perimembranous (pattern I), stippled cytoplasmic (pattern II), or diffuse cytoplasmic (pattern III).

2.5. Measurement of Biochemical Analytes in the Blood Serum

Blood was collected from the jugular vein on the day of the surgical excision, before any handling or medication. Clot activator tubes were used, in which the whole blood was left to rest for 20 min and then centrifuged for 10 min in 3000 rpm. Serum aliquots were harvested and stored at −80 °C until further analysis. All analyses were conducted in a blinded manner concerning the prognostic factors of the mast cell tumors (MCTs) to eliminate any potential bias in the evaluation of the results.

The paraoxonase-1 (PON-1) activity assay was performed to assess the enzyme's hydrolytic activity using 4-nitrophenyl acetate as the substrate as previously described [19]. PON-1 catalyzes the hydrolysis of 4-nitrophenyl acetate into 4-nitrophenol, which is measured spectrophotometrically at 405 nm. The increase in absorbance corresponds to the formation of 4-nitrophenol, reflecting PON-1 activity. Enzyme activity is expressed in units per liter (IU/mL), where one unit represents the amount of enzyme that hydrolyzes 1 µmol of 4-nitrophenyl acetate per minute under the assay conditions. An automated clinical biochemistry analyzer (Olympus AU400, Chemistry Analyzer, Beckman Coulter, Brea, CA, USA) was used for measurement.

The activity of butyrylcholinesterase (BChE) was measured using butyrylthiocholine as the substrate. BChE catalyzes the hydrolysis of butyrylthiocholine into thiocholine, which reacts with 5,5′-dithiobis(2-nitrobenzoic acid) (DTNB) to produce a yellow-colored compound, 5-thio-2-nitrobenzoate. The rate of the reaction was monitored spectrophotometrically at 412 nm, with the increase in absorbance being proportional to BChE activity. Results are expressed in micromoles per milliliter per minute (μmol/mL·min), representing the amount of enzyme needed to hydrolyze 1 μmol of butyrylthiocholine per minute under the assay conditions. An automated clinical biochemistry analyzer (Olympus AU400, Chemistry Analyzer, Beckman Coulter, Brea, CA, USA) was used for measurement.

The d-ROMs test, a commercially available assay (Diacron International, Grosseto, Italy) was used to assess oxidative stress by measuring the concentration of reactive oxygen metabolites in the sample according to the previously validated procedure [38]. This test is based on the principle that hydroperoxides, which are generated during oxidative processes, react with a chromogenic substrate (N,N-diethyl-p-phenylenediamine) in the presence of iron ions, forming a colored radical cation. The intensity of the color, measured spectrophotometrically at 505 nm using the Free Carpe Diem analyzer (Diacron International, Grosseto, Italy), is directly proportional to the concentration of ROMs in the sample, reflecting the level of oxidative stress. Results are expressed in Carratelli units (CARR U), where 1 CARR U corresponds to 0.08 mg/dL of hydrogen peroxide.

The total antioxidant capacity was evaluated using both the OXY-adsorbent assay and the CUPRAC method.

The CUPRAC assay involves the reduction in cupric ions (Cu^{2+}) to cuprous ions (Cu^{+}) by antioxidants in the sample using a validated automated assay [39]. In the presence of neocuproine, the reduced Cu^{+} forms a colored complex, which is measured spectrophotometrically at 450 nm. The intensity of the color is directly proportional to the antioxidant capacity. The results are expressed in mmol/L, reflecting the concentration of antioxidants capable of reducing copper ions in the sample. An automated clinical biochemistry analyzer (Olympus AU400, Chemistry Analyzer, Beckman Coulter, Brea, CA, USA) was used for measurement.

The commercially available OXY-adsorbent assay (Diacron International, Grosseto, Italy) is a spectrophotometric method to measure antioxidant capacity in serum samples, previously used in canine samples [40]. This approach involves the oxidation of physiological antioxidants, such as uric acid, glutathione, thiol groups, vitamins, glutathione peroxidase, superoxide dismutase, and catalase, by a high concentration of hypochlorous acid (HClO) in the serum. Following a 10 min incubation period, any remaining HClO reacts with an alkyl-substituted aromatic amine (A-NH2) dissolved in a chromogenic mixture. The reaction oxidizes the amine, generating a colored product that is quantified spectrophotometrically. The intensity of the color measured with the Free Carpe Diem analyzer (Diacron International, Grosseto, Italy) is inversely related to the sample's antioxidant capacity and directly proportional to the amount of HClO in the sample. The results are expressed as micromoles of HClO consumed per milliliter of sample (μmol HClO/mL).

2.6. Statistical Analysis

The dogs were divided into groups based on the histologic location of the neoplasm (cutaneous or subcutaneous). Cutaneous neoplasms were divided into further groups based on the Kiupel (high- and low-grade) and Patnaik (grade 1, 2 or 3) histologic grading. The patients were also grouped based on immunohistochemical staining for Ki67 (>23 or $\leq$23 positive nuclei per cm^2 grid) and KIT pattern (I or II–III). ANOVA and independent t-test were used for detecting differences in mean values of the measured variables among different groups with significance level of a = 0.05. All analyses were performed using R Statistical Software (R Core Team 2021).

3. Results

3.1. Epidemiological Data

A total of 39 dogs with MCT were included in the study, including 24 female and 15 male dogs, with a median age of 9 years (range: 3–14 years). They comprised 15 mixed-breed and 24 purebred dogs, including Pitbulls (n = 7), Boxers (n = 4), Maltese (n = 3) and 1 each of the following breeds: Labrador Retriever, Epagneul Breton, Golden Retriever, French Bulldog, Schnauzer, Cane Corso, Dogo Argentino, Yorkshire Terrier, Shar Pei, and Caucasian Shepherd. These data are summarized in Table 1.

Table 1. Epidemiological data of the dogs with mast cell tumors included in the study.

Characteristic	Details
Total number of dogs	39
Gender	24 Female (61.5%) 15 Male (38.5%)
Age	Median: 9 years Range: 3–14 years
Breed Distribution	Mixed-breed: 15 dogs (38.5%) Purebred: 24 dogs (61.5%)
Purebred Breakdown	Pitbull: 7 dogs (17.9%) Boxer: 4 dogs (10.3%) Maltese: 3 dogs (7.7%) Other Breeds (1 dog each): Labrador Retriever, Epagneul Breton, Golden Retriever, French Bulldog, Schnauzer, Cane Corso, Dogo Argentino, Yorkshire Terrier, Shar Pei, Caucasian Shepherd (2.6% each)

3.2. Distribution of Mast Cell Tumors According to Histologic Location, Clinical Staging, Histologic Grading, and Immunohistochemistry

In this study, a total of 33 mast cell tumors (MCTs) were classified according to the Kiupel system, with 25 classified as low-grade and 8 as high-grade. Based on the Patnaik classification, 1 MCT was categorized as grade 1, 25 as grade 2, and 7 as grade 3. Tumor histology also showed that 33 were cutaneous, while 6 were subcutaneous. Regarding metastasis status, 24 MCTs were non-metastatic, while 15 showed evidence of metastasis. Ki67 proliferation index revealed that 12 tumors had more than 23 positive nuclei per 1 cm^2 grid, and 27 had 23 or fewer. KIT immunohistochemistry showed that 23 tumors exhibited pattern I, 14 pattern II, and 2 pattern III. These findings are summarized in Table 2.

Table 2. Distribution of mast cell tumors (MCTs) by classification, location, metastatic status, Ki67 proliferation index, and KIT staining patterns.

Parameter	Number of Cases	Percentage (%) *
Kiupel Classification		
- Low-grade	25	64.1
- High-grade	8	20.5
- Subcutaneous tumors (grading not applicable)	6	15.4
Patnaik Classification		
- Grade 1	1	2.6
- Grade 2	25	64.1
- Grade 3	7	17.9
- Subcutaneous tumors (grading not applicable)	6	15.4
Tumor histologic location		
- Cutaneous	33	84.6
- Subcutaneous	6	15.4

Table 2. *Cont.*

Parameter	Number of Cases	Percentage (%) *
Metastatic status		
– Non-metastatic	24	61.5
– Metastatic	15	38.5
Ki67 Positive Nuclei per 1 cm^2 Grid		
– >23	12	30.8
– ≤23	27	69.2
KIT pattern		
– Pattern I	23	59.0
– Pattern II	14	35.9
– Pattern III	2	5.1

* Percentages are based on the total number of dogs (*n* = 39). Kiupel and Patnaik classifications are applied to 33 cutaneous tumors.

3.3. Comparison of the Biochemical Analytes Based on Kiupel Histologic Grading System

The mean (±SD) values of the measured analytes in dogs with low- and high-grade MCTs, according to the Kiupel classification, are presented in Table 3. The mean values of PON-1 were significantly higher in the low-grade neoplasms (Figure 1). No significant differences were found for the other redox analytes.

Table 3. Mean (±SD) values of biochemical analytes in 33 dogs with cutaneous mast cell tumors (MCTs) graded by the 2-tier Kiupel histologic system.

Kiupel Grade	PON-1 (IU/mL)	BCHE (μmol/mL·min)	CUPRAC (mmol/L)	d-ROMs (CARR U)	OXY-Adsorbent (μmol HClO/mL)
Low-grade (*n* = 25)	2.91 ± 0.62	4.83 ± 1.60	0.30 ± 0.05	93.96 ± 19.88	291.98 ± 48.80
High-grade (*n* = 8)	2.16 ± 0.72	4.36 ± 1.67	0.27 ± 0.04	91.38 ± 19.02	252.71 ± 50.22
p-value	0.022	0.502	0.066	0.746	0.077

Abbreviations of Table 3: PON-1: Paraoxonase-1, BCHE: Butyrylcholinesterase, CUPRAC: Cupric Reducing Antioxidant Capacity, d-ROMs: Diacron Reactive Oxygen Metabolites, OXY-Adsorbent: Diacron Oxygen Adsorbing Substances Assay.

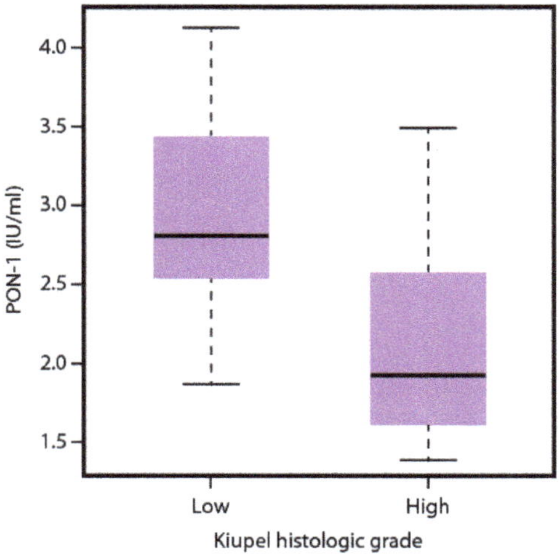

Figure 1. Boxplot illustrating Paraoxonase-1 (PON-1) activity in dogs with cutaneous (*n* = 33) mast cell tumors (MCTs) categorized by Kiupel histologic grading. A total of 25 dogs had low-grade MCTs, and 8 had high-grade MCTs. The mean PON-1 activity was significantly lower in high-grade MCTs compared to low-grade MCTs (*p* = 0.022).

3.4. Comparison of the Biochemical Analytes Based on Patnaik Histologic Grading System

The mean (±SD) values of the biochemical analytes in dogs with grades 1, 2, and 3 MCTs, according to Patnaik's classification, are presented in Table 4. The mean values of PON-1 differed significantly among grades, with lower values measured in dogs belonging to grade 3 (Figure 2). No significant differences were found for the other analytes.

Table 4. Mean (±SD) values of biochemical analytes in 33 dogs with cutaneous mast cell tumors (MCTs) graded by the 3-tier Patnaik histologic system.

Patnaik Grade	PON-1 (IU/mL)	BCHE (μmol/mL·min)	CUPRAC (mmol/L)	d-ROMs (CARR U)	OXY-Adsorbent (μmol HClO/mL)
Grade 1 (n = 1)	2.88 ± na	5.60 ± na	0.26 ± na	73.00 ± na	226.50 ± na
Grade 2 (n = 25)	2.94 ± 0.63	4.88 ± 1.65	0.30 ± 0.05	93.64 ± 20.30	291.42 ± 49.66
Grade 3 (n = 7)	1.96 ± 0.50	4.00 ± 1.42	0.27 ± 0.05	95.14 ± 17.01	258.46 ± 51.32
p-value	0.003	0.387	0.172	0.574	0.177

Abbreviations of Table 4: PON-1: Paraoxonase-1, BCHE: Butyrylcholinesterase, CUPRAC: Cupric Reducing Antioxidant Capacity, d-ROMs: Diacron Reactive Oxygen Metabolites, OXY-Adsorbent: Diacron Oxygen Adsorbing Substances Assay, na: Not Applicable.

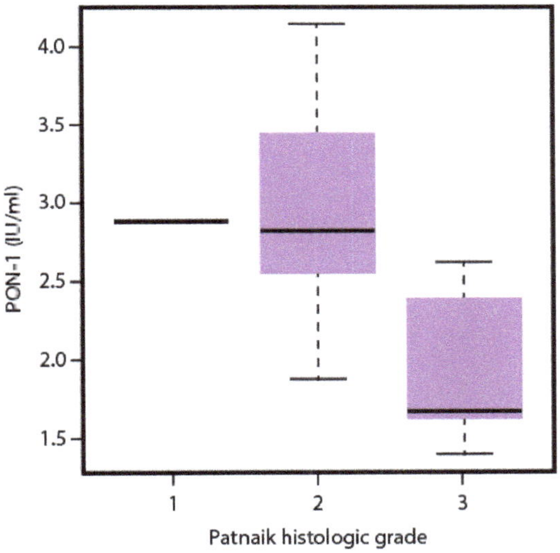

Figure 2. Boxplot illustrating Paraoxonase-1 (PON-1) activity in dogs with cutaneous (n = 33) mast cell tumors (MCTs) categorized by Patnaik histologic grading. In total, 1 dog had a grade 1 MCT, 25 had grade 2 MCTs, and 7 had grade 3 MCTs. The mean PON-1 activity was significantly lower in grade 3 MCTs (p = 0.003).

3.5. Comparison of the Biochemical Analytes Based on the Histologic Location of MCTs

The mean (±SD) values of the biochemical analytes in dogs with cutaneous (n = 33) and subcutaneous (n = 6) MCTs are presented in Table 5. Redox analytes did not differ between the two groups.

Table 5. Mean (±SD) values of biochemical analytes in dogs with cutaneous or subcutaneous mast cell tumors.

Histologic Location	PON-1 (IU/mL)	BCHE (μmol/mL·min)	CUPRAC (mmol/L)	d-ROMs (CARR U)	OXY-Adsorbent (μmol HClO/mL)
Cutaneous (*n* = 33)	2.73 ± 0.71	4.72 ± 1.60	0.30 ± 0.05	93.33 ± 19.41	282.46 ± 51.28
Subcutaneous (*n* = 6)	2.18 ± 0.57	3.60 ± 1.19	0.28 ± 0.07	96.17 ± 18.02	266.75 ± 35.23
p-value	0.070	0.079	0.668	0.736	0.377

Abbreviations of Table 5: PON-1: Paraoxonase-1, BCHE: Butyrylcholinesterase, CUPRAC: Cupric Reducing Antioxidant Capacity, d-ROMs: Diacron Reactive Oxygen Metabolites, OXY-Adsorbent: Diacron Oxygen Adsorbing Substances Assay.

3.6. Comparison of the Biochemical Analytes According to MCTs, Metastatic Status

The mean (±SD) values of the measured analytes with regard to the metastatic status of the tumors are included in Table 6. No significant differences were found in the redox status between dogs with metastatic and with no metastatic MCTs.

Table 6. Mean (±SD) values of biochemical analytes in dogs with metastatic and not metastatic cutaneous/subcutaneous mast cell tumors.

Metastatic Status	PON-1 (IU/mL)	BCHE (μmol/mL·min)	CUPRAC (mmol/L)	d-ROMs (CARR U)	OXY-Adsorbent (μmol HClO/mL)
Metastatic (*n* = 15)	2.74 ± 0.61	4.73 ± 1.35	0.29 ± 0.05	92.25 ± 21.06	284.06 ± 47.04
Non-metastatic (*n* = 24)	2.49 ± 0.85	4.24 ± 1.92	0.29 ± 0.06	96.20 ± 15.55	273.61 ± 53.26
p-value	0.318	0.393	0.887	0.506	0.538

Abbreviations of Table 6: PON-1: Paraoxonase-1, BCHE: Butyrylcholinesterase, CUPRAC: Cupric Reducing Antioxidant Capacity, d-ROMs: Diacron Reactive Oxygen Metabolites, OXY-Adsorbent: Diacron Oxygen Adsorbing Substances Assay.

3.7. Comparison of the Biochemical Analytes in MCTs Evaluated with the Ki67 Proliferation Index

Table 7 presents the mean values of the biochemical analytes in dogs with MCTs evaluated by the Ki67 proliferation index. No significant differences were found between dogs with normal and increased Ki67 labeled cells.

Table 7. Mean (±SD) values of biochemical analytes in dogs with cutaneous/subcutaneous mast cell tumors (MCTs) evaluated by the Ki67 index.

No of Ki67 Positive Nuclei per cm^2	PON-1 (IU/mL)	BCHE (μmol/mL·min)	CUPRAC (mmol/L)	d-ROMs (CARR U)	OXY-Adsorbent (μmol HClO/mL)
>23 (*n* = 12)	2.59 ± 0.70	4.28 ± 1.08	0.30 ± 0.06	89.41 ± 10.49	292.81 ± 48.01
<=23 (*n* = 27)	2.39 ± 0.77	4.18 ± 1.67	0.27 ± 0.04	90.54 ± 19.71	264.52 ± 50.61
p-value	0.464	0.856	0.887	0.854	0.133

Abbreviations of Table 7: PON-1: Paraoxonase-1, BCHE: Butyrylcholinesterase, CUPRAC: Cupric Reducing Antioxidant Capacity, d-ROMs: Diacron Reactive Oxygen Metabolites, OXY-Adsorbent: Diacron Oxygen Adsorbing Substances Assay.

3.8. Comparison of the Biochemical Analytes in Dogs with Different KIT Expression Patterns

The mean values of the biochemical analytes in MCTs with pattern I vs. patterns II–III are presented in Table 8. No significant differences were found based on the KIT expression pattern.

Table 8. Mean (±SD) values of biochemical analytes in dogs with cutaneous/subcutaneous mast cell tumors (MCTs) evaluated by the KIT expression patterns.

KIT Pattern	PON-1 (IU/mL)	BCHE (μmol/mL·min)	CUPRAC (mmol/L)	d-ROMs (CARR U)	OXY-Adsorbent (μmol HClO/mL)
I (n = 23)	2.69 ± 0.82	4.14 ± 1.36	0.30 ± 0.07	88.7 ± 10.29	300.81 ± 50.37
II–III (n = 16)	2.41 ± 0.67	4.29 ± 1.37	0.28 ± 0.05	90.5 ± 16.95	270.43 ± 48.41
p-value	0.364	0.780	0.364	0.721	0.133

Abbreviations of Table 8: PON-1: Paraoxonase-1, BCHE: Butyrylcholinesterase, CUPRAC: Cupric Reducing Antioxidant Capacity, d-ROMs: Diacron Reactive Oxygen Metabolites, OXY-Adsorbent: Diacron Oxygen Adsorbing Substances Assay.

4. Discussion

This study aimed to investigate analytes related to oxidative status and lipid metabolism in dogs with MCTs and explore their association with well-established prognostic factors of MCTs. Of the assessed panel of markers, only PON-1 activity showed a significant association with MCTs grading, being significantly reduced in dogs with high-grade MCTs.

The finding of decreased PON-1 activity in dogs with high-grade MCTs, according to both the Kiupel and Patnaik grading systems, highlights the potential role of oxidative stress in tumor progression, as well as the potential prognostic role of PON-1 levels in canine MCTs. Importantly, if validated, PON-1 could serve as a clinically relevant biomarker that can be measured in blood prior to surgery, aiding in preoperative risk stratification and treatment planning. PON-1 is an enzyme with known antioxidant properties, and its reduced activity suggests increased oxidative stress in dogs with more aggressive tumors. This result is consistent with findings from other studies, which show that oxidative stress is closely linked to tumor progression, DNA damage, and inflammation [41,42]. Multiple studies have demonstrated that oxidative stress correlates with more aggressive tumor behavior and poorer prognostic outcomes. In canine mammary carcinoma, dogs with tumors exhibited higher oxidative stress levels compared to healthy dogs, with significant reductions observed following surgical treatment [43,44]. Similarly, in cases of multicentric lymphoma, oxidative damage was elevated both before and after chemotherapy, particularly in advanced stages, with increased antioxidant capacity observed in dogs that responded well to treatment [45]. Another study highlighted an imbalance in oxidative and antioxidant markers in dogs with lymphoma, which normalized following clinical remission [46]. Overall, these findings emphasize the role of oxidative stress as a key factor in cancer prognosis.

The medical literature provides extensive evidence on the measurement of blood redox status in various human cancers. Oxidative stress, as measured by 8-hydroxydeoxyguanosine (8-OHdG), has been linked to the development of cancer, while elevated Malondialdehyde (MDA) and reduced vitamin E levels correlate with unfavorable breast cancer outcomes [29,30]. In women with ovarian carcinoma, elevated 8-OHdG concentrations are also associated with a poor prognosis [31]. Additionally, a study on 53 colorectal cancer patients, using d-ROMs to assess oxidative status, identified oxidative stress as a potential independent prognostic marker [47]. This evidence supports the idea that oxidative stress plays a critical role not only in cancer development but also in determining disease outcome.

Interestingly, no association was found between PON-1 concentration and MCT metastasis and IHC markers, despite the fact that they are associated with more advanced grading status. This may underline the fact that the best proxy of MCT behavior is the histologic grade rather than the remainder variables assessed in this study. The lack of correlation between PON-1 and metastasis or IHC markers suggests that oxidative stress as measured by PON-1 may be influenced by tumor biology in a manner independent of these commonly assessed factors. Furthermore, it highlights the complexity of MCT pathophysiology, where not all prognostic indicators may converge on the same mechanistic pathways.

Notably, there was also no association found between the other oxidative and lipid metabolism analytes evaluated in this study (BChE, d-ROMs, CUPRAC, oxy-adsorbent capacity) and tumor grading, metastasis, Ki67 index, and KIT pattern, likely indicating that they are of limited clinical importance as redox status indicators compared to PON-1 in dogs with MCTs. However, the limited sample size may have influenced these results. For instance, the CUPRAC and oxy-adsorbent assays demonstrated variation across histologic grades, but the observed differences did not reach statistical significance ($p = 0.066$ and $p = 0.077$, respectively). This discrepancy may also reflect the inherent differences in the nature of the markers. PON-1 is a relatively stable biomarker, offering insight into cumulative oxidative stress over time, while the other assays provide more transient, momentary snapshots of the oxidative and antioxidant status. Total antioxidant levels can change rapidly with dietary intake or acute stressors, whereas PON-1 activity may reflect a cumulative effect of oxidative stress over time [48]. Moreover, in conditions such as nephropathy and Crohn's disease, PON-1's levels have been shown to correlate with the severity of oxidative stress and inflammation, further supporting its role as a long-term biomarker [49,50]. This distinction may explain the stronger association of PON-1 with tumor grading and highlights its potential as a more robust and clinically relevant marker.

Previous reports have suggested that subcutaneous MCTs are generally less aggressive than their cutaneous counterparts [51]. However, the oxidative analytes assessed in this study did not reflect this biological difference, possibly due to the relatively small sample size of subcutaneous tumors.

Several limitations of this study should be acknowledged. First, the relatively small sample size, particularly in certain subgroups, such as subcutaneous MCTs and high-grade tumors, may have limited our ability to detect significant associations across all redox analytes. Larger studies would be required to confirm the findings and to explore the relationship between oxidative status and MCT progression more comprehensively, as well as examine the correlation of oxidative analytes with prognostic factors in subcutaneous MCTs [3,4] and metastatic lymph node grade [52]. Additionally, only a limited range of oxidative markers were assessed in this study. While PON-1 was significantly correlated with tumor grading, other oxidative stress markers such as d-ROMs did not show similar trends, suggesting the need for a broader evaluation of oxidative stress pathways and measurement of more stable analytes. Finally, this preliminary study did not take into account the time to relapse and median survival time of the affected animals. This would be crucial in the attempt to validate PON-1 activity as an independent prognostic factor in canine MCTs. Future studies are ongoing and will account for these variables and employ larger samples to better understand the role of oxidative stress in canine MCTs.

5. Conclusions

The results of this study suggest that while PON-1 may be an important marker of oxidative stress in high-grade MCTs, other oxidative and lipid metabolism analytes do not appear to be of clinical importance in tumor progression or prognosis. This highlights the need for a more targeted investigation of specific oxidative pathways that may contribute to tumor behavior in dogs with MCTs. Our findings suggest the potential role of PON-1 as a prognostic biomarker in canine MCTs, since it correlates significantly with histologic grading, the most important established prognostic factor. However, its utility as a prognostic tool requires further validation in larger-scale studies. Future research should address current limitations by including larger populations and longitudinal designs that assess time to relapse and survival time. Expanding the scope of investigation to explore additional oxidative stress markers and their interactions with tumor biology could also uncover novel insights into MCT progression. Further studies with a larger population that will include time to relapse and survival time are ongoing.

Author Contributions: Conceptualization, A.G. and Z.P.; methodology, A.G. and Z.P.; validation, A.G., A.T. (Asta Tvarijonaviciute), J.J.C. and Z.P.; formal analysis, A.T. (Androniki Tamvakis); investigation, A.G. and Z.P.; resources, A.G., M.E.M., D.P., E.L. and Z.P.; writing—original draft preparation, A.G and Z.P.; writing—review and editing, A.G., M.E.M., D.P., E.L., J.J.C. and Z.P.; visualization,

A.G. and Z.P.; supervision, Z.P.; project administration, Z.P. All authors have read and agreed to the published version of the manuscript.

Funding: This research received no external funding.

Institutional Review Board Statement: The study was conducted in accordance with the Declaration of Helsinki, and approved by the Ethics Committee of the Department of Veterinary Medicine, Aristotle University of Thessaloniki (protocol code 30583 and date of approval 8 December 2023).

Informed Consent Statement: Informed consent was obtained from all owners of animals involved in the study.

Data Availability Statement: The data presented in this study are available on request from the corresponding author due to ethical restrictions.

Conflicts of Interest: The authors declare no conflicts of interest.

References

1. Bostock, D.E. Neoplasms of the Skin and Subcutaneous Tissues in Dogs and Cats. *Br. Vet. J.* **1986**, *142*, 1–19. [CrossRef] [PubMed]
2. Kiupel, M.; Webster, J.D.; Bailey, K.L.; Best, S.; DeLay, J.; Detrisac, C.J.; Fitzgerald, S.D.; Gamble, D.; Ginn, P.E.; Goldschmidt, M.H.; et al. Proposal of a 2-tier histologic grading system for canine cutaneous mast cell tumors to more accurately predict biological behavior. *Vet. Pathol.* **2011**, *48*, 147–155. [CrossRef] [PubMed]
3. Thompson, J.J.; Pearl, D.L.; Yager, J.A.; Best, S.J.; Coomber, B.L.; Foster, R.A. Canine subcutaneous mast cell tumor: Characterization and prognostic indices. *Vet. Pathol.* **2011**, *48*, 156–168. [CrossRef] [PubMed]
4. Thompson, J.J.; Yager, J.A.; Best, S.J.; Pearl, D.L.; Coomber, B.L.; Torres, R.N.; Kiupel, M.; Foster, R.A. Canine subcutaneous mast cell tumors: Cellular proliferation and KIT expression as prognostic indices. *Vet. Pathol.* **2011**, *48*, 169–181. [CrossRef]
5. Romansik, E.M.; Reilly, C.M.; Kass, P.H.; Moore, P.F.; London, C.A. Mitotic index is predictive for survival for canine cutaneous mast cell tumors. *Vet. Pathol.* **2007**, *44*, 335–341. [CrossRef]
6. Kiupel, M.; Webster, J.D.; Kaneene, J.B.; Miller, R.; Yuzbasiyan-Gurkan, V. The use of KIT and tryptase expression patterns as prognostic tools for canine cutaneous mast cell tumors. *Vet. Pathol.* **2004**, *41*, 371–377. [CrossRef]
7. Scase, T.J.; Edwards, D.; Miller, J.; Henley, W.; Smith, K.; Blunden, A.; Murphy, S. Canine mast cell tumors: Correlation of apoptosis and proliferation markers with prognosis. *J. Vet. Intern. Med.* **2006**, *20*, 151–158. [CrossRef]
8. Ozaki, K.; Yamagami, T.; Nomura, K.; Narama, I. Prognostic Significance of Surgical Margin, Ki-67 and Cyclin D1 Protein Expression in Grade II Canine Cutaneous Mast Cell Tumor. *J. Vet. Med. Sci.* **2007**, *69*, 1117–1121. [CrossRef]
9. Webster, J.D.; Yuzbasiyan-Gurkan, V.; Miller, R.A.; Kaneene, J.B.; Kiupel, M. Cellular proliferation in canine cutaneous mast cell tumors: Associations with c-KIT and its role in prognostication. *Vet. Pathol.* **2007**, *44*, 298–308. [CrossRef]
10. Thamm, D.H.; Vail, D.M. Mast cell tumours. In *Small Animal Clinical Oncology*, 4th ed.; Withrow, S.J., Vail, D.M., Eds.; Saunders-Elsevier: St. Louis, MO, USA, 2007; pp. 402–424.
11. Horta, R.S.; LaValle, G.E.; Monteiro, L.N.; Souza, M.C.C.; Cassali, G.D.; Araújo, R.B. Assessment of Canine Mast Cell Tumor Mortality Risk Based on Clinical, Histologic, Immunohistochemical, and Molecular Features. *Vet. Pathol.* **2018**, *55*, 212–223. [CrossRef]
12. Sies, H.; Berndt, C.; Jones, D.P. Oxidative Stress. *Annu. Rev. Biochem.* **2017**, *86*, 715–748. [CrossRef]
13. Harwell, B. Biochemistry of oxidative stress. *Biochem. Soc. Trans.* **2007**, *35*, 1147–1150. [CrossRef]
14. Kilk, K.; Meitern, R.; Härmson, O.; Soomets, U.; Hõrak, P. Assessment of oxidative stress in serum by d-ROMs test. *Free Radic. Res.* **2014**, *48*, 883–889. [CrossRef]
15. Tsamesidis, I.; Egwu, C.O.; Samara, D.; Vogiatzi, D.; Lettas, A.; Lymperaki, E. Effects of Greek Honey and Propolis on Oxidative Stress and Biochemical Analytes in Regular Blood Donors. *J. Xenobiot.* **2022**, *12*, 13–20. [CrossRef]
16. Takaki, J. Associations of Job Stress Indicators with Oxidative Biomarkers in Japanese Men and Women. *Int. J. Environ. Res. Public Health* **2013**, *10*, 6662–6671. [CrossRef] [PubMed]
17. Katerji, M.; Filippova, M.; Duerksen-Hughes, P. Approaches and Methods to Measure Oxidative Stress in Clinical Samples: Research Applications in the Cancer Field. *Oxid. Med. Cell Longev.* **2019**, *2019*, 1279250. [CrossRef]
18. Oberacker, T.; Kraft, L.; Schanz, M.; Latus, J.; Schricker, S. The Importance of Thioredoxin-1 in Health and Disease. *Antioxidants* **2023**, *12*, 1078. [CrossRef]
19. Ceron, J.J.; Tecles, F.; Tvarijonaviciute, A. Serum paraoxonase 1 (PON1) measurement: An update. *BMC Vet. Res.* **2014**, *10*, 74. [CrossRef]
20. Nuhu, F.; Gordon, A.; Sturmey, R.; Seymour, A.-M.; Bhandari, S. Measurement of Glutathione as a Tool for Oxidative Stress Studies by High Performance Liquid Chromatography. *Molecules* **2020**, *25*, 4196. [CrossRef] [PubMed]
21. Ford, E.S.; Schleicher, R.L.; Mokdad, A.H.; Ajani, U.A.; Liu, S. Distribution of serum concentrations of alpha-tocopherol and gamma-tocopherol in the US population. *Am. J. Clin. Nutr.* **2006**, *84*, 375–383. [CrossRef] [PubMed]
22. Munteanu, I.G.; Apetrei, C. Analytical Methods Used in Determining Antioxidant Activity: A Review. *Int. J. Mol. Sci.* **2021**, *22*, 3380. [CrossRef] [PubMed]
23. Durrington, P.N.; Bashir, B.; Soran, H. Paraoxonase 1 and atherosclerosis. *Front. Cardiovasc. Med.* **2023**, *10*, 1065967. [CrossRef] [PubMed]
24. Soran, H.; Schofield, J.D.; Durrington, P.N. Antioxidant properties of HDL. *Front. Pharmacol.* **2015**, *6*, 222. [CrossRef] [PubMed]

25. Medina-Díaz, I.M.; Ponce-Ruíz, N.; Rojas-García, A.E.; Zambrano-Zargoza, J.F.; Bernal-Hernández, Y.Y.; González-Arias, C.A.; Barrón-Vivanco, B.S.; Herrera-Moreno, J.F. The Relationship between Cancer and Paraoxonase 1. *Antioxidants* **2022**, *11*, 697. [CrossRef]
26. Gensthaler, L.; Jomrich, G.; Brugger, J.; Kollmann, D.; Paireder, M.; Bologheanu, M.; Horn, A.; Riegler, F.M.; Asari, R.; Schoppmann, S.F. Preoperative BChE serves as a prognostic marker in patients with resectable AEG after neoadjuvant chemotherapy. *Langenbecks Arch. Surg.* **2023**, *408*, 227. [CrossRef]
27. Lampón, N.; Hermida-Cadahia, E.F.; Riveiro, A.; Tutor, J.C. Association between butyrylcholinesterase activity and low-grade systemic inflammation. *Ann. Hepatol.* **2012**, *11*, 356–363. [CrossRef]
28. Liu, J.; Tian, T.; Liu, X.; Cui, Z. BCHE as a Prognostic Biomarker in Endometrial Cancer and Its Correlation with Immunity. *J. Immunol. Res.* **2022**, *2022*, 6051092. [CrossRef] [PubMed]
29. Loft, S.; Olsen, A.; Møller, P.; Poulsen, H.E.; Tjønneland, A. Association between 8-oxo-7,8-dihydro-2′-deoxyguanosine excretion and risk of postmenopausal breast cancer: Nested case-control study. *Cancer Epidemiol. Biomark. Prev.* **2013**, *22*, 1289–1296. [CrossRef]
30. Saintot, M.; Mathieu-Daude, H.; Astre, C.; Grenier, J.; Simony-Lafontaine, J.; Gerber, M. Oxidant-antioxidant status in relation to survival among breast cancer patients. *Int. J. Cancer* **2002**, *97*, 574–579. [CrossRef]
31. Pylväs, M.; Puistola, U.; Laatio, L.; Kauppila, S.; Karihtala, P. Elevated serum 8-OHdG is associated with poor prognosis in epithelial ovarian cancer. *Anticancer Res.* **2011**, *31*, 1411–1415.
32. Rubio, C.P.; Martinez-Subiela, S.; Tvarijonaviciute, A.; Hernández-Ruiz, J.; Pardo-Marin, L.; Segarra, S.; Ceron, J.J. Changes in serum biomarkers of oxidative stress after treatment for canine leishmaniosis in sick dogs. *Comp. Immunol. Microbiol. Infect. Dis.* **2016**, *49*, 51–57. [CrossRef] [PubMed]
33. Rubio, C.P.; Martínez-Subiela, S.; Hernández-Ruiz, J.; Tvarijonaviciute, A.; Cerón, J.J.; Allenspach, K. Serum biomarkers of oxidative stress in dogs with idiopathic inflammatory bowel disease. *Vet. J.* **2017**, *221*, 56–61. [CrossRef]
34. Cucchi, A.; Ramoni, R.; Basini, G.; Bussolati, S.; Quintavalla, F. Oxidant–Antioxidant Status in Canine Multicentric Lymphoma and Primary Cutaneous Mastocytoma. *Processes* **2020**, *8*, 802. [CrossRef]
35. Finotello, R.; Pasquini, A.; Meucci, V.; Lippi, I.; Rota, A.; Guidi, G.; Marchetti, V. Redox status evaluation in dogs affected by mast cell tumour. *Vet. Comp. Oncol.* **2014**, *12*, 120–129. [CrossRef] [PubMed]
36. Book, A.P.; Fidel, J.; Wills, T.; Bryan, J.; Sellon, R.; Mattoon, J. Correlation of ultrasound findings, liver and spleen cytology, and prognosis in the clinical staging of high metastatic risk canine mast cell tumors. *Vet. Radiol. Ultrasound* **2011**, *52*, 548–554. [CrossRef] [PubMed]
37. Warland, J.; Amores-Fuster, I.; Newbury, W.; Brearley, M.; Dobson, J.M. The utility of staging in canine mast cell tumours. *Vet. Comp. Oncol.* **2012**, *12*, 287–298. [CrossRef]
38. Pasquini, A.; Luchetti, E.; Marchetti, V.; Cardini, G.; Iorio, E.L. Analytical performances of d-ROMs test and BAP test in canine plasma. Definition of the normal range in healthy Labrador dogs. *Vet. Res. Commun.* **2008**, *32*, 137–143. [CrossRef]
39. Rubio, C.P.; Tvarijonaviciute, A.; Martinez-Subiela, S.; Hernández-Ruiz, J.; Cerón, J.J. Validation of an automated assay for the measurement of cupric reducing antioxidant capacity in serum of dogs. *BMC Vet. Res.* **2016**, *12*, 137. [CrossRef]
40. Candellone, A.; Girolami, F.; Badino, P.; Jarriyawattanachaikul, W.; Odore, R. Changes in the Oxidative Stress Status of Dogs Affected by Acute Enteropathies. *Vet. Sci.* **2022**, *9*, 276. [CrossRef]
41. Nemec Svete, A.; Verk, B.; Čebulj-Kadunc, N.; Salobir, J.; Rezar, V.; Domanjko Petrič, A. Inflammation and its association with oxidative stress in dogs with heart failure. *BMC Vet. Res.* **2021**, *17*, 176. [CrossRef]
42. Poetsch, A.R. The genomics of oxidative DNA damage, repair, and resulting mutagenesis. *Comput. Struct. Biotechnol. J.* **2020**, *18*, 207–219. [CrossRef] [PubMed]
43. Machado, V.S.; Crivellenti, L.Z.; Bottari, N.B.; Tonin, A.A.; Pelinson, L.P.; Borin-Crivellenti, S.; Santana, A.E.; Torbitz, V.D.; Moresco, R.N.; Duarte, T.; et al. Oxidative stress and inflammatory response biomarkers in dogs with mammary carcinoma. *Pathol. Res. Pract.* **2015**, *211*, 677–681. [CrossRef] [PubMed]
44. Russo, C.; Simonelli, S.M.; Luz, M.B.; Carrera, A.C.; Moreno, I.F.; Bracarense, A.P.F.R.L. Oxidative stress in female dogs with mammary neoplasms. *Pesq. Vet. Bras.* **2021**, *41*, e06742. [CrossRef]
45. Bottari, N.B.; Munhoz, T.D.; Torbitz, V.D.; Tonin, A.A.; Anai, L.A.; Semolin, L.M.; Jark, P.C.; Bollick, Y.S.; Moresco, R.N.; França, R.T.; et al. Oxidative stress in dogs with multicentric lymphoma: Effect of chemotherapy on oxidative and antioxidant biomarkers. *Redox Rep.* **2015**, *20*, 267–274. [CrossRef] [PubMed]
46. Winter, J.L.; Barber, L.G.; Freeman, L.; Griessmayr, P.C.; Milbury, P.E.; Blumberg, J.B. Antioxidant status and biomarkers of oxidative stress in dogs with lymphoma. *J. Vet. Intern. Med.* **2009**, *23*, 311–316. [CrossRef]
47. Sugimoto, K.; Sakamoto, K.; Kawai, M.; Kawano, S.; Munakata, S.; Ishiyama, S.; Takahashi, M.; Kojima, Y.; Tomiki, Y. Serum oxidative stress is an independent prognostic marker in colorectal cancer. *Transl. Cancer Res.* **2019**, *8*, 1699–1708. [CrossRef]
48. Roxo, D.F.; Arcaro, C.A.; Gutierres, V.O.; Costa, M.C.; Oliveira, J.O.; Lima, T.F.O.; Assis, R.P.; Brunetti, I.L.; Baviera, A.M. Curcumin combined with metformin decreases glycemia and dyslipidemia, and increases paraoxonase activity in diabetic rats. *Diabetol. Metab. Syndr.* **2019**, *11*, 33. [CrossRef]
49. Szczeklik, K.; Mach, T.; Cibor, D.; Owczarek, D.; Sapa, J.; Papież, M.; Pytko-Polończyk, J.; Krzyściak, W. Correlation of Paraoxonase-1 with the Severity of Crohn's Disease. *Molecules* **2018**, *23*, 2603. [CrossRef]
50. Hashemi, M.; Sadeghi-Bojd, S.; Raeisi, M.; Moazeni-Roodi, A. Evaluation of paraoxonase activity in children with nephrotic syndrome. *Nephrourol. Mon.* **2013**, *5*, 978–982. [CrossRef]

51. de Nardi, A.B.; dos Santos Horta, R.; Fonseca-Alves, C.E.; de Paiva, F.N.; Linhares, L.C.M.; Firmo, B.F.; Ruiz Sueiro, F.A.; de Oliveira, K.D.; Lourenço, S.V.; De Francisco Strefezzi, R.; et al. Diagnosis, Prognosis and Treatment of Canine Cutaneous and Subcutaneous Mast Cell Tumors. *Cells* **2022**, *11*, 618. [CrossRef]
52. Weishaar, K.M.; Thamm, D.H.; Worley, D.R.; Kamstock, D.A. Correlation of nodal mast cells with clinical outcome in dogs with mast cell tumour and a proposed classification system for the evaluation of node metastasis. *J. Comp. Pathol.* **2014**, *151*, 329–338. [CrossRef] [PubMed]

MDPI AG
Grosspeteranlage 5
4052 Basel
Switzerland
Tel.: +41 61 683 77 34

Antioxidants Editorial Office
E-mail: antioxidants@mdpi.com
www.mdpi.com/journal/antioxidants

MDPI

www.ingramcontent.com/pod-product-compliance
Lightning Source LLC
LaVergne TN
LVHW070448061126
851858LV00011B/189